Nutritional Management of Hospitalized Patients

Nutritional Management of Hospitalized Patients

Editor: Natasha Parsons

AMERICAN
MEDICAL PUBLISHERS
www.americanmedicalpublishers.com

AMERICAN
MEDICAL PUBLISHERS
www.americanmedicalpublishers.com

Cataloging-in-Publication Data

Nutritional management of hospitalized patients / edited by Natasha Parsons.
p. cm.
Includes bibliographical references and index.
ISBN 978-1-63927-766-7
1. Hospital patients--Nutrition. 2. Diet therapy. 3. Diet in disease. 4. Diseases--Nutritional aspects.
5. Hospitals--Food service. 6. Hospital care. I. Parsons, Natasha.
RM216 .N88 2023
615.854--dc23

American Medical Publishers,
41 Flatbush Avenue,
1st Floor, New York,
NY 11217, USA

ISBN 978-1-63927-766-7 (Hardback)

Contents

Preface

The main aim of this book is to educate learners and enhance their research focus by presenting diverse topics covering this vast field. This is an advanced book which compiles significant studies by distinguished experts in the area of analysis. This book addresses successive solutions to the challenges arising in the area of application, along with it; the book provides scope for future developments.

Malnourishment refers to a condition, which occurs due to the consumption of a diet that has insufficient nutrients or consumption of the wrong type of diet. Hospitalized patients are often malnourished and this condition is often not diagnosed and treated. Studies have suggested that many medical inpatients who are malnourished suffer from multiple comorbidities. In clinical practice, most of the nutritional guidelines are developed taking into account a single disease, which makes it difficult to devise proper nutritional guidelines for polymorbid patients. Management of malnourishment involves providing nutritional supplementation that can improve functioning of muscle and increasing the weight. In case of patients whose daily nutritional demands cannot be fulfilled through oral diets, the medical practitioners may prescribe enteral nutrition (EN), wherein, nutrients are introduced in the body through a catheter or probe that is inserted into the gastric or intestinal region of the patients. The education and awareness of proper nutritional diet can also be helpful in improving the condition. This book presents the latest studies on the nutritional management of hospitalized patients. It will help new researchers by foregrounding their knowledge in this area of study.

It was a great honour to edit this book, though there were challenges, as it involved a lot of communication and networking between me and the editorial team. However, the end result was this all-inclusive book covering diverse themes in the field.

Finally, it is important to acknowledge the efforts of the contributors for their excellent chapters, through which a wide variety of issues have been addressed. I would also like to thank my colleagues for their valuable feedback during the making of this book.

Editor

1

Association between Selected Dietary Habits and Lipid Profiles of Patients with Cardiovascular Disease

Jana Kopčeková [1], Mária Holovičová [1], Martina Gažarová [1], Jana Mrázová [1], Marta Habánová [1], Lucia Mečiarová [1] and Monika Bronkowska [2,*]

1 Department of Human Nutrition, Faculty of Agrobiology and Food Resources, Slovak University of Agriculture in Nitra, 949 01 Nitra, Slovakia; jana.kopcekova@uniag.sk (J.K.); mariaholovicova23@gmail.com (M.H.); martina.gazarova@uniag.sk (M.G.); jana.mrazova@uniag.sk (J.M.); marta.habanova@uniag.sk (M.H.); lucia.meciarova@leanenterprise.sk (L.M.)

2 Department of Human Nutrition, Faculty of Biotechnology and Food Science, Wroclaw University of Environmental and Life Sciences, 51-630 Wroclaw, Poland

* Correspondence: monika.bronkowska@upwr.edu.pl

Abstract: This study evaluated the associations between selected dietary habits and lipid profiles in a group of 800 randomly selected patients hospitalized in the Nitra Cardio Center, Slovakia. Patients were aged 20–101 years (only men, the average age was 61.13 ± 10.47 years). The data necessary for the detection of dietary habits were obtained by a questionnaire method in closed-ended format. Data collection was carried out simultaneously with the somatometric and biochemical examinations of the respondents ensured by the Nitra Cardio Center. The following parameters were evaluated: total cholesterol (T-C), low-density lipoprotein cholesterol (LDL-C), high-density lipoprotein cholesterol (HDL-C), triglycerides, and blood glucose. Statistical comparisons between groups were performed using one-way analysis of variance (one-way ANOVA), followed by Tukey's post hoc test. We detected significant differences ($p < 0.05$) in the influence of the number of daily meals on T-C and LDL-C, which were higher in men who consumed 1–2 meals compared with 3–4 or 5–6 meals. In the consumption of meat, eggs, and fish, there was no significant effect on the biochemical parameters of blood ($p > 0.05$). We recorded a significant effect ($p < 0.001$) on T-C and LDL-C levels between low-fat and whole-fat milk consumption. Except for the impact of fruit consumption on the HDL-C level ($p < 0.001$), the different frequencies of fruit consumption showed non-significant changes for the lipid profile levels. We detected a significant effect ($p = 0.017$) of the consumption of vegetables 1–2 times/week on LDL-C in favor of daily consumption. Our results support that monitoring the lipid profile is an important determinant in the prevention and treatment of cardiovascular disease. The conducted research emphasizes the importance of diet dependence on the improvement of the quality of treatment and nutrition of people with this type of disease.

Keywords: cardiovascular disease; lipid profile; food frequency; dietary habits

1. Introduction

Currently, a substantial increase in cardiovascular disease (CVD) is noticeable all over the world; it is deemed to be the main cause of death in both developed and developing countries [1,2]. The proportion of deaths in Europe from CVD amongst men is 43% and 55% amongst women. It is estimated that 30% of people under the age of 65 on this continent die of CVD [3]. The main cause of CVD (which is the reason for high mortality in the population) is atherosclerosis. The causes and risk factors of atherosclerosis are still not fully known. In spite of this, some risk determinants have been identified that may increase the risk of developing atherosclerosis. Mainly, they include: high-serum total cholesterol (T-C), low-density lipoprotein cholesterol (LDL-C), and high-density lipoprotein cholesterol (HDL-C), as well as hypertension, smoking, diabetes, obesity, and sedentary lifestyle [4].

Numerous clinical and epidemiological experimental studies have shown that nutrition plays an important role in the prevention and secondary prevention of atherosclerosis [4]. It is assumed that as much as 80% of cardiovascular incidents could probably be avoided by implementing a proper lifestyle (weight control, avoiding alcohol and smoking, exercising, and balanced nutrition). It is also necessary to pay attention to adequate clinical care and biological risk factors [3]. The World Health Organization emphasizes that improper nutrition, a sedentary lifestyle, alcohol abuse, and smoking are the main modifiable risk factors for chronic diseases such as CVD, cancer, respiratory disorders, and metabolic diseases [5].

The first evidence of the association between diet/physical activity and well-being was found in the 1960s following the first results of a study named the "Seven Countries' Study" [6]. The first results from this study were surprising because they distinctly showed that the countries of the Mediterranean basin (Italy and Greece) had the lowest incidence of death from CVD and cancer compared to all other countries [6]. In the last two decades, considerable knowledge has been gained from intervention studies about food and nutrients that favorably or adversely affect the cardiovascular system [7,8].

While foods from animal sources contain important nutrients that may not be readily available from plant sources, high consumption of red meat is associated with a greater risk of morbidity and mortality from CVD. Such diets may contain high levels of total and saturated fats in addition to cholesterol. Numerous studies have demonstrated the benefits of diets high in fruit, vegetables, whole grains, and fish, as well as low in red meat, high-fat dairy products, and trans- and saturated fats. On the other hand, most recent meta-analyses of randomized trials and observational studies found no beneficial effects of reducing saturated fatty acid (SFA) intake on CVD and total mortality, and instead found protective effects against strokes [9].

High concentrations of T-C, LDL cholesterol, and triacylglycerols indicate that the individual is at risk for the onset of CVD [10]. Increased concentration of LDL cholesterol in the blood serum is a recognized risk factor for the development of heart disease. However, the relationship between the dietary cholesterol content and the serum LDL-C concentration is still unknown [11].

This study aimed to evaluate the associations between selected dietary habits and lipid profiles in a group of randomly selected patients hospitalized in the Nitra Cardio Center, Slovakia.

The research was approved by the Ethics Committee of Kardiocentrum Nitra and the Ethics Committee of the Specialized Hospital, St. Zoerardus Zobor, protocol number 10.6.2014.

2. Materials and Methods

We evaluated the relationship between selected dietary habits and lipid profiles in a group of 800 randomly selected men hospitalized in the Nitra Cardio Center, Slovakia. The study was approved by the Nitra Cardio Center, and all participants signed the written consent before participating in the study. Patients were aged 20–101 years (the average age was 61.13 ± 10.47 years). Patients were selected using the method of random selection. Respondents included in the study had either overcome myocardial infarction or were diagnosed with angina pectoris and hospitalized after undergoing catheterization. Data were collected during the years 2015–2018.

The data necessary for the detection of dietary habits were obtained by a questionnaire method in closed-ended format. The questionnaire was applied individually by a single interviewer. The questionnaire contained two parts. The first part included questions concerning the socio-demographic situation of the subjects, physical activity, use of tobacco, and medical history. The second part of the questionnaire concerned the analysis of selected dietary habits, including the number of the consumed meals, their regularity, snacking between meals, types of snacks consumed, and the eating frequency of selected groups of food products. The questionnaire was anonymous; its completion was voluntary, with only one response to be circled for each question. The questionnaire was compiled by the Department of Human Nutrition (Slovak University of Agriculture in Nitra) and approved by the Nitra Cardio Center.

Data collection was carried out simultaneously with the somatometric and biochemical examinations of the respondents ensured by the Nitra Cardio Center. The following parameters, considered to be major risk factors for CVD, were evaluated: T-C, LDL-C, HDL-C, triglycerides (TG), and blood glucose. Venous blood was collected in the morning after 8 h of fasting in a standard manner, using 2.5 mL EDTA (ethylenediaminetetraacetic acid) solution in a 7.5 mL serum gel tube. Following the separation of blood serum, the lipid profile was measured using the Automatic Biochemical Analyzer BioMajesty® JCA-BM6010/C (DiaSys Diagnostic System GmbH, Holzheim, Germany). The anthropometric parameters of body weight (kg) and height (cm) were measured on outpatient electronic medical scales (Tanita WB-3000, Tanita Co., Tokyo, Japan). The body mass index (BMI) was calculated by dividing the body weight in kilograms by the square of the height in meters.

The data were checked for normality. Assumptions for the normal distribution of data were tested using the Shapiro–Wilk test. Parametric statistics were used to evaluate differences in parameters that were characterized by a normal distribution (Food Frequency Questionnaire - FFQ). Statistical comparisons between groups were performed using one-way analysis of variance (ANOVA), followed by Tukey's post hoc test. For parameters inconsistent with the normal distribution, they were expressed as the median (Me) and the lower and upper quartiles (Q1, Q3). Here, nonparametric statistics and Spearman's rank order correlations were used to compare the differences. Two-sample non-parametric comparisons were performed using the Mann–Whitney U test. Significance was assumed when $p < 0.05$. Statistica Cz 10 (TIBCO Software, Inc., Palo Alto, CA, USA) and MS Excel 2007 (Microsoft Corporation, Redmond, WA, USA) were used.

3. Results

From the obtained individual values, we calculated the basic statistical characteristics. These characteristics of the study participants are shown in Table 1. The demographic characteristics of study participants are shown in Table 2.

Table 1. Characteristics of study participants ($n = 800$).

Characteristic	Me	Q1	Q3
Age (years)	61.00	56.00	68.00
BMI (kg/m^2)	29.05	26.73	31.78
TC (mmol/L)	4.65	3.80	5.55
LDL-C (mmol/L)	2.85	2.19	3.52
HDL-C (mmol/L)	1.11	0.92	4.01
TG (mmol/L)	1.51	1.07	2.21
Glucose (mmol/L)	5.94	5.30	7.28

Abbreviations: Me: median; Q1: lower quartile; Q3: upper quartile; BMI: body mass index; T-C: total cholesterol; LDL-C: low-density lipoprotein cholesterol; HDL-C: high-density lipoprotein cholesterol; TG: triglycerides.

In the prevention of obesity and lipid metabolism disorders, attention is paid to the regular consumption of meals, with appropriate time intervals between them. This statement is supported by the fact that people who consume low-quantity food doses per day had increased levels of T-C and a higher prevalence of obesity and CVD [12], which was also confirmed by our results. It turned out that most of the respondents (69.25%) consumed 3–4 meals a day (Table 3). Only 25.3% of participants reported 5–6 meals a day. We detected significant differences ($p < 0.05$) between the influence of the number of daily meals on T-C and LDL-C, which were higher in men who consumed 1–2 meals compared with 3–4 or 5–6 meals (Table 3). Previous studies have shown that a higher daily eating frequency is associated with an increased intake of energy, which comes mainly from carbohydrates and not from fats or proteins. Such studies also found a positive relationship between a higher daily eating frequency and the consumption of nutrients such as dietary fiber, vitamin C, folic acid, calcium, magnesium, and iron [13].

Table 2. Demographic characteristics of study participants (n = 800).

Characteristics	n	%	Characteristics	n	%
Social status			Family status		
employed	273	34.2	married	582	72.7
unemployed	127	15.7	divorced	111	13.9
retired	400	50.1	widowed	107	13.4
Age categories (years)			Education		
<40	30	3.7	basic	98	12.2
40–49	65	8.1	apprenticeship	234	29.4
50–59	229	28.6	secondary	302	37.7
60–69	315	39.4	higher	166	20.7
70–79	147	18.4	Physical activity		
≥80	14	1.8	15–30 min/day	285	35.6
BMI (kg/m^2)			30–60 min/day	161	20.1
<18.5	3	0.3	>60 min/day	354	44.3
18.5–25	93	11.6	Smoker		
25–30	402	50.2	Yes	251	31.4
≥30	302	37.9	No	549	68.6

Table 3. Effect of the number of daily meals on lipid profile (mmol/L).

Number of Daily Meals	n (%)	T-C (Average ± SD)	LDL-C (Average ± SD)	HDL-C (Average ± SD)	TG (Average ± SD)
1–2	76 (9.5)	4.92 ± 1.13	3.14 ± 0.84	1.19 ± 0.42	1.59 ± 0.80
3–4	522 (65.2)	4.73 ± 1.20	2.98 ± 1.02	1.16 ± 0.40	1.77 ± 1.03
5–6	202 (25.3)	4.34 ± 1.12	2.65 ± 0.90	1.11 ± 0.35	1.64 ± 0.94
p-value		0.031 [a]; 0.033 [b]	0.032 [a]; 0.031 [b]	>0.05	>0.05

Abbreviations: T-C: total cholesterol; LDL-C: LDL cholesterol; HDL-C: HDL cholesterol; TG: triglycerides. [a] Significant difference between 1–2 and 5–6 daily meals. [b] Significant difference between 3–4 and 5–6 daily meals.

Although consumption of red meat is valuable as a source of protein, iron, vitamin B_{12}, and other B vitamins in the human diet [14], its excessive consumption, as seen in many Western nations, may be associated with obesity, CVD, some types of oncological diseases, diabetes, and other non-communicable diseases [15–17]. The link between meat consumption and the incidence of chronic diseases and mortality has been evaluated in hundreds of observational epidemiological studies over the last few decades. Despite these substantial data, it is not yet clear whether the increased intake of certain groups of meat (e.g., total, unprocessed, or processed red meat) or certain species (e.g., beef or pork) contribute independently to the risk of the disease [18].

We found that pork is the most popular; 72.7% of respondents reported consuming it 1–2 times/week (Table 4). Escriba-Perez et al. [19] monitored the consumption of meat in 800 respondents aged 25–75 years. The most common was chicken, which was consumed by up to 90.87% of respondents at least once a week. The second most frequently consumed was beef (63.62%), and third was pork (52.62%). Escriba-Perez et al. [19] also stated that red meat consumption frequency also differed between the sexes. Beef was consumed more frequently by males, while females consumed more chicken than red meat. The results of the effect of the frequency of red meat consumption on the lipid profiles of participants in the current study are shown in Table 4. The highest T-C and LDL-C values were seen in men who consumed red meat 3–4 times/week. For the consumption of pork and beef, there was no significant effect on the blood biochemical parameters ($p > 0.05$). Only pork consumption had a significant effect on TG ($p = 0.046$). Kontogianni et al. [20] found that a high intake of red meat (more than eight servings/month) was associated with an increased risk of acute coronary syndromes, but low intake (less than four servings/month) showed no association.

Table 4. Effect of the frequency of consumption of red meat on lipid profile (mmol/L).

Frequency of Meat Consumption	*n* (%)	T-C (Average ± SD)	LDL-C (Average ± SD)	HDL-C (Average ± SD)	TG (Average ± SD)
Pork					
1–2 times/week	582 (72.7)	4.57 ± 1.11	2.82 ± 0.93	1.19 ± 0.46	1.68 ± 0.82
3–4 times/week	94 (11.7)	4.78 ± 1.07	2.87 ± 0.88	1.14 ± 0.33	2.02 ± 0.98
1–2 times/month	112 (14.0)	4.77 ± 1.33	2.92 ± 0.98	1.17 ± 0.28	1.94 ± 1.08
no consumption	12 (1.6)	4.58 ± 1.09	2.78 ± 0.87	1.18 ± 0.09	1.96 ± 0.37
p-value		>0.05	>0.05	>0.05	0.046 [a], 0.039 [b]
Beef					
1–2 times/week	370 (46.2)	4.62 ± 1.14	2.84 ± 0.91	1.17 ± 0.38	1.68 ± 0.77
3–4 times/week	44 (5.5)	4.52 ± 0.78	2.70 ± 0.38	1.07 ± 0.29	1.99 ± 1.23
1–2 times/month	374 (46.7)	4.51 ± 1.16	2.79 ± 1.01	1.21 ± 0.49	1.77 ± 0.88
no consumption	12 (1.6)	4.53 ± 0.18	3.08 ± 0.78	1.17 ± 0.06	1.87 ± 0.13
p-value		>0.05	>0.05	>0.05	>0.05

Abbreviations: T-C: total cholesterol; LDL-C: LDL cholesterol; HDL-C: HDL cholesterol; TG: triglycerides. [a] Significant difference between 1–2 times/week and 3–4 times/week. [b] Significant difference between 1–2 times/week and 1–2 times/month.

Our results show that most respondents (60.5%) consume 1–5 eggs weekly (Table 5). This consumption rate is associated with non-significantly lower T-C and LDL-C ($p > 0.05$). The significant effect ($p < 0.001$) was observed on the TG levels, which were highest at the consumption of >10 eggs per week. Consumption of more eggs was non-significantly associated with higher T-C and LDL-C and lower HDL-C values. Baumgartner et al. [21] found that in 57 healthy volunteers (32 females and 25 men) aged 18–65 years, the consumption of one egg/day increased T-C by 0.63 mmol/L and LDL-C by 0.59 mmol/L relative to the control group. On the contrary, in a cohort study with 7216 participants, Díez-Espino et al. [22] found that consumption of 2–4 eggs/week was not associated with high cardiovascular risk. From a meta-analysis based on randomized controlled trials, with intervention periods ranging between 3 and 20 weeks and changes in cholesterol intakes between 137 and 897 mg/day, it was estimated that each 100 mg increase in dietary cholesterol intake increased the serum LDL-C concentration by 0.050 mmol/L [23].

Table 5. Effect of consumption of eggs on lipid profile (mmol/L).

Number of Eggs/Week	*n* (%)	T-C (Average ± SD)	LDL-C (Average ± SD)	HDL-C (Average ± SD)	TG (Average ± SD)
no consumption	162 (20.2)	4.06 ± 1.02	2.43 ± 0.94	1.16 ± 0.31	1.45 ± 0.64
1–5	484 (60.5)	4.59 ± 1.10	2.77 ± 0.88	1.17 ± 0.34	1.74 ± 0.88
6–10	134 (16.7)	4.81 ± 1.16	2.92 ± 0.78	1.19 ± 0.44	2.01 ± 1.00
>10	20 (2.6)	5.30 ± 0.57	3.34 ± 0.28	0.97 ± 1.11	3.81 ± 1.06
p-value		>0.05	>0.05	>0.05	<0.001 [a,b]

Abbreviations: T-C: total cholesterol; LDL-C: LDL cholesterol; HDL-C: HDL cholesterol; TG: triglycerides. [a] Significant difference between 1–5 eggs and more than 10 eggs/week. [b] Significant difference between 6–10 eggs and more than 10 eggs/week.

In our group of respondents, the consumption of fish (sea or freshwater, 1–2 times/week) was recorded in only 35% and 43.1% of men, respectively (Table 6). Alarmingly, up to 24% of the patients consumed sea fish only 1–2 times/month. The different frequencies of fish consumption showed non-significant changes regarding the lipid profile. A meta-analysis of 17 cohort studies showed that both low (one serving/week) and moderate (2–4 servings/week) fish consumption were inversely associated with coronary heart disease (CHD) mortality, while no additional benefits were seen at higher intakes [24].

Table 6. Effect of the frequency of consumption of fish on lipid profile.

Frequency of Consumption	n (%)	T-C (Average ± SD)	LDL-C (Average ± SD)	HDL-C (Average ± SD)	TG (Average ± SD)
Sea fish					
1–2 times/week	280 (35.0)	4.64 ± 1.23	2.80 ± 0.97	1.23 ± 0.53	1.70 ± 0.82
1–2 times/month	192 (24.0)	4.48 ± 1.20	2.89 ± 0.97	1.20 ± 0.30	1.54 ± 0.81
sometimes	136 (17.0)	4.49 ± 0.97	2.69 ± 0.79	1.17 ± 0.39	1.78 ± 0.90
no consumption	192 (24.0)	4.65 ± 1.14	2.96 ± 0.98	1.15 ± 0.26	1.98 ± 0.96
p-value		>0.05	>0.05	>0.05	0.001 [a], 0.022 [b]
Freshwater fish					
1–2 times/week	345 (43.1)	4.70 ± 1.26	2.97 ± 1.03	1.15 ± 0.40	1.70 ± 1.08
1–2 times/month	293 (36.6)	4.73 ± 1.16	2.97 ±1.00	1.15 ± 0.39	1.67 ± 0.91
sometimes	105 (13.1)	4.53 ± 1.10	2.76 ± 0.98	1.15 ± 0.36	1.94 ± 0.98
no consumption	57 (7.2)	4.21 ± 0.99	2.54 ± 0.69	1.11 ± 0.31	1.79 ± 0.83
p-value		>0.05	>0.05	>0.05	>0.05

Abbreviations: T-C: total cholesterol; LDL-C: LDL cholesterol; HDL-C: HDL cholesterol; TG: triglycerides. [a] Significant difference between 1–2 times/month and no consumption. [b] Significant difference between 1–2 times/week and no consumption.

The daily consumption of milk and milk products was recorded in 45.2% of our patients (Table 7). The results indicated that T-C, LDL-C, and TG values were highest in patients who consumed medium-fat milk. We recorded a significant effect of milk type on the T-C and LDL-C levels.

Table 7. Effect of milk type and frequency of consumption of milk and dairy products on lipid profile.

Parameter	n (%)	T-C (Average ± SD)	LDL-C (Average ± SD)	HDL-C (Average ± SD)	TG (Average ± SD)
Type of Milk					
low-fat	86 (10.7)	4.41 ± 1.26	3.32 ± 1.03	1.20 ± 0.45	1.82 ± 1.06
medium-fat	334 (41.7)	4.52 ± 1.15	2.77 ± 0.97	1.13 ± 0.39	1.59 ± 0.83
whole-fat	173 (21.6)	4.42 ± 1.16	2.64 ± 0.98	1.16 ± 0.42	1.67 ± 0.84
no consumption	207 (26.0)	4.60 ± 1.17	2.87 ± 0.96	1.19 ± 0.37	1.83 ± 1.06
p-value		<0.001 [a,b], 0.006 [c]	0.002 [a], <0.001 [b], 0.015 [c]	>0.05	>0.05
Frequency of Dairy Product Consumption					
daily	362 (45.2)	4.90 ± 1.22	2.81 ± 1.01	1.49 ± 0.57	1.70 ± 1.37
3–4 times/week	166 (20.7)	4.52 ± 0.99	2.48 ± 0.97	1.38 ± 0.30	1.44 ± 0.65
1–2 times/week	248 (31.0)	4.82 ± 1.52	2.82 ± 1.12	1.45 ± 0.42	1.59 ± 0.90
no consumption	24 (3.1)	5.03 ± 0.93	3.01 ± 0.65	1.21 ± 0.44	2.40 ± 1.54
p-value		>0.05	>0.05	>0.05	>0.05

Abbreviations: T-C: total cholesterol; LDL-C: LDL cholesterol; HDL-C: HDL cholesterol; TG: triglycerides. [a] Significant difference between medium- fat and low-fat milk. [b] Significant difference between whole-fat and low-fat milk. [c] Significant difference between no consumption and low-fat milk.

Among the 800 participants in our study, 64.7% ate fruit and 54.7% ate vegetables as part of their daily diet (Table 8). Respondents who consumed fruits and vegetables daily had higher T-C and LDL-C values. Except for the impact of fruit consumption on HDL-C levels ($p < 0.001$), the different frequencies of fruit consumption showed non-significant changes in the lipid levels. We detected a significant effect ($p = 0.017$) of the consumption of vegetables 1–2 times/week on LDL-C in favor of daily consumption.

Table 8. Effect of the frequency of consumption of fruit and vegetables on lipid profile.

Type of Food	*n* (%)	T-C (Average ± SD)	LDL-C (Average ± SD)	HDL-C (Average ± SD)	TG (Average ± SD)
Fruit					
daily	518 (64.7)	4.60 ± 1.17	2.89 ± 0.98	1.13 ± 0.37	1.63 ± 0.83
3–4 times/week	146 (18.2)	4.55 ± 1.22	2.80 ± 0.94	1.14 ± 0.37	1.71 ± 0.82
1–2 times/week	120 (15.0)	4.64 ± 1.49	2.64 ± 1.20	1.43 ± 0.43	1.38 ± 0.95
no consumption	16 (2.1)	4.20 ± 0.61	2.57 ± 0.62	1.20 ± 0.27	1.53 ± 0.62
p-value		>0.05	>0.05	<0.001 [a,b]	>0.05
Vegetable					
daily	438 (54.7)	4.79 ± 1.12	2.72 ± 0.89	1.45 ± 0.51	1.76 ± 1.11
3–4 times/week	170 (21.3)	5.02 ± 1.32	3.02 ± 1.13	1.43 ± 0.37	1.40 ± 0.63
1–2 times/week	137 (17.1)	5.14 ± 1.37	3.09 ± 1.15	1.49 ± 0.37	1.46 ± 1.22
no consumption	55 (6.9)	4.58 ± 1.30	2.70 ± 0.99	1.20 ± 0.32	1.78 ± 0.59
p-value		>0.05	0.017 [a]	>0.05	>0.05

Abbreviations: T-C: total cholesterol; LDL-C: LDL cholesterol; HDL-C: HDL cholesterol; TG: triglycerides. [a] Significant difference between daily and 1–2 times/week. [b] Significant difference between 3–4 times/week and 1–2 times/week.

The study group also analyzed the correlation of Spearman's rank order (r) with division into age groups, BMI value, and smoking status. Significance was assumed when $p < 0.05$.

Table 9 presents the Kruskal–Wallis rank ANOVA by age group. No statistically significant correlation was found in this analysis.

Table 9. Kruskal–Wallis rank analysis of variance (ANOVA) by age group.

Age	*n*	Glucose Me (Q1; Q3)	T-C Me (Q1; Q3)	LDL-C Me (Q1; Q3)	HDL-C Me (Q1; Q3)	TG Me (Q1; Q3)	BMI Me (Q1; Q3)
<30	8	5.34 (4.77; 7.15)	3.13 (3.00; 5.05)	2.05 (1.95; 3.24)	0.79 (0.72; 1.05)	1.31 (1.01; 2.58)	26.77 (17.90; 28.06)
31–55	105	5.95 (5.31; 7.20)	5.95 (5.31; 7.20)	5.95 (5.31; 7.20)	5.95 (5.31; 7.20)	5.95 (5.31; 7.20)	5.95 (5.31; 7.20)
56–75	616	5.93 (5.31; 7.27)	4.60 (3.79; 5.54)	2.84 (2.19; 3.48)	1.10 (0.91; 1.34)	1.51 (1.10; 2.21)	29.06 (26.83; 31.38)
>75	71	6.00 (5.18; 7.40)	4.83 (3.92; 5.99)	3.11 (2.15; 3.72)	1.10 (0.91; 1.34)	1.39 (0.88; 2.18)	29.05 (26.85; 30.45)
p-value		>0.05	>0.05	>0.05	>0.05	>0.05	>0.05

Abbreviations: Me: median; Q1: lower quartile; Q3: upper quartile; BMI: body mass index; T-C: total cholesterol; LDL-C: LDL cholesterol; HDL-C: HDL cholesterol; TG: triglycerides.

Next, an ANOVA of the Kruskal–Wallis ranks was performed with the division of the BMI index range (Table 10). Significance was assumed when $p < 0.05$. No statistically significant correlation was found in this analysis.

Table 10. Kruskal–Wallis rank ANOVA analysis by BMI group.

BMI	*n*	Glucose Me (Q1; Q3)	T-C Me (Q1; Q3)	LDL-C Me (Q1; Q3)	HDL-C Me (Q1; Q3)	TG Me (Q1; Q3)
<18.49	3	4.77 (4.77; 5.30)	3.13 (3.13; 6.93)	2.05 (2.05; 3.85)	0.72 (0.72; 1.13)	1.24 (1.24; 3.48)
18.5–24.99	93	6.40 (5.22; 7.20)	5.95 (5.31; 7.20)	5.95 (5.31; 7.20)	5.95 (5.31; 7.20)	5.95 (5.31; 7.20)
25–29.99	401	6.00 (5.31; 7.27)	4.60 (3.79; 5.54)	2.84 (2.19; 3.48)	1.10 (0.91; 1.34)	1.51 (1.10; 2.21)
>30	303	5.90 (5.31; 7.20)	4.72 (3.83; 5.55)	2.83 (2.20; 3.73)	1.10 (0.89; 1.36)	1.66 (1.16; 2.35)
p-value		>0.05	>0.05	>0.05	>0.05	>0.05

Abbreviations: Me: median; Q1: lower quartile; Q3: upper quartile; BMI: body mass index; T-C: total cholesterol; LDL-C: LDL cholesterol; HDL-C: HDL cholesterol; TG: triglycerides.

Next, an ANOVA of the Kruskal–Wallis ranks was performed with the sample divided into smokers and non-smokers (Table 11). Significance was assumed when $p < 0.05$. No statistically significant correlation was found in this analysis.

Table 11. Kruskal–Wallis rank ANOVA analysis by smoker group.

Smoker	*n*	Glucose Me (Q1; Q3)	T-C Me (Q1; Q3)	LDL-C Me (Q1; Q3)	HDL-C Me (Q1; Q3)	TG Me (Q1; Q3)
no	532	5.88 (5.38; 7.20) *	4.71 (3.83; 5.57)	2.87 (2.21; 3.54)	1.11 (0.94; 1.36)	1.52 (1.05; 2.27)
yes	268	6.14 (5.22; 7.40) *	4.50 (3.79; 5.46)	2.83 (2.12; 3.45)	1.09 (0.91; 1.36)	1.46 (1.13; 2.04)
p-value		<0.03 *	>0.05	>0.05	>0.05	>0.05

Abbreviations: Me: median; Q1: lower quartile; Q3: upper quartile; BMI: body mass index; T-C: total cholesterol; LDL-C: LDL cholesterol; HDL-C: HDL cholesterol; TG: triglycerides; * Kruskal–Wallis ranks.

In the next stage, the Mann–Whitney U test was carried out, taking into account the status of smoking cigarettes. Significance was assumed when $p < 0.05$. There were statistically significant differences in glucose concentration between smokers and non-smokers (Table 11).

Table 12 shows the results of the significance of Spearman's rank correlation (r > 0.5) by group. Significance was assumed when $p < 0.05$. Spearman's rank correlations were found to be statistically significant (r > 0.5).

Table 12. Correlations by Spearman's rank.

	Glucose	T-C	LDL-C	HDL-C	TG
Glucose	-	−0.047	−0.032	**−0.21** *	0.067
T-C	−0.047	-	**0.87** *	**0.27** *	**0.26** *
LDL-C	−0.032	**0.87** *	-	**0.10** *	**0.16** *
HDL-C	**−0.21** *	**0.27** *	**0.10** *	-	**−0.26** *
TG	0.067	**0.26** *	**0.16** *	**−0.26** *	-

Spearman's rank correlations. Significance was assumed when $p < 0.05$ *; Bold, the correlations statistically significant in the analysis of Spearman's rank correlation at the significance level $p > 0.5$.

It was found that there were statistically significant correlations between the selected biochemical indices. With the increase in glucose, the concentration of HDL-cholesterol fraction drops statistically significantly (r = −0.21). As the concentration of triglycerides increases, the concentration of the HDL cholesterol ratio decreases (r = −0.26).

Due to the fact that in the age/BMI/smoker groups, no equal variances were found, the research hypothesis did not allow for a two-factor analysis.

4. Discussion

The European Prospective Investigation into Cancer and Nutrition (EPIC) study included nearly 500,000 participants across 10 European countries and more than 5000 cardiovascular events. It confirmed that the consumption of processed meat is strongly associated with CVD risk and that the consumption of unprocessed red meat has little to no association [25].

In a meta-analysis of 20 studies (17 prospective cohorts and three case–control studies) that included 1,218,380 individuals, Micha et al. [26] concluded that intake of processed, but not red, meat was associated with an increased incidence of CHD. The authors further speculated that the higher sodium and nitrate content of processed meat might contribute to its impact on CVD.

Since the discovery that eggs, and especially egg yolks, contain a notable quantity of cholesterol, numerous studies have tried to investigate the effect of egg consumption on the risk of CVD. Following the results of these studies, it is now widely known that dietary cholesterol intake does not noticeably affect fasting plasma lipid profile, and some studies showed that eggs might even have anti-atherogenic properties [27]. Although eggs are a major source of dietary cholesterol, they are also an inexpensive source of unsaturated fat, high-quality protein, folate, and other vitamins and minerals [28].

Many studies suggest that increasing fish consumption is recommended for the intake of omega-3 fatty acids and also to confer benefits for CVD risk reduction [29]. In a prospective analysis on 20,969 subjects free from CVD at baseline, Bonaccio et al. [30] detected that fish was consumed by almost all subjects in the cohort (99.5%). Beyond promoting a healthy dietary lifestyle overall, dietary guidelines recommend eating fish at least twice (two servings) a week [30] because of the well-documented inverse association with risk of developing CVD (supported by several meta-analyses). Mean total fish intake in the study sample was 44.6 g/day, and mean frequency of fish intake was 2.4 times/week.

The results of the observational study, regardless of the level of milk fat, have not found a link between milk product intake and increased risk of CHD, stroke, or other heart and vessel diseases. Short-term intervention studies have shown that whole milk and butter increase not only LDL-C, but also HDL-C, and, therefore, may not affect plasma levels (or could reduce T-C to HDL-C) [31]. Milk and dairy products are a source of energy and high-quality protein, and they also contain important trace elements in our diet [32]. Consumption of milk and its products is one of the key elements of a rational, balanced diet. In the case of mammals, milk is the first food that provides energy and all the necessary nutrients to ensure proper growth and development. This highlights the very important role of milk and its products as a source of calcium, which plays a key role in the formation of bone mass. However, there is some controversy about the consumption of dairy and dairy products in adulthood, especially concerning non-human milk. Despite these controversies, epidemiological studies support the possible role of its consumption in preventing many chronic diseases, such as CVD, some forms of cancer, obesity, and diabetes [33]. The association of milk or dairy product consumption with CVD is still controversial [34,35].

Milk and dairy products have been shown to have a beneficial effect on lowering blood pressure and increasing HDL-C, which is associated with a reduced risk of CVD [32]. Most dietary guidelines recommend 2–3 servings of dairy products/day [36,37]. More recently, Drouin-Chartier et al. [38] conducted a randomized control trial involving 76 patients with mild to moderate hypertension. It was found that consuming a total of three servings per day of milk (low-fat), yoghurt (low-fat), and cheese (regular-fat) significantly reduced the mean daytime systolic blood pressure (2 mmHg; $p = 0.05$) in men but not in women when compared with a dairy-free control diet. In terms of cardiovascular health, however, the fat content of these products is important [31].

Fruits and vegetables are highly nutritious products, containing large amounts of dietary fiber, vitamins, and minerals, and are also characterized by a high antioxidant potential. It is believed that higher consumption of these product groups reduces the risk of developing chronic diseases, including diseases of the cardiovascular system. Therefore, it is recommended to include five portions of fruits and vegetables in daily food rations [39]. From randomized controlled studies, fruits and vegetables were shown to have a favorable effect on several risk factors, including: blood pressure, lipid concentration, insulin resistance, inflammatory biomarker concentrations, endothelial function, and weight control [40,41].

He et al. [41] reported that the average fruit and vegetable intake in most developed countries is three portions/day, which is below the recommended amount of at least five portions/day. Pérez [42] states that women consume fruits and vegetables more often than men, and men with diagnosed cancer, heart disease, high blood pressure, or diabetes mellitus tend to consume these foods more often than healthy men.

Although this study provided new insight into the relationship between selected eating habits and the lipid profiles of patients with cardiovascular disease, it has some limitations. First, the study was conducted only on the population of one country, so it provides detailed information only about that particular population, and should be reproduced in other countries. Moreover, the study only looked at men, while, in fact, the relationship between eating habits is, of course, also relevant among women. In subsequent studies, it is worth conducting similar studies among people of both sexes. Additionally, comparisons of the results obtained by gender would probably be very valuable. Another limitation of the publication may also be unequal age groups, unequal groups, and a very large discrepancy within the group when it comes to the respondents. Finally, the study only assessed the declared behaviors, which were not verified by direct observational research techniques.

5. Conclusions

In our study, we observed the associations between selected dietary habits and lipid profiles in a group of randomly selected patients with CVD. Our results showed a positive relationship between a higher daily eating frequency and lower levels of T-C and LDL-C. We have not confirmed the effect of more frequent consumption of red meat on higher T-C and LDL-C levels. Consumption of more than 10 eggs was associated with higher T-C, LDL-C, and lower HDL-C levels. We recorded a significant difference between the effect of low-fat and whole-fat milk consumption on the T-C and LDL-C levels. Except for the impact of fruit consumption on HDL-C level, the different frequencies of consumption of fruit showed non-significant changes regarding the profile of lipid levels. We found a positive effect of daily consumption of vegetables on LDL-C, compared with consumption 1–2 times/week. Our results support the hypothesis that diet is one of the most important determinants in CVD and its associated risk factors.

Author Contributions: Conceptualization, J.K. and M.H. (Marta Habánová); methodology, J.K.; software, J.M. and M.G.; validation, J.K., M.H. (Marta Habánová), and M.H. (Mária Holovičová); formal analysis, J.K.; investigation, M.H. (Mária Holovičová); resources, M.G. and L.M.; data curation, M.H. (Marta Habánová); writing—original draft preparation, J.K.; writing—review and editing, M.B.; visualization, J.M.; supervision, M.H. (Marta Habánová); project administration, J.K.; funding acquisition, M.B. All authors have read and agreed to the published version of the manuscript.

Acknowledgments: We express our gratitude to the participants for their contributions to the study, and also to the Nitra Cardio Center, APVV-18-0227.

References

1. Gaziano, T.A.; Bitton, A.; Anand, S.; Abrahams-Gessel, S.; Murphy, A. Growing epidemic of coronary heart disease in low- and middle-income countries. *Curr. Probl. Cardiol.* **2010**, *35*, 72–115. [CrossRef]
2. Mittal, B.V.; Singh, A.K. Hypertension in the developing world: Challenges and opportunities. *Am. J. Kidney Dis.* **2010**, *55*, 590–598. [CrossRef]
3. Carpentier, Y.A.; Komsa-Penkova, R.S. The place of nutrition in the prevention of cardiovascular diseases (CVDs). *e-SPEN Eur. e-J. Clin. Nutr. Metab.* **2011**, *6*, e272–e282. [CrossRef]
4. Torres, N.; Guevara-Cruz, M.; Velázquez-Villegas, L.A.; Tovar, A.R. Nutrition and atherosclerosis. *Arch. Med. Res.* **2015**, *46*, 408–426. [CrossRef]
5. Sofi, F.; Macchi, C.; Abbate, R.; Gensini, G.F.; Casini, A. Mediterranean diet and health status: An updated meta-analysis and a proposal for a literature-based adherence score. *J. Health Nutr.* **2014**, *17*, 2769–2782. [CrossRef] [PubMed]
6. Keys, A.; Mienotti, A.; Karvonen, M.J.; Aravanis, C.; Blackburn, H.; Buzina, R.; Djordjevic, B.S.; Dontas, A.S.; Fidanza, F.; Keys, M.H.; et al. The diet and 15-year death rate in the Seven Countries Study. *Am. J. Epidemiol.* **1986**, *124*, 903–915. [CrossRef]
7. Keller, K.; López, S.R.; Moreno, M.C.; Cantero, P.A. Associations between food consumption habits with meal intake behaviour in Spanish adults. *Appetite* **2014**, *83*, 63–68. [CrossRef]
8. Ambrosini, G.L.; Huang, R.C.; Mori, T.A.; Hands, B.P.; O'Sullivan, T.A.; de Klerk, N.H.; Beilin, L.J.; Oddy, W.H. Dietary patterns and markers for the metabolic syndrome in Australian adolescents. *Nutr. Metab. Cardiovasc. Dis.* **2010**, *20*, 274–283. [CrossRef]
9. Astrup, A.; Magkos, F.; Bier, D.M.; Brenna, J.T.; Otto, M.C.O.; Hill, J.O.; King, J.C.; Mente, A.; Ordovas, J.M.; Volek, J.S.; et al. Saturated fats and health: A reassessment and proposal for food-based recommendations. *J. Am. Coll. Cardiol.* **2020**, *76*, 844–857. [CrossRef]

10. Wooton, A.K.; Melchior, L.M. Obesity and type 2 diabetes in our youth: A recipe for cardiovascular disease. *J. Nurse Pract.* **2017**, *13*, 222–227. [CrossRef]
11. Clayton, Z.S.; Fusco, E.; Kern, M. Egg consumption and heart health: A review. *Nutrition* **2017**, *37*, 79–85. [CrossRef]
12. Jurkovičová, J. *We're Aware of Healthy Living? The Health Condition of Slovak Population of 1999–2004 and the Prevention of Cardiovascular and Diseases of Civilization*, 1st ed.; Comenius University in Bratislava: Bratislava, Slovakia, 2005; ISBN 80-223-2132-X.
13. Kerver, J.M.; Yang, E.J.; Obayashi, S.; Bianchi, L.; Song, W.O. Meal and snack patterns are associated with dietary intake of energy and nutrients in US adults. *J. Am. Diet. Assoc.* **2006**, *106*, 46–53. [CrossRef]
14. de Castro Cardoso Pereira, P.M.; dos Reis Baltazar Vicente, A.F. Meat nutritional composition and nutritive role in the human diet. *Meat Sci.* **2013**, *93*, 586–592. [CrossRef] [PubMed]
15. Huang, T.; Yang, B.; Zheng, J.; Li, G.; Wahlqvist, M.; Li, D. Cardiovascular disease mortality and cancer incidence in vegetarians: A meta-analysis and systematic review. *Ann. Nutr. Metab.* **2012**, *60*, 233–240. [CrossRef]
16. Pan, A.; Sun, Q.; Bernstein, A.M.; Schulze, M.B.; Manson, J.E.; Stampfer, M.J.; Willett, W.C.; Hu, F.B. Red meat consumption and mortality: Results from 2 prospective cohort studies. *Arch. Intern. Med.* **2012**, *172*, 555–563. [CrossRef]
17. McAfee, A.J.; McSorley, E.M.; Cuskelly, G.J.; Moss, B.W.; Wallace, J.M.W.; Bonham, M.P.; Fearon, A.M. Red meat consumption: An overview of the risks and benefits. *Meat Sci.* **2010**, *84*, 1–13. [CrossRef]
18. Micha, R.; Michas, G.; Lajous, M.; Mozaffarian, D. Processing of meats and cardiovascular risk: Time to focus on preservatives. *BMC Med.* **2013**, *11*, 136. [CrossRef]
19. Escriba-Perez, C.; Baviera-Puig, A.; Buitrago-Vera, J.; Montero-Vicente, L. Consumer profile analysis for different types of meat in Spain. *Meat Sci.* **2017**, *129*, 120–126. [CrossRef]
20. Kontogianni, M.D.; Panagiotakos, D.B.; Pitsavos, C.; Chrysohoou, C.; Stefanadis, C. Relationship between meat intake and the development of acute coronary syndromes: The CARDIO2000 case-control study. *Eur. J. Clin. Nutr.* **2008**, *62*, 171–177. [CrossRef]
21. Baumgartner, S.; Kelly, E.R.; van der Made, S.; Berendschot, T.T.J.M.; Husche, C.; Lütjohann, D.; Plat, J. The influence of consuming an egg or an egg-yolk buttermilk drink for 12 wk on serum lipids, inflammation, and liver function markers in human volunteers. *Nutrition* **2013**, *29*, 1237–1244. [CrossRef]
22. Díez-Espino, J.; Basterra-Gortari, F.J.; Salas-Salvadó, J.; Buil-Cosiales, P.; Corella, D.; Schröder, H.; Estruch, R.; Ros, E.; Gómez-Gracia, E.; Arós, F.; et al. Egg consumption and cardiovascular disease according to diabetic status: The PREDIMED study. *Clin. Nutr.* **2017**, *36*, 1015–1021. [CrossRef] [PubMed]
23. Weggemans, R.M.; Zock, P.L.; Katan, M.B. Dietary cholesterol from eggs increases the ratio of total cholesterol to high-density lipoprotein cholesterol in humans: A meta-analysis. *Am. J. Clin. Nutr.* **2001**, *73*, 885–891. [CrossRef]
24. Zheng, J.; Huang, T.; Yu, Y.; Hu, X.; Yang, B.; Li, D. Fish consumption and CHD mortality: An updated meta-analysis of seventeen cohort studies. *Public Health Nutr.* **2012**, *15*, 725–737. [CrossRef]
25. Rohrmann, S.; Overvad, K.; Bueno-de-Mesquita, H.B.; Jakobsen, M.U.; Egeberg, R.; Tjønneland, A.; Nailler, L.; Boutron-Ruault, B.-C.; Clavel-Chapelon, F.; Palli, D.; et al. Meat consumption and mortality—Results from the European Prospective Investigation into Cancer and Nutrition. *BMC Med.* **2013**, *11*, 63. [CrossRef]
26. Micha, R.; Wallace, S.K.; Mozaffarian, D. Red and processed meat consumption and risk of incident coronary heart disease, stroke, and diabetes mellitus: A systematic review and meta-analysis. *Circulation* **2010**, *121*, 2271–2283. [CrossRef]
27. Fernandez, M.L. Rethinking dietary cholesterol. *Curr. Opin. Clin. Nutr. Metab. Care* **2012**, *15*, 117–121. [CrossRef]
28. Song, W.O.; Kerver, J.M. Nutritional contribution of eggs to American diets. *J. Am. Coll. Nutr.* **2000**, *19*, 556S–562S. [CrossRef]
29. Raatz, S.K.; Silverstein, J.T.; Jahns, L.; Picklo, M.J., Sr. Issues of fish consumption for cardiovascular disease risk reduction. *Nutrients* **2013**, *5*, 1081–1097. [CrossRef]
30. Bonaccio, M.; Ruggiero, E.; Castelnuovo, A.D.; Costanzo, S.; Persichillo, M.; De Curtis, A.; Cerletti, C.; Donati, M.B.; de Gaetano, G.; Iacoviello, L. Fish intake is associated with lower cardiovascular risk in a Mediterranean population: Prospective results from the Moli-sani study. *Nutr. Metab. Cardiovasc. Dis.* **2017**, *27*, 865–873. [CrossRef]

31. Huth, P.J.; Park, K.M. Influence of dairy product and milk fat consumption on cardiovascular disease risk: A review of the evidence. *Adv. Nutr.* **2012**, *3*, 266–285. [CrossRef] [PubMed]
32. German, J.B.; Gibson, R.A.; Krauss, R.M.; Nestel, P.; Lamarche, B.; van Staveren, W.A.; Steijns, J.M.; de Groot, L.C.P.G.M.; Lock, A.L.; Destaillats, F. A reappraisal of impact of dairy foods and milk fat on cardiovascular disease risk. *Eur. J. Nutr.* **2009**, *48*, 191–203. [CrossRef]
33. Pereira, P.C. Milk nutritional composition and its role in human health. *Nutrition* **2014**, *30*, 619–627. [CrossRef] [PubMed]
34. Lamarche, B.; Givens, D.I.; Soedamah-Muthu, S.; Krauss, R.M.; Jakobsen, M.U.; Bischoff-Ferrari, H.A.; Pan, A.; Després, J.P. Does milk consumption contribute to cardiometabolic health and overall diet quality? *Can. J. Cardiol.* **2016**, *32*, 1026–1032. [CrossRef]
35. Alexander, D.D.; Bylsma, L.C.; Vargas, A.J.; Cohen, S.S.; Doucette, A.; Mohamed, M.; Irvin, S.R.; Miller, P.E.; Watson, H.; Fryzek, J.P. Dairy consumption and CVD: A systematic review and meta-analysis. *Br. J. Nutr.* **2016**, *115*, 737–750. [CrossRef]
36. Doidge, J.C.; Segal, L. Most Australians do not meet recommendations for dairy consumption: Findings of a new technique to analyse nutrition surveys. *Aust. N. Z. J. Public Health* **2012**, *36*, 236–240. [CrossRef]
37. Da Silva, M.S.; Rudkowska, I. Dairy products on metabolic health: Current research and clinical implications. *Maturitas* **2014**, *77*, 221–228. [CrossRef]
38. Drouin-Chartier, J.P.; Gagnon, J.; Labonté, M.È.; Desroches, S.; Charest, A.; Grenier, G.; Dodin, S.; Lemieux, S.; Couture, P.; Lamarche, B. Impact of milk consumption on cardiometabolic risk in postmenopausal women with abdominal obesity. *Nutr. J.* **2015**, *14*, 12. [CrossRef]
39. Berciano, S.; Ordovás, J.M. Nutrition and cardiovascular health. *Rev. Española Cardiol. (Engl. Ed.)* **2014**, *67*, 738–747. [CrossRef]
40. Olatona, F.A.; Onabanjo, O.O.; Ugbaja, R.N.; Nnoaham, K.E.; Adelekan, D.A. Dietary habits and metabolic risk factors for non-communicable diseases in a university undergraduate population. *J. Health Popul. Nutr.* **2018**, *37*, 21. [CrossRef]
41. He, F.J.; Nowson, C.A.; Macgregor, G.A. Fruit and vegetable consumption and stroke: Meta-analysis of cohort studies. *Lancet* **2006**, *367*, 320–326. [CrossRef]
42. Pérez, C.E. Fruit and vegetable consumption. *Health Rep.* **2002**, *13*, 23–31.

2

The Effects of the Dietary Approaches to Stop Hypertension (DASH) Diet on Metabolic Syndrome in Hospitalized Schizophrenic Patients

Tamara Sorić [1,*], Mladen Mavar [1] and Ivana Rumbak [2]

1 Psychiatric Hospital Ugljan, Otočkih dragovoljaca 42, 23275 Ugljan, Croatia; ravnatelj@pbu.hr
2 Faculty of Food Technology and Biotechnology, University of Zagreb, 10000 Zagreb, Croatia; ivana.rumbak@pbf.hr
* Correspondence: tamara.novoselic@pbu.hr

Abstract: The relationship between the Dietary Approaches to Stop Hypertension (DASH) diet and metabolic syndrome (MetS) in people with schizophrenia is unknown and remains to be investigated. Therefore, we have conducted a three-month parallel-group randomized controlled trial. Sixty-seven hospitalized schizophrenic patients with MetS [$n = 33$ in the intervention group (IG) and $n = 34$ in the control group (CG)] completed the intervention. The IG followed the DASH diet with the caloric restriction of approximately 1673.6 kJ/day (400 kcal/day) when compared to the standard hospital diet followed by the CG. Simultaneously, both groups participated in a nutrition counseling program. Anthropometric and biochemical parameters and blood pressure were measured at the baseline and after three months, while nutrient intakes during the intervention were assessed using three non-consecutive 24-hour dietary recalls. The analyses were carried out based on the per-protocol approach. At three months, the MetS prevalence significantly decreased in both the IG and the CG (75.8%, $p = 0.002$, and 67.7%, $p = 0.0003$, respectively; odds ratio = 0.9; 95% confidence interval = 0.43–1.87). No significant differences in the prevalence of MetS and its features were found between the groups.

Keywords: DASH diet; diet quality; metabolic syndrome; nutrition counseling; schizophrenia

---

1. Introduction

The metabolic syndrome (MetS) is a complex medical condition consisting of several interconnected parameters including abdominal obesity, elevated serum triglycerides (TG), decreased levels of high-density lipoprotein cholesterol (HDL-C), elevated blood pressure (BP), and increased levels of fasting blood glucose (GLC) [1], and is considered as one of the major predictors for the development of cardiovascular diseases and type 2 diabetes mellitus [1,2]. Due to continuous increase in MetS prevalence during the last few decades [3], it has become one of the leading global public health problems [4]. However, in certain population groups, including people with serious mental illnesses such as schizophrenia, MetS prevalence is estimated to be much higher than among people without mental disorders [5]. According to the results of numerous previously conducted studies, the MetS prevalence in people with schizophrenia is approximately 1.5–2 times higher than among the mentally healthy people [6,7]. Furthermore, it is already well-known that people suffering from schizophrenia have reduced life expectancy and increased mortality rate when compared to the general population [8], which is largely due to the presence of MetS [9].

Because of the aforementioned, the syndrome itself and the identification of possible mechanisms for its prevention and treatment have been in the focus of numerous researches in the field of psychiatry. Despite the scientific interest, the exact reasons for a higher occurrence of MetS among people with schizophrenia have not yet been completely clarified [9]. Although atypical antipsychotics are considered to be the major contributor [10], there is a growing body of evidence suggesting that unhealthy dietary habits, common for individuals suffering from schizophrenia, have a significant role in its development [9,11]. Previously published studies conducted among people with schizophrenia reported higher intake of salt, total sugars, and fats, primarily saturated fatty acids (SFA), along with the lower intake of dietary fiber and fruits when compared to the general population [12–15]. Even though such dietary habits are generally associated with unfavorable health implications [16–19], there is still no consensus on the most effective nutrition therapy for the MetS [20]. Therefore, it is of an utmost importance to develop an adequate nutritional intervention program that would be effective in its treatment.

The Dietary Approaches to Stop Hypertension (DASH) is a diet primarily designed to lower BP [21,22]. In a DASH dietary pattern, a special emphasis has been put on low-fat milk and dairy products, whole grains, lean meat, fruits, and vegetables, together with the reduction of sodium intake [23]. Although primarily intended for individuals with the diagnosis of hypertension, according to Hill et al., it could also be beneficial in treating MetS [24]. Until today, several randomized controlled trials (RCTs) examined the impact of the DASH diet on MetS or some of its features in different population groups, and the results mostly showed amelioration of the studied parameters [25–27]. Beneficial effects of the DASH dietary pattern on cardiometabolic parameters in people with and without diabetes mellitus were also confirmed in the recently conducted umbrella review by Chiavaroli et al. [28]. However, studies on the relationship between the DASH diet and different health outcomes in people with schizophrenia are still insufficient and limited [29] and, to the best of our knowledge, there are no published RCTs evaluating the effects of the DASH diet on MetS in this specific population group.

Therefore, the main purpose of the present study was to examine the effects of the DASH diet on MetS and its features in hospitalized schizophrenic patients. In addition, we also examined the effects of this specific dietary pattern on other studied anthropometric and biochemical parameters and on the diet quality. We hypothesized that the application of the DASH diet would result in significant improvements in all of the studied health parameters, as well as in the diet quality.

2. Materials and Methods

2.1. Study Participants and Setting

The present three-month parallel-group RCT was conducted between May 2, 2017 and December 20, 2017 in the Psychiatric Hospital Ugljan, Croatia.

Hospitalized individuals, both men and women, aged between 18–67, with the diagnosis of schizophrenia (F20.0–F20.9) according to the 10th Revision of the International Classification of Diseases and without any physical or cognitive impairments that could disable full participation in the study were screened after providing written informed consent to verify whether they meet all of the other inclusion criteria for the participation in the RCT. All the study participants had previously been hospitalized and were residing in the Psychiatric Hospital Ugljan prior to commencement of the study because of the exacerbation in their mental illness, and were considered eligible to enter the study only if they were in a stable phase of schizophrenia (defined by the fact that the prescribed antipsychotic therapy has not changed significantly in the previous month). Other inclusion criteria were as follows: having a diagnosis of MetS according to the Joint Interim Statement definition [30], taking antipsychotic medications for the last six months or longer, and providing a written informed consent for the participation in the RCT. On the other hand, individuals were considered ineligible to participate in the RCT if they followed one of the specific hospital diets with restrictions in the intake of specific food items, groups and/or nutrients, if they were currently taking weight loss pharmacotherapy, or if they experienced a significant body weight (BW) loss in the last three months. Participants were also excluded from the study for one or more of the following reasons: personal request, exacerbation in mental condition, the appearance of a new illness that could disable full participation or could have an impact on the study outcomes, a significant change in pharmacotherapy, cognitive deteriorations that disable full participation, disinterest and refusal to fully participate, or hospital discharge. The researcher (hospital nutritionist) recruited all the study participants by word-of-mouth.

Sample size calculation was performed using a module Power analysis Sample Size Calculation of the statistical software Statistica, version 6.1. (StatSoft Inc, Tulsa, OK, USA) [31]. The calculation was based on the impact of nutritional intervention on MetS and its components, for the two intervention arms. The MetS prevalence at three months was the primary endpoint for the sample size calculation and the calculation was based on the expectation that the three-month intervention program would result in the reduction of MetS prevalence from 100% to 57% in the intervention group (IG) and in the reduction of MetS prevalence from 100% to 90% in the control group (CG). Sample size calculation was also based on the fact that between-group and within-group difference of 10% in the following parameters is considered clinically significant: BP, TG, HDL-C, low-density lipoprotein cholesterol (LDL-C), total cholesterol (TC), and GLC. With the estimated magnitude of significant difference of 10%, a standard deviation of 15%, and with a type I error rate (alpha) 0.05 and a power goal of 0.80, the threshold was 33 participants per group. The obtained value was increased by 15%–20% due to the assumed drop-outs.

2.2. *Randomization*

The participants who met all the inclusion criteria were randomized to the IG or the CG using computer-generated random numbers (Excel RAND function). In a stratified randomization scheme, the study participants were block-randomized by age, sex, body mass index (BMI), and waist circumference (WC) at a ratio of 1:1. The randomization process was performed by an independent statistician and the randomization list was then provided to the researcher who assigned participants to the study groups. Both the researcher and the participants were not blinded to the study allocation.

2.3. *Ethics*

Participation in the study was entirely voluntary and all participants had to provide written informed consents, separately for participation in the pre-enrollment screening and in the RCT. Out of 79 randomized participants, 22 participants ($n = 11$ in the IG and $n = 11$ in the CG) were deprived of legal capacity. For those participants, written informed consents were provided from both the participants and their legal guardians. The number of participants deprived of legal capacity who have completed the three-month intervention is presented in Table 1. Prior to signing of the informed consent, the researcher thoroughly explained the study procedures, aims, and potential outcomes individually to each participant and his legal guardian, where applicable. The study was approved by the Ethics Committee of the Psychiatric Hospital Ugljan (approval number: 01-552/01-16; approval date: November 21, 2016) and the Central Ethics Committee of the Medical School, University of Zagreb (approval number: 380-59-10106-17-100/56; approval date: February 23, 2017). All the study procedures were performed following the principles of the Declaration of Helsinki. The clinical trial was registered in ClinicalTrials.gov (NCT04025073).

2.4. *Study Design*

During the three-month intervention period, the IG was requested to follow the DASH diet. The caloric intake of the prescribed diet was reduced by approximately 1673.6 kJ/day (400 kcal/day) when compared to the standard hospital diet (SHD). Higher caloric restriction, even though it could lead to better outcomes, was circumvented in order to prevent its potential negative psychological side effects. The diet was planned by the researcher according to the specific DASH diet recommendations and prescribed macronutrient and micronutrient contents [23]. The average daily intakes of the most important components of the prescribed DASH diet were: energy intake 8067.6 kJ (1928.2 kcal), total fat 24.5%, SFA 5.8%, protein 19.4%, carbohydrates 55.7%, cholesterol 111.8 mg, sodium 2170.1 mg, potassium 4769.3 mg, calcium 1262.6 mg, magnesium 501.1 mg, and dietary fiber 31.0 g. Simultaneously, the CG continued to follow the SHD planned according to the requirements determined by the decision on the nutritional standard for hospitalized patients in Croatia [32]. The calculated average daily intakes of the same nutrition components indicated for the DASH diet were as follows: energy intake 9770.1 kJ (2335.1 kcal), total fat 28.3%, SFA 7.8%, protein 16.8%, carbohydrates 54.8%, cholesterol 222.3 mg, sodium 3905.5 mg, potassium 3866.7 mg, calcium 1284.23 mg, magnesium 359.4 mg, and dietary fiber 24.6 g. Besides the aforementioned, in the DASH diet the refined cereals (white bread, white rice, and white pasta) were replaced with whole grains (whole-grain bread, brown rice, and whole-wheat pasta), while low-fat dairy products (0.9% fat content) replaced those with 2.8% fat content. Nuts and seeds, together with fruits and vegetables occupied an important place in the DASH daily menus. For meal planning and nutrient composition analyses computer software Program Prehrane 5.0 (IG PROG, Rijeka, Croatia) has been used. Meal planning and nutrient composition analyses were conducted by the researcher.

Additionally, both the IG and the CG participants joined the nutrition counseling program designed to give them all relevant information about healthy eating. The program included the following four lectures: MyPlate dietary guidelines [33]; The basic principles of healthy, balanced nutrition; How to read and understand food labels?, and Diet and chronic diseases—prevention and treatment. Because of the interactive character, the lectures were organized in groups of up to 10 participants. At the end of the program, participants were given the brochures summarizing the most important information covered by the lectures.

2.5. Data Collection and Outcome Measures

Participants' basic socio-demographic and lifestyle characteristics were gathered by the researcher in a form of face-to-face interviews, while the relevant medical history details were provided by the hospital personnel. The global severity of the psychotic illness was evaluated at the baseline by hospital psychiatrists using the Signs and Symptoms of Psychotic Illness (SSPI) scale [34]. In order to estimate an additional daily energy intake in the previous month, the participants were asked to report the consumption frequency, along with an estimated quantity and name of the manufacturer, of all the foods and beverages individually purchased and consumed in addition to the ones regularly provided by the hospital. The interviews lasted approximately 15 minutes and were carried out by the researcher at the beginning of the intervention. All the gathered information was subsequently checked with the medical personnel of the departments where the participants were located. The calculations of additional daily energy intakes were done using the computer software Program Prehrane 5.0.

During the intervention, compliance with the prescribed diets (both the DASH diet and the SHD) was assessed using three non-consecutive 24-hour dietary recalls (24-h DRs) (two weekdays and one weekend day) for each participant. DRs were administered by the researcher, and the participants were asked to recall all the foods and beverages, regardless of whether they were provided by the hospital or individually purchased, together with their estimated quantities, consumed in the previous day. Standard household measures such as cups, spoons, and serving sizes were used to help participants estimate the amounts of foods and beverages consumed. The average duration of the single interview was approximately 20 minutes. On average, three 24-h DRs were conducted daily in order to cover as much intervention days as possible. For each participant, one 24-h DR was assessed per month. Due to the additional consumption of the purchased foods and beverages, which could not be restricted, when conducting the 24-h DRs, it was of the utmost importance that the participants were adherent to either the DASH diet or the SHD. Those participants refusing the prescribed diets provided by the hospital would have been excluded from the study. The analyses of the 24-h DRs were performed by the researcher using the computer software Program Prehrane 5.0. As the intervention was conducted in an inpatient setting, knowing the meal recipes was material for precise quantification of the consumed food portions and for the calculation of nutritional intakes. For the items not present in the Program Prehrane 5.0 database, the food composition data provided on food labels were used.

Furthermore, basic anthropometric measurements including measurements of BW, body height (BH), WC, hip circumference (HC), and % body fat (% BF) were carried out by the researcher following the standard instructions [35]. BW and BH were measured using a digital medical scale with stadiometer Seca 799 (Vogel & Halke GmbH & Co., Hamburg, Germany). BMI was calculated using the following formula: BW (kg) / BH (m^2). WC and HC were measured using a non-stretchable measuring tape and the measured values were used for the calculation of the WHR by the formula: WC (cm) / HC (cm). The OMRON BF500 analyzer (Omron Healthcare, Vernon Hills, IL, USA) was used for the determination of % BF.

Blood samples were taken after an overnight fast from the antecubital vein and all the relevant concentrations were determined on the day of the blood sampling. Blood GLC concentration was measured using the enzymatic reference method with hexokinase. Serum TG and TC levels were measured using the enzymatic colorimetric method, while the homogeneous enzymatic colorimetric test has been used for the determination of serum HDL-C concentrations. The analyses were performed using commercially available enzymatic reagents on the Cobas c 111 analyzer (Roche Diagnostics Ltd., Rotkreuz, Switzerland). LDL-C concentrations were calculated using the Fiedewald formula [36]. Blood samplings, together with blood sample analyses and calculations were carried out by laboratory personnel in the Department of Medical Biochemistry, Psychiatric Hospital Ugljan.

Two trained nurses from the Department of Psychosomatic Medicine, Psychiatric Hospital Ugljan performed two consecutive readings of BP with the five-minute interval between the readings using the aneroid BP gauge Riester Ri-san (Rudolf Riester GmbH, Jungingen, Germany). The readings were carried out following the standard instructions [37]. For the analysis, the mean value of the two readings has been used.

Anthropometric measurements, blood sampling, blood sample analysis, and BP assessment were conducted both at the baseline and at the end of the intervention.

According to the Joint Interim Statement definition [30], participants were determined to have MetS if they had at least three of the following components: (1) elevated WC (cut-off points for Europids: ≥94 cm for men, ≥80 cm for women); (2) elevated TG (≥1.7 mmol/L) or drug treatment for elevated TG; (3) reduced HDL-C (<1.0 mmol/L for men, <1.3 mmol/L for women) or drug treatment for reduced HDL-C; (4) elevated BP [systolic blood pressure (SBP) ≥130 mmHg and/or diastolic blood pressure (DBP) ≥85 mmHg] or antihypertensive drug treatment in a patient with a history of hypertension; (5) elevated fasting GLC (≥5.6 mmol/L) or drug treatment for elevated GLC.

2.6. *Statistical Analysis*

Statistical analyses were performed using statistical software Statistica, version 6.1 (StatSoft Inc, Tulsa, OK, USA). The assumption of normality was investigated with the Kolmogorov–Smirnov test and the Shapiro–Wilk W-test. Due to the drop-outs, the analyses were carried out based on the per-protocol approach.

Participants' basic characteristics, medical history details, and nutrient intakes were presented as means and standard deviations (SD) (metric data) or as numbers of participants and percentages (nominal/ordinal data). Pre- and post-intervention numerical results were shown as means and SD, along with 95% confidence intervals (CIs), while pre- and post-intervention categorical data were presented as numbers of participants and percentages, along with 95% CIs for one proportion calculated using the Pearson Chi-square test. To understand the size of changes found, estimated effects and the respective 95% CIs were calculated. To evaluate the between-group differences in basic characteristics and medical history details, the paired samples t-test and Mann–Whitney U test were used for numerical variables, and the Pearson Chi-square test was used for categorical variables. Pre- and post-intervention numerical data were compared within the groups using a paired samples t-test and between the groups using an independent samples t-test. For the comparison of pre- and post-intervention categorical data within and between the groups, a Pearson Chi-square test or a Fischer's exact test were used. To analyze the between-group differences in the nutrient intakes, a paired samples t-test was used. The threshold of significance for all the analyses was $p < 0.05$.

3. Results

Out of 79 participants allocated either to the IG or the CG, a total of 67 participants (33 participants in the IG and 34 participants in the CG) completed the three-month intervention. The reasons for participants' drop-out were hospital discharge ($n = 11$) and death ($n = 1$) (Figure 1). The participation in the present study could not influence the length of hospital stay and the participants "ready to go home" were discharged regardless of the MetS and their participation in the RCT. Discharged participants were excluded from analysis because all the relevant data were not obtained prior to hospital discharge. During the intervention, there were no unintended effects reported.

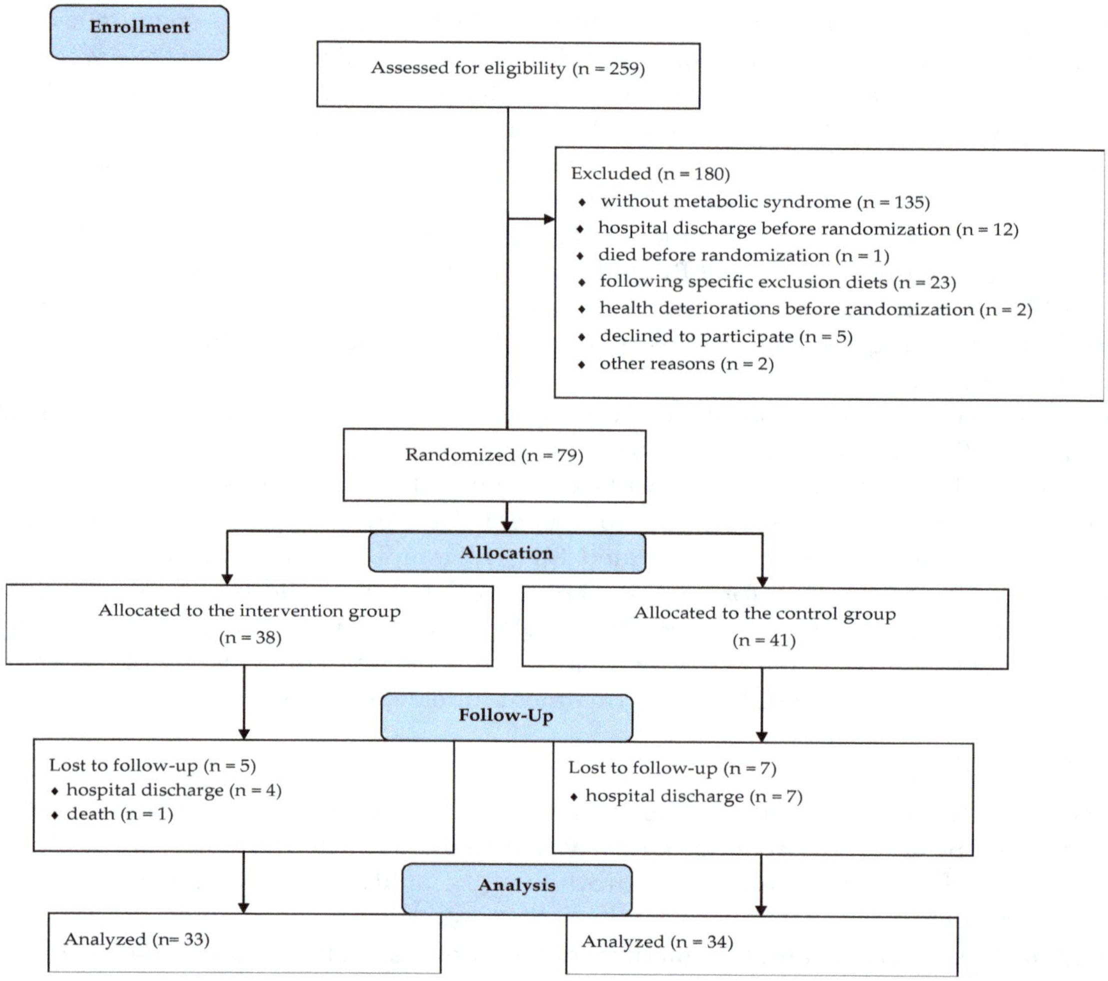

Figure 1. The CONSORT flow diagram showing the progression by stages of a randomized controlled trial.

Participants' basic characteristics and medical history details are summarized in Table 1. The vast majority of the participants were men [28 participants (84.8%) in the IG and 29 participants (85.3%) in the CG]. The mean age of the IG participants was 53.2 ± 8.9 years and of the CG participants 50.7 ± 8.0 years. There were no significant differences detected between the IG and the CG regarding any of the studied parameters listed in Table 1, except for taking hyperglycemia medications ($p = 0.028$).

Table 1. Basic characteristics and medical history details of the study participants.

Characteristics	IG (n = 33) n (%) or Mean (SD)	CG (n = 34) n (%) or Mean (SD)	p
Sex			
male	28 (84.8)	29 (85.3)	0.959 [a]
female	5 (15.2)	5 (14.7)	
Age (years)	53.2 (8.9)	50.7 (8.0)	0.228 [b]
Educational level			
no formal education or primary education	12 (36.4)	7 (20.6)	0.568 [a]
secondary education or higher	21 (63.6)	27 (79.4)	
Working status			
employed	0 (0) [d]	1 (2.9) [d]	0.450 [a]
unemployed	15 (45.5)	11 (32.4)	
retired	17 (51.5)	19 (55.9)	
receiver of social welfare	1 (3.0)	3 (8.8)	
Marital status			
single	29 (87.9)	31 (91.2)	0.967 [a]
married/in a relationship	4 (12.1)	3 (8.8)	
Residential area			
urban	18 (54.5)	11 (32.4)	0.113 [a]
rural	15 (45.5)	23 (67.6)	
Illness duration (years)	17.6 (12.7)	17.9 (12.6)	0.808 [c]
Type of schizophrenia			
paranoid	22 (66.7)	27 (79.4)	0.171 [a]
residual	11 (33.3)	5 (14.7)	
other	0 (0) [d]	2 (5.9) [d]	
Deprivation of legal capacity			
yes	10 (30.3)	10 (29.4)	0.851 [a]
no	23 (69.7)	24 (70.6)	
Number of antipsychotics			
1	3 (9.1)	9 (26.5)	0.199 [c]
2–3	27 (81.8)	22 (64.7)	
>3	3 (9.1)	3 (8.8)	
Type of antipsychotics			
typical	1 (3.0)	2 (5.9)	0.511 [a]
atypical	20 (60.6)	16 (47.1)	
both	12 (36.4)	16 (47.1)	
Taking antidepressants			
yes	3 (9.1)	4 (11.8)	0.721 [a]
no	30 (90.9)	30 (88.2)	
Taking mood stabilizers			
yes	13 (39.4)	13 (38.2)	0.926 [a]
no	20 (60.6)	21 (61.8)	
Taking antiepileptics			
yes	2 (6.1)	4 (11.8)	0.414 [a]
no	31 (93.9)	30 (88.2)	
Taking anxiolytics			
yes	19 (57.6)	21 (61.8)	0.727 [a]
no	14 (42.4)	13 (38.2)	
Taking antiparkinsonics			
yes	11 (33.3)	9 (26.5)	0.539 [a]
no	22 (66.7)	25 (73.5)	
Taking antihypertensive drug therapy			
yes	11 (33.3)	8 (23.5)	0.373 [a]
no	22 (66.7)	26 (76.5)	
Taking hypertriglyceridemia medications			
yes	5 (15.2)	4 (11.8)	0.900 [a]
no	28 (84.8)	30 (88.2)	
Taking hyperglycemia medications			
yes	0 (0)	5 (14.7)	0.028 [a,e]
no	33 (100.0)	29 (85.3)	

Table 1. *Cont.*

Characteristics	IG (n = 33) n (%) or Mean (SD)	CG (n = 34) n (%) or Mean (SD)	p
Smoking status			
current smokers	24 (72.7)	24 (70.6)	0.934 [a]
ex-smokers/never smokers	9 (27.3)	10 (29.4)	
Alcohol consumption			
yes	2 (6.1)	3 (8.8)	0.972 [a]
no	31 (93.9)	31 (91.2)	
Physical activity			
inactive	22 (66.7)	24 (70.6)	
moderate activity	11 (33.3)	9 (26.5)	0.789 [a]
high activity	0 (0) [d]	1 (2.9) [d]	
Additional daily energy intake (kJ/kcal)	2259.8/540.1 (2278.2/544.5)	1812.9/433.3 (2279.9/544.9)	0.425 [c]
The overall SSPI score [f]	26.5 (13.1)	30.0 (10.9)	0.236 [b]

IG, intervention group; CG, control group; n, number of participants; SD, standard deviation; SSPI scale, Signs and Symptoms of Psychotic Illness scale; [a] Pearson Chi-square test (statistically significant $p < 0.05$); [b] paired samples t-test (statistically significant $p < 0.05$); [c] Mann–Whitney U test (statistically significant $p < 0.05$); [d] values not included in the analysis; [e] statistically verified that the exclusion of participants taking hyperglycemia medications would not change significantly the blood glucose levels ($p = 0.143$; paired samples t-test); [f] the SSPI scale consists of 20 different signs and symptoms of psychotic illness. For each item a score in a range of 0–4 is assigned. The overall score represents the sum of all the subscale scores with 80 being the highest overall score.

The impact of the DASH diet vs. the SHD on studied anthropometric and biochemical parameters and BP are summarized in Table 2. Compliance with the DASH diet resulted in significant decrease in BW (mean difference (MD) ± SD = 2.43 ± 3.14; 95% CI = 1.36–3.50; $p < 0.001$), BMI (MD ± SD = 0.79 ± 1.08; 95% CI = 0.43–1.16; $p < 0.001$), WC (MD ± SD = 3.54 ± 3.84; 95% CI = 2.23–4.85; $p < 0.001$), HC (MD ± SD = 1.76 ± 2.44; 95% CI = 0.92–2.59; $p < 0.001$), WHR (MD ± SD = 0.02 ± 0.04; 95% CI = 0.004–0.03; $p = 0.015$), and DBP (MD ± SD = 5.30 ± 9.78; 95% CI = 1.97–8.64; $p = 0.004$) in the IG. On the other hand, following the SHD resulted in significant decrease in the values of the following parameters among the CG participants: BW (MD ± SD = 1.65 ± 3.85; 95% CI = 0.35–2.94; $p = 0.018$), BMI (MD ± SD = 0.50 ± 1.19; 95% CI = 0.10–0.90; $p = 0.019$), WC (MD ± SD = 2.45 ± 4.18; 95% CI = 1.05–3.86; $p = 0.002$), and WHR (MD ± SD = 0.01 ± 0.03; 95% CI = 0.01–0.02; $p = 0.006$). When comparing the two groups, there were no significant differences detected for any of the parameters listed in Table 2, both at the baseline and at the end of the intervention period.

The impact of the DASH diet on the prevalence of MetS and its features are shown in Table 3. At three months, a significant decrease in MetS prevalence was observed in both the IG and the CG (75.8%, $p = 0.002$ and 67.7%, $p = 0.0003$, respectively; OR = 0.9; 95% CI = 0.43–1.87). However, we did not detect any significant between-group differences in the prevalence of MetS and its features after the intervention.

Finally, we have examined the impact of the intervention on diet quality. Compliance with the DASH diet and the SHD was assessed using a total of 201 24-h DRs (99 for the compliance with the DASH diet and 102 for the compliance with the SHD). For both the IG and the CG, the average daily intakes of the most important nutrient components in the DASH dietary pattern are presented in Figure 2. During the intervention, total daily intakes of energy, cholesterol, and sodium were significantly lower in the IG, when compared to the CG (all $p < 0.001$). Furthermore, the participants in the IG consumed significantly more dietary fiber, potassium, and magnesium (all $p < 0.001$) than in the CG. Regarding the percentages of energy from macronutrients, the diet of the IG participants had a significantly lower percentage of energy derived from total fats and SFA (all $p < 0.001$), along with a significantly higher percentage of energy from carbohydrates ($p < 0.001$) and protein ($p = 0.001$). For the total daily intake of calcium, no significant difference was noted between the two studied groups ($p = 0.946$).

Table 2. The impact of the DASH diet vs. the SHD on anthropometric parameters, BP, and biochemical parameters in hospitalized schizophrenic patients with MetS.

Parameter	IG (n = 33)				CG (n = 34)					
	Baseline	At 3 Months	EE (%) (95% CI) [a]	p [b]	Baseline	At 3 Months	EE (%) (95% CI) [a]	p [b]	p [c]	p [d]
	Mean (SD) (95% CI)	Mean (SD) (95% CI)			Mean (SD) (95% CI)	Mean (SD) (95% CI)				
BW (kg)	89.60 (15.81) (83.99–95.21)	87.17 (15.52) (81.67–92.67)	15.7 (14.6–16.7)	<0.001	88.56 (13.97) (83.69–93.43)	86.92 (13.93) (82.06–91.78)	11.8 (10.5–13.1)	0.018	0.776	0.943
BMI (kg/m^2)	28.95 (5.21) (27.1–30.8)	28.16 (5.04) (26.37–29.95)	15.7 (15.3–16.1)	<0.001	27.47 (3.90) (26.11–28.83)	26.96 (3.95) (25.58–28.34)	12.8 (12.3–13.2)	0.019	0.189	0.281
WC (cm)	109.09 (12.25) (104.75–113.43)	105.55 (12.22) (101.22–109.88)	29.0 (27.7–30.3)	<0.001	106.92 (9.40) (103.64–110.2)	104.47 (9.75) (101.07–107.87)	25.1 (23.7–26.6)	0.002	0.417	0.690
HC (cm)	107.89 (10.55) (104.15–111.63)	106.14 (10.21) (102.52–109.76)	17.2 (16.3–18.0)	<0.001	106.57 (6.90) (104.16–108.98)	105.64 (7.20) (103.13–108.15)	13.0 (11.9–14.1)	0.098	0.546	0.817
WHR	1.01 (0.05) (0.99–1.03)	0.99 (0.06) (0.97–1.01)	27.2 (27.2–27.2)	0.015	1.00 (0.05) (0.98–1.02)	0.99 (0.05) (0.97–1.01)	27.7 (27.7–27.7)	0.006	0.531	0.684
% BF [e]	28.32 (9.22) (25.05–31.59)	28.34 (8.76) (25.18–31.50)	6.9 (6.1–7.7)	0.165	26.79 (7.97) (23.97–29.61)	27.54 (8.22) (24.62–30.46)	−9.1 (−10.1 to −8.0)	0.185	0.472	0.703
SBP (mmHg)	130.38 (15.53) (124.87–135.89)	126.52 (13.05) (121.89–131.15)	29.6 (24.6–34.7)	0.144	129.41 (19.98) (122.44–136.38)	126.25 (17.90) (120.00–132.5)	17.7 (10.3–25.0)	0.399	0.826	0.945
DBP (mmHg)	85.53 (9.31) (82.23–88.83)	80.23 (9.93) (76.71–83.75)	53.4 (50.1–56.7)	0.004	84.34 (9.70) (80.95–87.72)	82.72 (10.03) (79.22–86.22)	16.1 (12.9–19.4)	0.332	0.610	0.310
TG (mmol/L)	2.15 (0.92) (1.83–2.47)	2.32 (1.21) (1.89–2.75)	−14.1 (−14.4 to −13.8)	0.276	1.81 (0.82) (1.52–2.10)	1.83 (0.79) (1.56–2.10)	−3.0 (−3.3 to −2.7)	0.890	0.118	0.056
HDL-C (mmol/L)	0.92 (0.31) (0.81–1.03)	0.95 (0.30) (0.84–1.06)	−11.1 (−11.2 to −11.1)	0.169	0.93 (0.19) (0.86–1.00)	1.00 (0.29) (0.90–1.10)	−25.0 (−25.1 to −24.9)	0.085	0.859	0.481
LDL-C (mmol/L) [f]	3.19 (1.11) (2.79–3.59)	3.04 (0.86) (2.73–3.35)	17.0 (16.7–17.3)	0.336	3.07 (0.90) (2.76–3.38)	3.27 (0.78) (3.00–3.54)	−25.5 (−25.8 to −25.2)	0.188	0.646	0.255
TC (mmol/L)	5.08 (1.25) (4.64–5.52)	5.02 (1.07) (4.64–5.40)	5.4 (5.0–5.7)	0.746	4.83 (1.08) (4.45–5.21)	5.09 (1.03) (4.73–5.45)	−25.2 (−25.5 to −24.8)	0.195	0.386	0.795
GLC (mmol/L)	5.59 (0.78) (5.32–5.86)	5.34 (0.53) (5.15–5.53)	47.3 (47.1–47.6)	0.101	6.21 (1.73) (5.61–6.81)	5.69 (1.69) (5.10–6.28)	30.8 (30.1–31.4)	0.146	0.061	0.254

DASH, Dietary Approaches to Stop Hypertension; SHD, standard hospital diet; BP, blood pressure; MetS, metabolic syndrome; IG, intervention group; CG, control group; n, number of participants; SD, standard deviation; CI, confidence interval; EE, estimated effect; BW, body weight; BMI, body mass index; WC, waist circumference; HC, hip circumference; WHR, waist-to-hip ratio; % BF, % body fat; SBP, systolic blood pressure; DBP, diastolic blood pressure; TG, triglycerides; HDL-C, high-density lipoprotein cholesterol; LDL-C, low-density lipoprotein cholesterol; TC, total cholesterol; GLC, glucose; [a] standardized effect size; represents the ratio of the mean difference and the standard deviation, calculated according to the following formula: (mean difference/standard deviation) * 100; [b] comparison of differences within groups using a paired samples t-test; [c] comparison of differences between groups at the baseline using an independent samples t-test; [d] comparison of differences between groups at three months using an independent samples t-test; [e] due to tremor it was not possible to measure % BF at three months for one participant in the IG and both at the baseline and at three months for one participant in the CG; [f] both at the baseline and at three months, the LDL-C for one participant in the IG could not be calculated using Fiedewald formula due to TG levels being >4.6 mmol/L.

Table 3. The impact of the DASH diet vs. the SHD on the prevalence of MetS and its features in hospitalized schizophrenic patients with MetS (using Joint Interim Statement diagnostic criteria).

Parameter (95% CI for 1 Proportion) [a]	IG (n = 33)		p [b]	CG (n = 34)		p [b]	p [c]	p [d]	OR (95% CI)
	Baseline n (%)	At 3 Months n (%)		Baseline n (%)	At 3 Months n (%)				
elevated WC (≥94 cm men; ≥80 cm women)	31 (93.9) (0.80–0.99)	29 (87.9) (0.72–0.97)	0.391	34 (100.0) (0.90–1.00)	32 (94.1) (0.80–0.99)	0.151 [e]	0.238 [e]	0.371	1.0 (0.50–2.03)
elevated TG (≥1.7 mmol/L) or pharmacotherapy for elevated TG	27 (81.8) (0.65–0.93)	24 (72.7) (0.54–0.87)	0.378	19 (55.9) (0.38–0.73)	19 (55.9) (0.38–0.73)	1.000	0.022	0.150	1.1 (0.49–2.61)
low HDL-C (<1.0 mmol/L men; <1.3 mmol/L women) or pharmacotherapy for low HDL-C	26 (78.8) (0.61–0.91)	21 (63.6) (0.45–0.80)	0.174	24 (70.6) (0.53–0.85)	17 (50.0) (0.32–0.68)	0.082	0.440	0.260	0.9 (0.38–2.04)
elevated BP (SBP ≥130 mmHg and/or DBP ≥85 mmHg) or pharmacotherapy for elevated BP	8 (24.2) (0.11–0.42)	10 (30.3) (0.16–0.49)	0.580	8 (23.5) (0.11–0.41)	17 (50.0) (0.32–0.68)	0.023	0.945	0.100	1.7 (0.49–5.95)
elevated fasting GLC (≥5.6 mmol/L) or pharmacotherapy for elevated fasting GLC	15 (45.5) (0.28–0.64)	10 (30.3) (0.16–0.49)	0.204	19 (55.9) (0.38–0.73)	18 (52.9) (0.35–0.70)	0.807	0.393	0.060	1.4 (0.51–3.97)
MetS	33 (100.0) (0.89–1.00)	25 (75.8) (0.58–0.89)	0.002 [e]	34 (100.0) (0.90–1.00)	23 (67.7) (0.49–0.83)	0.0003 [e]	1.000	0.461	0.9 (0.43–1.87)

DASH, Dietary Approaches to Stop Hypertension; SHD, standard hospital diet; MetS, metabolic syndrome; IG, intervention group; CG, control group; n, number of participants; OR, odds ratio; WC, waist circumference; TG, triglycerides; HDL-C, high-density lipoprotein cholesterol; BP, blood pressure; SBP, systolic blood pressure; DBP, diastolic blood pressure; GLC, glucose; [a] calculated using Pearson Chi-square test; [b] comparison of differences within groups using Pearson Chi-square test or Fisher's exact test ([e]); [c] comparison of differences between groups at the baseline using Pearson Chi-square test or Fisher's exact test ([e]).;[d] comparison of differences between groups after three months using Pearson Chi-square test.

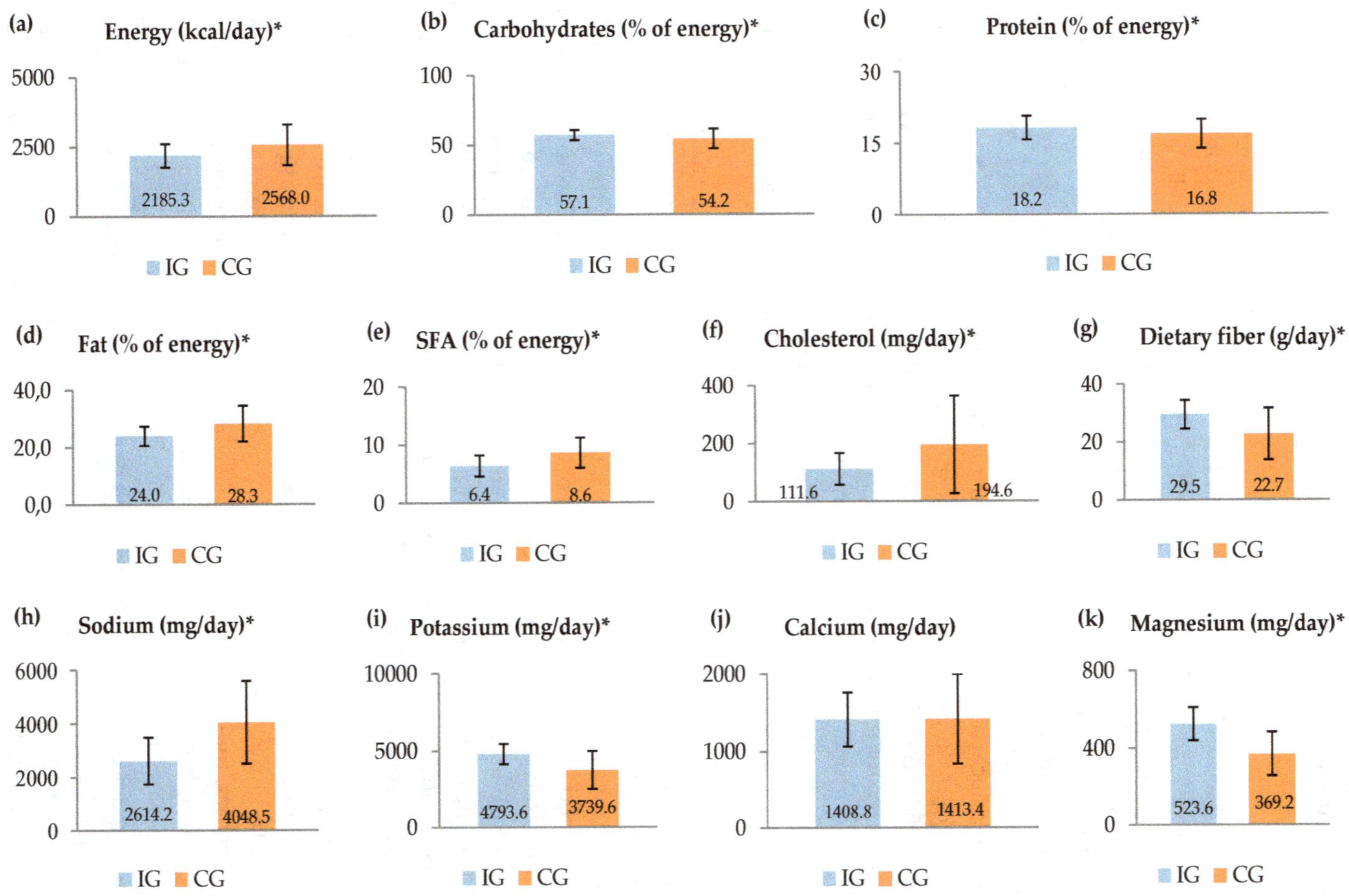

Figure 2. Nutrient intakes of the intervention group (IG = 33) and the control group (CG = 34) during the three-month intervention. Nutrient intakes are presented as means with standard deviations within bars. The first graph shows the energy intake in kcal/day. The values are equal to 9143.3 ± 1748.2 kJ/day and 10744.6 ± 3091.0 kJ/day, respectively (conversion factor: 1 kcal = 4.184 kJ). * significant difference ($p < 0.05$; calculated using a paired samples t-test): **(a)** $p < 0.001$; **(b)** $p < 0.001$; (c) $p = 0.001$; **(d)** $p < 0.001$; **(e)** $p < 0.001$, **(f)** $p < 0.001$; **(g)** $p < 0.001$, **(h)** $p < 0.001$; **(i)** $p < 0.001$; **(j)** $p = 0.946$; **(k)** $p < 0.001$.

4. Discussion

The present research, which was based on the per-protocol approach, showed no significant differences in the prevalence of MetS and its features between the IG and the CG. In addition, we have found that the application of the DASH diet, when compared to the SHD, significantly improved the diet quality of hospitalized schizophrenic patients with MetS. To the best of our knowledge, this is the first RCT which aimed to evaluate the impact of the DASH diet on MetS and its features in hospitalized schizophrenic patients.

Due to its high prevalence and numerous proven negative health implications, MetS represents one of the major concerns among people suffering from schizophrenia. Although the occurrence of MetS in people with schizophrenia has been mainly associated with antipsychotic treatment and characteristics of the psychotic illness, several general factors, including inadequate dietary habits, are also known for enhancing MetS predispositions [38]. Thus, asserting healthy dietary habits needs to be considered as one of the key factors in the treatment of MetS among people with schizophrenia. However, the RCTs examining the effects of nutritional interventions on MetS in people with schizophrenia are lacking and inconsistent, and it is, therefore, still unclear what would be the most appropriate nutritional approach for its treatment. In the last few decades, the DASH dietary pattern has been in the focus of numerous researches which have confirmed its favorable effects not only on BP, but also on MetS features in different population groups [25,26,39]. Nevertheless, no RCTs on the association between the DASH diet and MetS and its features in hospitalized schizophrenic patients have been published so far. In the present study we have detected significant improvements in several anthropometric parameters, including BW, BMI, WC, and WHR, in both the IG and the CG. These results are of great importance because the improvement in all of the aforementioned anthropometric parameters is crucial for the effective treatment of MetS [40].

After three months, significant decrease in DBP was observed among the participants in the IG, when compared to the baseline values. On the other hand, we failed to detect significant improvements in the SBP. When compared to the CG, there were no significant differences in the DBP and SBP levels at the end of the intervention. Our results are, therefore, not fully consistent with the findings of Saneei et al. [25]. In their RCT conducted on adolescents, Saneei et al. revealed that following the DASH diet recommendations, when compared to the general dietary advice, prevented the increase in DBP, while at the same time not affecting SBP levels [25]. Contrary to what we hypothesized at the beginning, we have failed to find significant improvements in the serum glucose levels and blood lipid profile in the IG after completing the three-month intervention. Thus, the aforementioned results are inconsistent with those of previously conducted studies [26,41,42].

The IG experienced a significant reduction in the MetS prevalence after three months. Surprisingly, what it was not expected is that the present study would result in the significant reduction of the MetS prevalence among the CG participants as well. As numerous confounding factors (Table 1) were taken in consideration, the improvements observed in the CG could potentially be due to the impact of some nonspecific factors, including the awareness of the study participants about the special emphasis being put on their diet, higher intention provided to participants during the intervention, and the desire to please the researcher [43]. Unfortunately, the present study concept did not allow us to conclude whether the impact of the aforementioned nonspecific factors influenced the positive outcomes observed in the CG.

In the CG, the prevalence of elevated BP significantly increased by the end of the intervention. Even though the between-group difference in the prevalence of elevated BP was not statistically significant, the results suggest that the DASH diet could potentially slow down the development of hypertension. Beneficial effects of the DASH diet on the prevalence of MetS and its features have been confirmed in several studies conducted on other population groups. Following the DASH diet recommendations in the population of adolescent girls resulted with significant reductions in the prevalence of elevated BP and MetS [25]. Specifically speaking, in the terms of the MetS prevalence, following the DASH dietary advice for six weeks reduced the prevalence from 56.7% to 46.7%, while the prevalence of the participants following usual dietary guidelines has not changed (53.3% both at baseline and at 6th week). Furthermore, the within-group change in the prevalence of the high BP did not reach statistical significance among the adolescent girls following the DASH diet (35% at baseline vs. 30% at 6th week), but when comparing the prevalence from the DASH diet group and the group following usual dietary guidelines the difference was statistically significant after six weeks (30% vs. 43%, respectively) [25]. In another RCT conducted on adult outpatients with the diagnosis of MetS, the adherence to the individually prescribed DASH diet led to the significant decrease in MetS prevalence (from 100% at baseline to 65% at six months), along with the significant ameliorations in MetS features when compared to the control diet and standard weight-reducing diet. The group following the weigh-reducing diet decreased the prevalence of MetS from 100% at baseline to 81% at six months, while the group following the control diet experienced no changes in the MetS prevalence [26]. Contrary to the findings of the aforementioned studies, the effectiveness of the DASH diet, when compared to the SHD, was not proven in the present study.

The results of the 24-h DRs have shown certain deviations from the prescribed nutrient intakes in both the IG and the CG. The observed discrepancies were mainly caused by the consumption of individually purchased food items. During the RCT, those purchasing habits of both groups had not changed significantly in the terms of the additional daily energy intake observed before the beginning of the intervention (the data not shown in the present study). Despite the observed deviations, the average daily energy intake of the IG remained reduced by approximately 1601.2 kJ (382.7 kcal) when compared to the average daily energy intake of the CG. Along with the energy intake, we have found that the application of the DASH diet, when compared to the SHD, led to significant reductions in the total daily intake of cholesterol, sodium, and percentages of energy from total fats and SFA, while it significantly increased the intake of dietary fiber, potassium, and magnesium. Despite the imperfect compliance, nutrient intakes of the IG and the CG remained significantly different in all of the main features that constitute the DASH diet, except for the intake of calcium (both the IG and the CG have reached the DASH goal for calcium intake). Therefore, the aforementioned findings suggest that this type of nutritional intervention is a beneficial tool for diet quality improvement in people with schizophrenia. Similar to our findings, in the research conducted by Teasdale et al. [44], a 12-week dietary intervention led to significant reductions in the daily intakes of energy and sodium in young people with first-episode psychosis, while Baker et al.'s [45] telephone intervention program significantly improved the overall diet quality in people with psychotic disorders.

The very nature of the participants' mental illness is of relevance for the interpretation of the obtained results. People with schizophrenia are generally less motivated to change unhealthy lifestyle patterns, including poor dietary habits. Hence, this could represent one of the possible reasons for discrepancies found between the prescribed and actual nutrient intakes which could consequently affect the main outcomes of the present study.

The key strength of our study is that it was conducted in an inpatient psychiatric setting where all the participants were provided with fully prepared meals throughout the intervention, and which has, in a great extent, reduced a participation burden. There were no significant differences between the IG and the CG considering a wide range of parameters (Table 1) that could potentially have an impact on the study outcomes. Therefore, the confounding effects of the selected parameters on the study outcomes are unlikely. Additionally, the design of the intervention program enables its reproduction in a large variety of hospital and nursing home facilities which would allow for results to be verified.

There are few study limitations that ought to be considered. Although some of the previously conducted studies [25,42] resulted in significant improvements over even a shorter period of time, the key reason for the absence of significant differences between the studied groups at the end of the intervention period in this study might have been due to a limited time duration of three months. Furthermore, even though the RCT was conducted in a controlled hospital environment, we could not restrict participants' individual purchasing of foods and beverages that were consumed in addition to the ones provided as a part of the intervention program. Additional energy intake was considered as one of the confounding factors, however we have not determined to what extent deviations caused by additional foods and beverages consumption influenced the final results. Finally, the present study did not account for some nonspecific factors mentioned earlier in the Discussion that could potentially explain the improvements observed in the CG and the absence of significant results between the groups.

Future studies with longer intervention duration are needed. Those studies should include additional study group that will receive neither the DASH diet nor the nutrition counseling in order to precisely assess their separated impacts on MetS and its features. For future studies it is also of essential importance to take in consideration all the nonspecific factors that could have the impact on the study's findings. Additionally, in those studies, a personal nutritional approach should be considered, as the adjusting of energy and nutrient requirements at the individual level are likely to lead to better results.

5. Conclusions

In conclusion, the DASH diet, when compared to the SHD, did not significantly affect MetS and its features, while it significantly improved the diet quality of hospitalized schizophrenic patients with MetS.

Author Contributions: Conceptualization, T.S., M.M., and I.R.; methodology, T.S., M.M., and I.R.; formal analysis, T.S.; investigation, T.S.; data curation, T.S.; writing—original draft preparation, T.S.; writing—review and editing, T.S., M.M., and I.R.; supervision, T.S., M.M., and I.R.; project administration, T.S. All authors read and approved the final version of the manuscript.

Acknowledgments: The authors would like to thank all the study participants. We are grateful to the personnel of the Psychiatric Hospital Ugljan for their support and cooperation during the research.

References

1. Kassi, E.; Pervanidou, P.; Kaltsas, G.; Chrousos, G. Metabolic syndrome: Definitions and controversies. *BMC Med.* **2011**, *9*, 48. [CrossRef] [PubMed]
2. Xu, H.; Li, X.; Adams, H.; Kubena, K.; Guo, S. Etiology of metabolic syndrome and dietary intervention. *Int. J. Mol. Sci.* **2019**, *20*, 128. [CrossRef] [PubMed]
3. Saklayen, M.G. The global epidemic of the metabolic syndrome. *Curr. Hypertens. Rep.* **2018**, *20*, 12. [CrossRef] [PubMed]
4. Li, R.; Li, W.; Lun, Z.; Zhang, H.; Sun, Z.; Kanu, J.S.; Qiu, S.; Cheng, Y.; Liu, Y. Prevalence of metabolic syndrome in Mainland China: A meta-analysis of published studies. *BMC Public Health* **2016**, *16*, 296. [CrossRef]
5. Malhotra, N.; Grover, S.; Chakrabarti, S.; Kulhara, P. Metabolic syndrome in schizophrenia. *Indian J. Psychol. Med.* **2013**, *35*, 227–240. [CrossRef]
6. Khalil, R.B. The metabolic syndrome and schizophrenia: A comorbidity or an association? *J. Pharmacol. Pharmacother.* **2013**, *4*, 174–175.
7. Martynikhin, I.; Tanyanskiy, D.; Rotar, O.; Solntsev, V.; Sokolian, N.; Neznanov, N.; Konradi, A.; Shlyakhto, E.; Denisenko, A. Risk of metabolic syndrome in patients with schizophrenia: Comparative study with population of bank employees in Russia. *Arch. Psychiatry Psychother.* **2013**, *2*, 15–20. [CrossRef]
8. Capasso, R.M.; Lineberry, T.W.; Bostwick, J.M.; Decker, P.A.; St Sauver, J. Mortality in schizophrenia and schizoaffective disorder: An Olmsted County, Minnesota cohort: 1950–2005. *Schizophr. Res.* **2008**, *98*, 287–294. [CrossRef]
9. Dipasquale, S.; Pariante, C.M.; Dazzan, P.; Aguglia, E.; McGuire, P.; Mondelli, V. The dietary pattern of patients with schizophrenia: A systematic review. *J. Psychiatr. Res.* **2013**, *47*, 197–207. [CrossRef]
10. Patel, J.K.; Buckley, P.F.; Woolson, S.; Hamer, R.M.; McEvoy, J.P.; Perkins, D.O.; Lieberman, J.A. CAFE Investigators. Metabolic profiles of second-generation antipsychotics in early psychosis: Findings from the CAFE study. *Schizophr. Res.* **2009**, *111*, 9–16. [CrossRef]

11. Kim, E.J.; Lim, S.Y.; Lee, H.J.; Lee, J.Y.; Choi, S.; Kim, S.Y.; Kim, J.M.; Shin, I.S.; Yoon, J.S.; Yang, S.J.; et al. Low dietary intake of n-3 fatty acids, niacin, folate, and vitamin C in Korean patients with schizophrenia and the development of dietary guidelines for schizophrenia. *Nutr. Res.* **2017**, *45*, 10–18. [CrossRef]
12. Ratliff, J.C.; Palmese, L.B.; Reutenauer, E.L.; Liskov, E.; Grilo, C.M.; Tek, C. The effect of dietary and physical activity pattern on metabolic profile in individuals with schizophrenia: A cross-sectional study. *Compr. Psychiatry* **2012**, *53*, 1028–1033. [CrossRef]
13. Brown, S.; Birtwistle, J.; Roe, L.; Thompson, C. The unhealthy lifestyle of people with schizophrenia. *Psychol. Med.* **1999**, *29*, 697–701. [CrossRef]
14. Simonelli-Muñoz, A.J.; Fortea, M.I.; Salorio, P.; Gallego-Gomez, J.I.; Sánchez-Bautista, S.; Balanza, S. Dietary habits of patients with schizophrenia: A self-reported questionnaire survey. *Int. J. Ment. Health Nurs.* **2012**, *21*, 220–228. [CrossRef]
15. Ito, H.; Kumagai, T.; Kimura, M.; Koike, S.; Shimizu, T. Dietary intake in body mass index differences in community-based Japanese patients with schizophrenia. *Iran. J. Public Health* **2015**, *44*, 639–645.
16. Siri-Tarino, P.W.; Sun, Q.; Hu, F.B.; Krauss, R.M. Saturated fat, carbohydrate, and cardiovascular disease. *Am. J. Clin. Nutr.* **2010**, *91*, 502–509. [CrossRef]
17. Hu, F.B.; Willett, W.C. Optimal diets for prevention of coronary heart disease. *JAMA* **2002**, *288*, 2569–2578. [CrossRef]
18. Delzenne, N.M.; Cani, P.D. A place for dietary fibre in the management of the metabolic syndrome. *Curr. Opin. Clin. Nutr. Metab. Care* **2005**, *8*, 636–640. [CrossRef]
19. Rust, P.; Ekmekcioglu, C. Impact of salt intake on the pathogenesis and treatment of hypertension. *Adv. Exp. Med. Biol.* **2017**, *956*, 61–84. [CrossRef]
20. Leão, L.S.; de Moraes, M.M.; de Carvalho, G.X.; Koifman, R.J. Nutritional interventions in metabolic syndrome: A systematic review. *Arq. Bras. Cardiol.* **2011**, *97*, 260–265. [CrossRef]
21. Sacks, F.M.; Svetkey, L.P.; Vollmer, W.M.; Appel, L.J.; Bray, G.A.; Harsha, D.; Obarzanek, E.; Conlin, P.R.; Miller, E.R.; Simons-Morton, D.G.; et al. DASH—Sodium Collaborative Research Group. Effects on blood pressure of reduced dietary sodium and the Dietary Approaches to Stop Hypertension (DASH) diet. DASH-Sodium Collaborative Research Group. *N. Engl. J. Med.* **2001**, *344*, 3–10. [CrossRef] [PubMed]
22. Blumenthal, J.A.; Babyak, M.A.; Hinderliter, A.; Watkins, L.L.; Craighead, L.; Lin, P.H.; Caccia, C.; Johnson, J.; Waugh, R.; Sherwood, A. Effects of the DASH diet alone and in combination with exercise and weight loss on blood pressure and cardiovascular biomarkers in men and women with high blood pressure: The ENCORE study. *Arch. Intern. Med.* **2010**, *170*, 126–135. [CrossRef] [PubMed]
23. U.S. Department of Health and Human Sciences, National Institutes of Health, National Heart, Lung, and Blood Institute. DASH Eating Plan. Available online: https://www.nhlbi.nih.gov/files/docs/public/heart/new_dash.pdf (accessed on 25 July 2019).
24. Hill, A.M.; Harris Jackson, K.A.; Roussell, M.A.; West, S.G.; Kris-Etherton, P.M. Type and amount of dietary protein in the treatment of metabolic syndrome: A randomized controlled trial. *Am. J. Clin. Nutr.* **2015**, *102*, 757–770. [CrossRef] [PubMed]
25. Saneei, P.; Hashemipour, M.; Kelishadi, R.; Rajaei, S.; Esmaillzadeh, A. Effects of recommendations to follow the Dietary Approaches to Stop Hypertension (DASH) diet v. usual dietary advice on childhood metabolic syndrome: A randomised cross-over clinical trial. *Br. J. Nutr.* **2013**, *110*, 2250–2259. [CrossRef]
26. Azadbakht, L.; Mirmiran, P.; Esmaillzadeh, A.; Azizi, T.; Azizi, F. Beneficial effects of a Dietary Approaches to Stop Hypertension eating plan on features of the metabolic syndrome. *Diabetes Care* **2005**, *28*, 2823–2831. [CrossRef]
27. Shenoy, S.F.; Poston, W.S.; Reeves, R.S.; Kazaks, A.G.; Holt, R.R.; Keen, C.L.; Chen, H.J.; Haddock, C.K.; Winters, B.L.; Khoo, C.S.; et al. Weight loss in individuals with metabolic syndrome given DASH diet counseling when provided a low sodium vegetable juice: A randomized controlled trial. *Nutr. J.* **2010**, *9*, 8. [CrossRef]
28. Chiavaroli, L.; Viquiliouk, E.; Nishi, S.K.; Blanco Mejia, S.; Rahelić, D.; Kahleová, H.; Salas-Salvadó, J.; Kendall, C.W.; Sievenpiper, J.L. DASH dietary pattern and cardiometabolic outcomes: An umbrella review of systematic reviews and meta-analyses. *Nutrients* **2019**, *11*, 338. [CrossRef]
29. Joseph, J.; Depp, C.; Shih, P.B.; Chadenhead, K.S.; Schmid-Schönbein, G. Modified Mediterranean diet for enrichment of short chain fatty acids: Potential adjunctive therapeutic to target immune and metabolic dysfunction in schizophrenia? *Front. Neurosci.* **2017**, *11*, 155. [CrossRef]

30. Alberti, K.G.; Eckel, R.H.; Grundy, S.M.; Zimmet, P.Z.; Cleeman, J.I.; Donato, K.A.; Fruchart, J.C.; James, W.P.; Loria, C.M.; Smith, S.C., Jr.; et al. Harmonizing the metabolic syndrome: A joint interim statement of the International Diabetes Federation Task Force on Epidemiology and Prevention; National Heart, Lung, and Blood Institute; American Heart Association; World Heart Federation; International Atherosclerosis Society; and International Association for the Study of Obesity. *Circulation* **2009**, *120*, 1640–1645. [CrossRef]
31. StatSoft, Inc. Electronic Statistics Textbook. Available online: http://www.statsoft.com/Textbook/Power-Analysis (accessed on 14 November 2019).
32. Ministry of Health. *Odluka o Standardu Prehrane Bolesnika u Bolnicama. [The Decision on the Nutritional Standard for Hospitalized Patients]*; Official Gazette of Croatia: Zagreb, Croatia, 2015. (In Croatian)
33. United States Department of Agriculture. Choose MyPlate. Available online: https://www.choosemyplate.gov (accessed on 10 August 2019).
34. Liddle, P.F.; Ngan, E.T.; Duffield, G.; Kho, K.; Warren, A.J. Signs and symptoms of psychotic illness (SSPI): A rating scale. *Br. J. Psychiatry* **2002**, *180*, 45–50. [CrossRef]
35. Lee, R.D.; Nieman, D.C. Anthropometry. In *Nutritional Assessment*, 5th ed.; McGraw-Hill: New York, NY, USA, 2010; pp. 160–213.
36. Fiedewald, W.T.; Levy, R.I.; Fredrickson, D.S. Estimation of the concentration of low-density lipoprotein cholesterol in plasma, without use of the preparative ultracentrifuge. *Clin. Chem.* **1972**, *18*, 499–502.
37. Frese, E.M.; Fick, A.; Sadowsky, H.S. Blood pressure measurement guidelines for physical therapists. *Cardiopulm. Phys. Ther. J.* **2011**, *22*, 5–12. [CrossRef]
38. De Hert, M.; Schreurs, V.; Vancampfort, D.; Van Winkel, R. Metabolic syndrome in people with schizophrenia: A review. *World Psychiatry* **2009**, *8*, 15–22. [CrossRef]
39. Esfandiari, S.; Bahadoran, Z.; Mirmiran, P.; Tohidi, M.; Azizi, F. Adherence to the dietary approaches to stop hypertension trial (DASH) diet is inversely associated with incidence of insulin resistance in adults: The Tehran lipid and glucose study. *J. Clin. Biochem. Nutr.* **2017**, *61*, 123–129. [CrossRef]
40. Gelli, C.; Tarocchi, M.; Abenavoli, L.; Di Renzo, L.; Galli, A.; De Lorenzo, A. Effect of a counseling-supported treatment with the Mediterranean diet and physical activity on the severity of the non-alcoholic fatty liver disease. *World J. Gastroenterol.* **2017**, *23*, 3150–3162. [CrossRef]
41. Obarzanek, E.; Sacks, F.M.; Vollmer, W.M.; Bray, G.A.; Miller, E.R., 3rd; Lin, P.H.; Karanja, N.M.; Most-Windhauser, M.M.; Moore, T.J.; Swain, J.F.; et al. DASH Research Group. Effects on blood lipids of a blood pressure-lowering diet: The Dietary Approaches to Stop Hypertension (DASH) Trial. *Am. J. Clin. Nutr.* **2001**, *74*, 80–89. [CrossRef]
42. Razavi Zade, M.; Telkabadi, M.H.; Bahmani, F.; Salehi, B.; Farshbaf, S.; Asemi, Z. The effects of DASH diet on weight loss and metabolic status in adults with non-alcoholic fatty liver disease: A randomized clinical trial. *Liver Int.* **2016**, *36*, 563–571. [CrossRef]
43. Nichols, L.O.; Martindale-Adams, J.L.; Burns, R.; Graney, M.J.; Zuber, J.K.; Kennedy, S.E. Potential explanations for control group benefit. *Clin. Trials* **2012**, *9*, 588–595. [CrossRef]
44. Teasdale, S.B.; Ward, P.B.; Rosenbaum, S.; Watkins, A.; Curtis, J.; Kalucy, M.; Samaras, K. A nutrition intervention is effective in improving dietary components linked to cardiometabolic risk in youth with first-episode psychosis. *Br. J. Nutr.* **2016**, *115*, 1987–1993. [CrossRef]
45. Baker, A.L.; Turner, A.; Kelly, P.J.; Spring, B.; Callister, R.; Collins, C.E.; Woodcock, K.L.; Kay-Lambkin, F.J.; Devir, H.; Lewin, T.J. 'Better Health Choices' by telephone: A feasibility trial of improving diet and physical activity in people diagnosed with psychotic disorders. *Psychiatry Res.* **2014**, *220*, 63–70. [CrossRef]

3

Comparison of Feeding Efficiency and Hospital Mortality between Small Bowel and Nasogastric Tube Feeding in Critically Ill Patients at High Nutritional Risk

Wei-Ning Wang [1,†], Chen-Yu Wang [2,3], Chiann-Yi Hsu [4] and Pin-Kuei Fu [2,5,6,*,†]

1 Department of Food and Nutrition, Taichung Veterans General Hospital, Taichung 40705, Taiwan; sherry@vghtc.gov.tw
2 Department of Critical Care Medicine, Taichung Veterans General Hospital, Taichung 40705, Taiwan; chestmen@gmail.com
3 Department of Nursing, Hungkuang University, Taichung 43302, Taiwan
4 Biostatistics Task Force of Taichung Veterans General Hospital, Taichung 40705, Taiwan; chiann@vghtc.gov.tw
5 College of Human Science and Social Innovation, Hungkuang University, Taichung 43302, Taiwan
6 Department of Computer Science, Tunghai University, Taichung 40705, Taiwan
* Correspondence: yetquen@gmail.com
† These authors contributed equally to this work.

Abstract: Nasogastric tube enteral nutrition (NGEN) should be initiated within 48 h for patients at high nutritional risk. However, whether small bowel enteral nutrition (SBEN) should be routinely used instead of NGEN to improve hospital mortality remains unclear. We retrospectively analyzed 113 critically ill patients with modified Nutrition Risk in Critically Ill (mNUTRIC) score ≥ 5 and feeding volume < 750 mL/day in the first week of their stay in the intensive care unit (ICU). Age, sex, mNUTRIC score, and Acute Physiology and Chronic Health Evaluation II (APACHE II) score were matched in the SBEN (n = 48) and NGEN (n = 65) groups. Through a univariate analysis, factors associated with hospital mortality were SBEN group (hazard ratio (HR), 0.56; 95% confidence interval (CI), 0.31–1.00), Simplified Organ Failure Assessment (SOFA) score on day 7 (HR, 1.12; 95% CI, 1.03–1.22), and energy intake achievement rate < 65% (HR, 2.53; 95% CI, 1.25–5.11). A multivariate analysis indicated that energy intake achievement rate < 65% on the third follow-up day (HR, 2.29; 95% CI, 1.12–4.69) was the only factor independently associated with mortality. We suggest initiation of SBEN on the seventh ICU day before parenteral nutrition initiation for critically ill patients at high nutrition risk.

Keywords: critically ill patients; feeding efficiency; high nutritional risk; hospital mortality; small bowel enteral nutrition

---

1. Introduction

Malnutrition and undernutrition have been recognized as a highly prevalent problem during intensive care unit (ICU) stays [1,2]. Up to 50–60% of critically ill patients are reported to experience energy and protein deficits during their ICU stay, which are correlated with morbidity and mortality [3,4]. No consensus exists regarding a gold standard tool for identifying ICU patients who are at high risk and are malnourished [5]. However, screening tools such as the Nutritional Risk Score, Nutrition Risk in Critically Ill (NUTRIC) assessment score, and modified NUTRIC (mNUTRIC) score have been widely applied to identify high-risk patients and enable initiation of early enteral nutrition (EN) therapy in the ICU [6–12]. Patients with mNUTRIC scores of more than 5 points are identified as being at high nutritional risk and urgently requiring additional energy support to reduce the likelihood of mortality [8,13,14]. In our previous study, an energy achievement rate of lower than 65% in patients admitted to ICU was associated with a higher risk of mortality [15], and targeted energy intake was also a mortality predictor in this population [13]. Therefore, a systemic approach to recognizing ICU patients at high nutritional risk and initiating early EN in these patients has become the standard of care for decreasing morbidity, pneumonia incidence, and even hospital mortality in critically ill patients [5–7,16–18].

The current guidelines recommend that early nasogastric tube enteral nutrition (NGEN) should be initiated within 48 h of ICU admission because this route is easier to facilitate initiation of EN as soon as possible [5–7,11]. However, small bowel EN (SBEN) has theoretical advantages over stomach EN because it not only decreases the risks of gastroesophageal reflux and aspiration pneumonia, but also delivers more nutrients than does NGEN [19–23]. The current guidelines including the European Society for Clinical Nutrition and Metabolism (ESPEN), the American Society for Parenteral and Enteral Nutrition (ASPEN), and the Society of Critical Care Medicine (SCCM) guidelines strongly recommend NGEN for EN initiation in critically ill patients at high risk and a shift to SBEN when the patient has developed intolerance of NGEN despite the administration of prokinetic agents [5–7]. For patients unable to meet the >60% achievement rate for protein and energy intake through the EN alone, supplemental parenteral nutrition (PN) can be considered after 7–10 days of EN [6,7].

Our previous study suggested the evaluation of the role of SBEN on the seventh day of the ICU stay for those with energy achievement rates of less than 60% [9]. We demonstrated that the feeding volume and achievement rates (%) of protein and energy intake were significantly higher after SBEN on the 10th day of the ICU stay [8]. We also found that an energy achievement rate lower than 65% on the third day after SBEN (the 10th day of the ICU stay) increased the mortality risk by a factor of 4.97 [8]. However, whether SBEN should be routinely used instead of NGEN for undernourished critically ill patients and to improve the hospital mortality remains unclear. The current retrospective study compared the feeding efficiency and hospital mortality of two feeding routes (maintaining NGEN or shifting to SBEN) on the seventh ICU day in ICU patients who were undernourished and at high nutritional risk.

2. Materials and Methods

2.1. Study Design and Ethic Approval

This retrospective, case–control study was conducted in the respiratory intensive care unit (RICU) of Taichung Veterans General Hospital from January 2014 to December 2015 in Central Taiwan. The Institutional Review Board of Taichung Veterans General Hospital reviewed and approved the study protocol (IRB number, CE16028A; date of approval, 29 January 2016). The current study waived the requirement for informed patient consent due to the availability of all delinked data from an electronic medical record system and the study design was a retrospective analysis.

2.2. Patient, Clinical Setting, Nutrition Evaluation, and Routine

The RICU is an adult medical ICU with 24 beds servicing patients with pneumonia accompanied by various conditions—such as septic shock and acute respiratory distress syndrome—of various severities. It has a full-time registered dietitian to conduct nutritional risk and target evaluation and provide suggestions for routine application. Serial information including mNUTRIC score, nutritional goals, and the achievement rate of energy target are routinely determined for each critically ill patient by the full-time dietitian. The mNUTRIC score has five components: age, number of comorbidities, Simplified Organ Failure Assessment (SOFA) score, Acute Physiology and Chronic Health Evaluation II (APACHE II) score, and days in hospital before ICU admission [24]. For every patient admitted to the RICU, the dietitian determines their mNUTRIC score (0–9 points) within 48 h of ICU admission and records it in the electronic medical record, as described in our previous study [8,13,15]. The target energy requirement was 25–30 kcal/kg/day and the protein intake target was 1.2 g/kg/day in accordance with the 2016 ASPEN/SCCM guidelines [6,7].The achievement rate (%) of energy was defined as follows: (actual energy intake/estimated energy requirement) × 100; the achievement rate (%) of protein was adjusted as follows: (actual protein intake/estimated protein requirement) × 100 [8,13,15].

Early EN was initiated on the first day for all patients admitted to the RICU except in some clinical contraindications. On the seventh ICU day, a transpyloric tube for SBEN was an option in patients with high nutritional risk (mNUTRIC ≥ 5) and severe malnutrition (energy target achievement rate < 30% or feeding volume < 750 mL/day) after trying prokinetic agents. Some of these patients were shifted to SBEN, but NGEN feeding was retained for others, because the use of SBEN for undernourished patients on the seventh ICU day is not mandatory according to the current guidelines. These clinical situations thus enabled us to analyze the two feeding routes on the seventh ICU day and their effects on feeding efficiency and mortality. From January 2014 to December 2015, a total of 113 patients with malnutrition and at high nutritional risk were retrospectively enrolled in the analysis and were classified into SBEN (n = 48) and NGEN (n = 65) groups through matching according to age, sex, mNUTRIC score, and APACHE II score (Supplementary Figure S1 revealed the study flow.).

2.3. *Data Collection, Adjustment, and Outcome Measures*

Data were collected on age, sex, body mass index (BMI), severity of illness (SOFA and APACHE II scores), mNUTRIC score, major comorbidities, and Charlson Comorbidity Index (CCI). The primary outcome was feeding efficiency, including average energy intake achievement rate (%); hospital mortality was the secondary outcome. The index date was the seventh day of the ICU stay, which was the day defining whether a patient with critical illness and malnutrition was placed in the SBEN or NGEN group. Those who had received transpyloric tube insertion were enrolled into the SBEN group. Daily energy intake was recorded from the index day (the seventh ICU day) until 7 days later (the 14th ICU day). As in our previous report [8], the serial nutrition parameters 3 days after the index date were employed to compare the feeding efficiency of the SBEN and NGEN groups. Feeding efficiency was evaluated by the following six parameters: (1) actual feeding volume (mL/day), (2) actual energy intake (kcal/day), (3) actual protein intake (g/day), (4) actual protein intake (g/kg/body weight (BW)), (5) energy intake achievement rate (%), and (6) protein intake achievement rate (%). The primary outcome was the comparison of feeding efficiency between the SBEN and NGEN groups. The secondary outcome was factors associated with hospital mortality in ICU patients with mNUTRIC score ≥ 5 and feeding volume < 750 mL/day. We also validated the power of hospital mortality prediction in this setting because an energy achievement rate of < 65% on the third day after the index date (the 10th ICU day) was demonstrated to be an outcome predictor in our other study [8].

2.4. *Statistical Analysis*

Categorical variables are presented as frequencies and percentages. The chi-squared test was used to determine significance. The Mann–Whitney U test was applied to determine differences between groups for data with nonparametric distribution, and the results are presented as the median and interquartile range (IQR). Factors associated with hospital mortality were assessed through Cox regression analysis. The strength of an association is presented as the hazard ratio (HR) and 95% confidence interval (CI). All tests were two sided, with $p < 0.05$ considered significant. The SPSS statistical software package (version 24.0; International Business Machines Corp, Armonk, NY, USA) was used for all statistical analyses.

3. Results

Table 1 reveals a comparison of demographic characteristics, severity scores, comorbidities, energy intake, and hospital mortality between the SBEN and NGEN groups. The median mNUTRIC score of the cohort was 7 (IQR, 5.25–8 in the SBEN group and 5.5–8 in the NGEN group), indicating that these patients were at high nutritional risk. The APACHE II (27.0 and 30.0 for the SBEN and NGEN groups, respectively) and SOFA (10 and 10 for the SBEN and NGEN groups, respectively) scores also indicated the high clinical severity of disease in this cohort. However, cardiovascular disease (64.58% and 26.15% in the SBEN and NGEN groups, respectively, $p < 0.001$) and cancer (45.83% and 12.31% in the SBEN and NGEN groups, respectively, $p < 0.001$) were more common in the SBEN group than the NGEN group; liver cirrhosis (22.92% and 55.38% in the SBEN and NGEN groups, respectively, $p = 0.001$) was less common in the SBEN group. The overall hospital mortality rate exhibited no significant difference between these two groups (43.75% and 43.08% in the SBEN and NGEN groups, respectively, $p > 0.05$). The achievement rate (%) of daily average energy intake on days 2–7 was significantly higher in the SBEN group than the NGEN group on each observation day. As shown in Table 1, the average energy achievement rate was higher than 60% in the SBEN group on the fourth day, but remained lower than 60% until the seventh day in the NGEN group. Using the energy achievement index parameter of more than 65% on the third day (the 10th ICU day) as the objective goal, 45.83% of patients achieved the goal in the SBEN group, but only 26.15% reached the goal in the NGEN group, a significant difference ($p = 0.048$).

Table 1. Demographic characteristics, severity scores, comorbidities, and clinical outcomes for all malnourished patients in the intensive care unit (ICU).

Variables	SBEN Group (n = 48)	NGEN Group (n = 65)	p-Value
Age (year)	70.45 (59.75–79.94)	74.17 (54.63–85.12)	0.423
Gender—Male (n, %) [a]	31 (64.58%)	48 (73.85%)	0.393
Body mass index (kg/m^2)	23.62 (21.29–27.32)	22.77 (21.1–25.05)	0.238
mNUTRIC score	7.00 (5.25–8)	7.0 (5.5–8)	0.491
APACHE II score	27.00 (24–32.75)	30.00 (27–33)	0.156
SOFA-day 1	10.00 (8–12.75)	10.00 (6.5–13)	0.875
SOFA—day 3 (n = 47 vs. 64)	9.00 (6–12)	10.00 (8–13)	0.172
SOFA—day 7 (n = 46 vs. 64)	8.5 (5–11)	9.0 (7–11)	0.490
CCI	2.5 (1–4)	0.0 (0–2)	<0.001 **
Comorbidity (n, %) [a]			
Diabetes mellitus	13 (27.08%)	20 (30.77%)	0.828
Chronic kidney disease	9 (18.75%)	14 (21.54%)	0.898
Cardiovascular disease	31 (64.58%)	17 (26.15%)	<0.001 **
Cancer	22 (45.83%)	8 (12.31%)	<0.001 **
Liver cirrhosis	11 (22.92%)	36 (55.38%)	0.001 **
Average energy intake achievement rate (%) after enrollment			1.000
2nd day	57.16 (36.29–70.69)	41.35 (30.16–65.12)	
3rd day	55.91 (41.5–75.49)	44.16 (30.85–64.41)	0.039 *
4th day	60.29 (41.29–75.11)	49.02 (32.36–66.74)	0.015 *
5th day	63.36 (43.2–78.62)	49.45 (32.05–69.46)	0.026 *
6th day	63.63 (45.5–81.01)	51.12 (32.24–71.99)	0.015 *
7th day	65.20 (48.91–84.47)	55.12 (32.57–75.35)	0.022 *
Average energy intake achievement rate (%) ≥ 65% (3 days after the index day) (n, %) [a]	22 (45.83%)	17 (26.15%)	0.031 *
Hospital mortality (n, %) [a]	21 (43.75%)	28 (43.08%)	0.048 *

[a] Chi-squared test or Mann–Whitney U test, * $p < 0.05$, ** $p < 0.01$. SBEN, small bowel enteral nutrition; NGEN, nasogastric tube enteral nutrition; mNUTRIC, modified Nutrition Risk in Critically Ill; APACHE II, Acute Physiology and Chronic Health Evaluation II; SOFA, Sequential Organ Failure Assessment; CCI, Charlson Comorbidity Index. Categorical variables are presented as frequencies and percentages (%).

Table 2 presents a comparison of the feeding efficiency of the SBEN and NGEN groups. Actual daily energy parameters represent the feeding efficiency on the third observation day, including actual feeding volume (mL/day), actual energy intake (kcal/day), actual protein intake (g/day), actual protein intake (g/kg/BW), energy intake achievement rate (%), and protein achievement rate (%). All feeding parameters were significantly higher in the SBEN group than the NGEN group (Table 2). The energy intake achievement rate (%) in the SBEN group significantly increased day by day compared with that in the NGEN group ($p = 0.021$; Figure 1).

Table 2. Comparison of feeding efficiency between SBEN and NGEN groups on the third day after enrollment in malnourished, critically ill, ICU patients.

Variables	SBEN Group ($n = 48$)	NGEN Group ($n = 65$)	*p*-Value
Actual feeding volume (mL/day)	992.88 (706.44–1191.38)	824.50 (541.38–1054.88) *	0.025 *
Actual energy intake (kcal/day)	921.15 (635.79–1172.81)	707.40 (487.24–949.39) **	0.004 **
Actual protein intake (g/day)	36.37 (25.43–46.91)	28.30 (19.49–37.98) **	0.005 **
Actual protein intake (g/kg/BW)	0.60 (0.41–0.74)	0.49 (0.31–0.69) *	0.029 *
Energy intake achievement rate (%)	60.29 (41.29–75.11)	49.02 (32.36–66.74) *	0.026 *
Protein intake achievement rate (%)	49.63 (34.16–62.01)	40.85 (25.78–57.18) *	0.029 *

Values are median (interquartile range (IQR)). Mann–Whitney U test. * $p < 0.05$, ** $p < 0.01$.

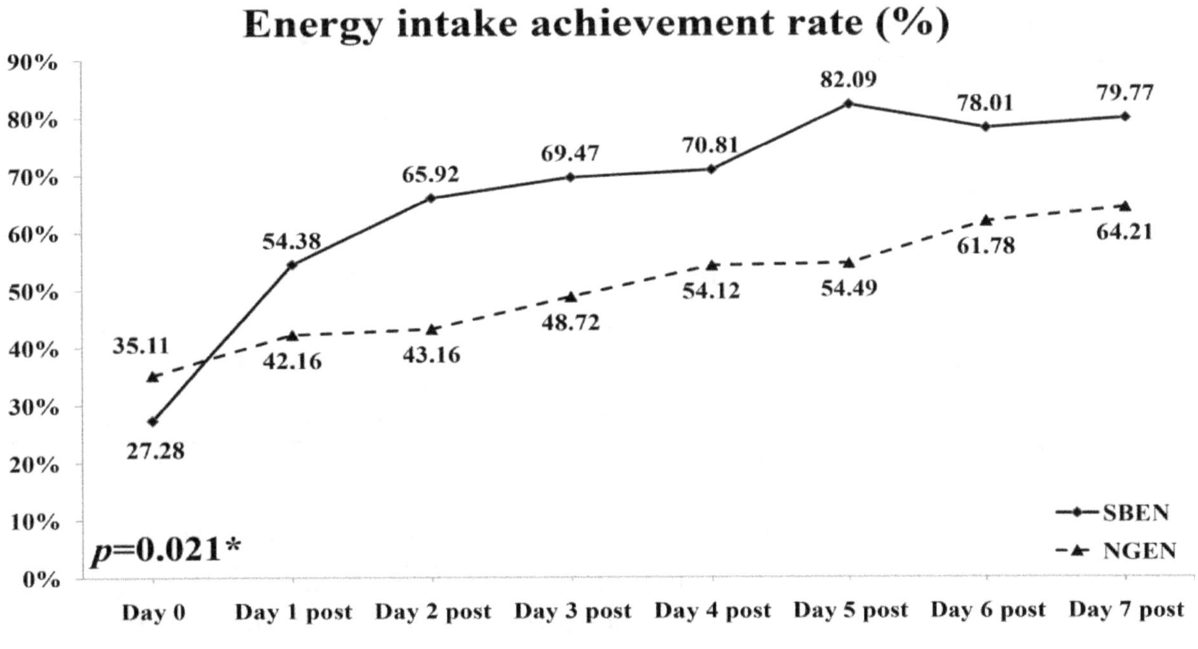

Figure 1. Achievement rate of energy intake for SBEN and NGEN groups. $p = 0.021$

The parameters of surviving and nonsurviving patients were compared (Table 3). The nonsurviving patients had higher SOFA scores on the seventh ICU day and lower energy intake achievement rates (%) on each day subsequent to the enrollment day. Age, sex, BMI, mNUTRIC score, APACHEII score, and comorbidities were not significantly different between the survival and nonsurvival groups. In the survival group, the median energy intake was 60% on the fourth day (the 11th ICU day). By contrast, the median energy intake achievement in the nonsurvival group remained at lower than 50%, even on the seventh day after enrollment (the 14th ICU day; Table 3).

Factors associated with mortality by Cox regression analysis are shown in Table 4. A univariate analysis identified only three factors associated with mortality: SBNE group (HR, 0.56; 95% CI, 0.31–0.997; $p = 0.049$), SOFA score on the seventh ICU day (HR, 1.12; 95% CI, 1.03–1.22; $p = 0.009$), and energy achievement rate < 65% on the third day after enrollment (the 10th ICU day; HR, 2.53; 95% CI, 1.25–5.11; $p = 0.01$). A multivariate analysis indicated that energy intake achievement rate < 65% on the third day after enrollment (HR, 2.29; 95% CI, 1.12–4.69) was the only predictive factor that differed significantly between the survival and nonsurvival groups. In this cohort, an energy achievement rate > 65% was associated with lower 60-day, 90-day, and hospital mortality after adjustment for age, sex, BMI, and SOFA and APACHE II scores in patients at high nutritional risk (mNUTRIC ≥ 5; Figure 2).

Table 3. Comparison of survivors and nonsurvivors according to hospital mortality in malnourished, critically ill, ICU patients.

Variables	Nonsurvival (n = 49)	Survival (n = 64)	p-Value
Group (n, %) [a]			1.000
SBEN group	37 (75.51%)	27 (42.19%)	
NGEN group	22.59 (57.14%)	37 (57.81%)	
Age (year)	72.13 (55.47–83.26)	73.03 (60.54–82.22)	0.498
Gender—Male (n, %) [a]	37 (75.51%)	42 (65.63%)	0.353
Body mass index (kg/m^2)	22.59 (20.44–26.67)	23.52 (21.41–26.21)	0.412
mNUTRIC score	7.00 (6–8)	7.00 (5–8)	0.255
APACHE II score	30.00 (26.5–34)	28.00 (24–32)	0.176
SOFA—day 1	10.00 (8–13.5)	10.00 (6–12.75)	0.257
SOFA—day 3	11.00 (8–13)	9.00 (6–12)	0.082
SOFA—day 7	10.00 (7–13)	8.00 (6–10) **	0.007 **
CCI	1.00 (0–3)	2.00 (0–3.75)	0.333
Comorbidity (n,%) [a]			
Diabetes mellitus	11 (22.45%)	22 (34.38%)	0.241
Chronic kidney disease	13 (26.53%)	10 (15.63%)	0.234
Cardiovascular disease	20 (40.82%)	28 (43.75%)	0.904
Cancer	12 (24.49%)	18 (28.13%)	0.827
Liver cirrhosis	19 (38.78%)	28 (43.75%)	0.735
Obstructive pulmonary disease	17 (34.69%)	20 (31.25%)	0.854
Average of energy intake achievement rate (%) post-enrollment			
2nd day	43.69 (24.9–58.88)	49.44 (35.44–70.69) *	0.042 *
3rd day	40.63 (24.43–63.04)	55.91 (38.98–72.22) **	0.009 **
4th day	41.45 (27.78–66.7)	59.76 (40.3–76.73) **	0.005 **
5th day	44.55 (26.86–68.16)	60.80 (44.13–84.31) **	0.002 **
6th day	45.97 (24.78–66.57)	63.45 (48.93–83.84) **	0.001 **
7th day	48.99 (25.01–67.34)	66.07 (50.68–84.47) **	<0.001 **

Values are median (IQR). Mann–Whitney U test. [a] Chi-squared test. * $p < 0.05$, ** $p < 0.01$.

Table 4. Cox regression analysis for factors associated with hospital mortality.

Variables	Univariate Analysis	Multivariate Analysis
	HR (95% CI)	HR (95% CI)
Age (year)	0.99 (0.98–1.01)	
Group (SBEN vs. NGEN)	0.56 (0.31–0.997) *	0.65 (0.36–1.18)
Gender (Female vs. Male)	0.62 (0.32–1.20)	
Body mass index (kg/m2)	0.97 (0.91–1.04)	
mNUTRIC score	0.91 (0.72–1.14)	
APACHE II score	1.01 (0.96–1.06)	
SOFA—day 1	0.99 (0.92–1.07)	
SOFA—day 3	1.05 (0.97–1.13)	
SOFA—day 7	1.12 (1.03–1.22) **	
Energy intake achievement rate (%) (3 days after the index day) (<65% vs. ≥65%)	2.53 (1.25–5.11) *	2.29 (1.12–4.69) *

Cox regression. * $p < 0.05$, ** $p < 0.01$.

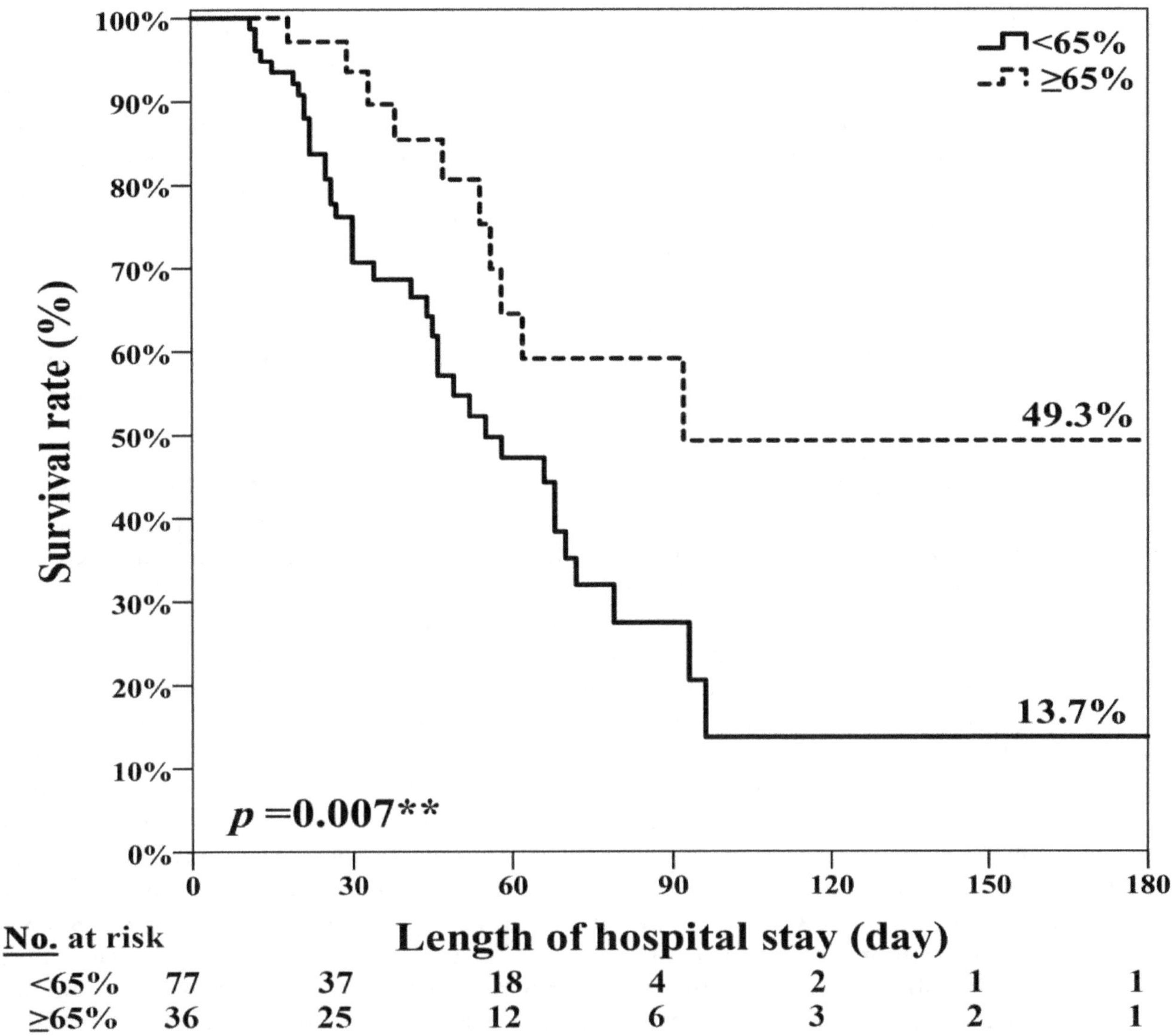

Figure 2. Energy achievement rate ≥ 65% on the 10th ICU day was significantly associated with lower hospital mortality in patients at high nutritional risk. ** $p = 0.007$.

4. Discussion

The present study reports three major findings regarding critically ill patients admitted to the ICU with malnourishment and high nutritional risk. First, after 7 days of stomach EN, the initiation of adjuvant SBEN improved energy delivery and had potential benefits in relation to hospital mortality compared with continued stomach EN. Second, the feeding efficiency increased significantly after SBEN initiation and resulted in the nutritional goal being achieved within 3 days. Third, achievement of 65% of the energy requirements by day 3 after SBEN initiation (on the 10th ICU day) was the key factor associated with survival. If a patient does not reach the goal within 3 days of SBEN initiation, we suggest that PN should be considered to improve the energy intake achievement rate.

The current guidelines—including the ASPEN/SCCM and ESPEN guidelines and the consensus statement of the Asia-Pacific and Middle East regions—recommend that every critically ill patient staying in the ICU for more than 48 h should be considered as being at risk of malnutrition, and a systemic approach to, as well as evaluation of, nutritional risk is suggested [5,6,11]. EN should be initiated within 48 h to provide nutritional support to critically ill patients who are unable to maintain volitional intake [5–7]. The current evidence does not suggest routine feeding through SBEN [19]. Accordingly, NGEN is recommended as the standard approach for early EN, and SBEN can be used as adjuvant therapy for those with gastric feeding intolerance that cannot be resolved with prokinetic agents [5–7]. In fact, studies have demonstrated that SBEN provides greater feeding efficiency than NGEN [19–21,23]. However, the right time to shift from NGEN to SBEN remains unclear in the current guidelines. Regarding actual clinical practice, we conduct a feeding protocol to evaluate the energy intake achievement rate at the end of the first week of an ICU stay, and this evaluation enables initiation of SBEN on the eighth ICU day as an option in ICU care [8]. Therefore, all patients enrolled in the present cohort had high mNUTRIC score (median mNUTRIC score, 7; IQR, 5.25–8) and low energy intake achievement rate (<50% of the target goal or feeding volume < 750 mL/day) even though NGEN was started within 48 h of ICU admission. To the best of our knowledge, the present study, which initiated SBEN as adjuvant therapy on the 7th ICU day to improve energy delivery compared with maintenance of NGEN, is the first data-based report to examine critically ill, ICU patients at high nutritional risk.

Another major issue overlooked in the guidelines is the optimal time at which to decide that the SBEN approach has failed and feeding route should be switched from SBEN to supplemental PN or total PN. Our previous study suggested that on the third day after SBEN initiation, the optimal energy intake achievement rate was higher than 65% [8]. For critically ill patients for whom NGEN has failed and have been shifted to SBEN on the eighth ICU day, an energy achievement rate of <65% 3 days after SBEN initiation was significantly associated with increased mortality (odds ratio, 4.97; 95% CI, 1.44–17.07) [8]. The 2019 ESPEN guidelines recommend that PN should not be started until all strategies to maximize EN tolerance have been attempted [5]. Heidegger et al. suggested that starting supplementary PN on the fourth day after ICU admission may reduce nosocomial infections and improve clinical outcomes in patients for whom EN is insufficient [25]. Some studies have suggested initiating EN plus PN between the fourth and seventh days in the ICU [26–28]. However, the 2016 ASPEN/SCCM guidelines recommend considering the initiation of supplemental PN only if >60% energy and protein intake achievement are not achieved after 7–10 days of EN because initiating PN before this time has no benefits [6,7]. Braunschweig et al. published research on the timing and doses of energy received by patients with acute lung injury, inferring that higher later (days ≥ 8) energy intake may reduce the mortality risk [29]. Therefore, the optimal time point for administration of supplementary PN with the aim of meeting full energy requirements and whether SBEN should be attempted before a patient is shifted to PN remain unclear. Our data suggest that for critically ill patients with mNUTRIC score ≥ 5 and poor feeding achievement rate (<50% of target goal or feeding volume < 750 mL/day) using gastric tube feeding, SBEN for 3 days is an option prior to PN initiation.

The final point that merits discussion is whether SBEN has advantages in terms of mortality. The literature shows that adequate nutritional support has a significant mortality benefit in those at high risk of malnutrition and who are critically ill [14,30]. Our study conducted in 2019 also suggested that energy requirements achieving <65% within 3 days of SBEN initiation is the independent factor associated with mortality (OR, 4.97; 95% CI, 1.44–17.07) in malnourished and high nutritional risk populations [8]. Our previous studies suggested that critically ill patients at high nutritional risk who receive at least 65% of their energy intake requirements and consume at least 800 kcal/day exhibit significantly lower 14-day, 28-day, and hospital mortality rates [13,15]. However, in populations at low nutritional risk (mNUTRIC score < 5), copious evidence indicates no survival benefits from full nutritional support [13,24,30–32]. This phenomenon is due to the strong correlation of suboptimal energy delivery with increased nosocomial infection, longer duration of ventilator dependency, and longer ICU and hospital stays—these factors contribute to greater mortality [14,15,33]. The current study enrolled patients from ICUs who were elderly, had high disease severity, and were at high nutrition risk. Most were admitted to the RICU because of pneumonia-related sepsis, septic shock, acute respiratory failure, or acute respiratory distress syndrome. Therefore, adequate nutritional support played a major role in their survival. The nutritional intake cut-off value for distinguishing survival from nonsurvival was 65%, the same as that indicated by our other research [8,13]. The univariate analysis revealed that the SBEN group experienced mortality benefits, but had a higher SOFA score on the seventh ICU day, and energy intake achievement rate < 65% on the 10th ICU day was significantly associated with hospital mortality. However, in the multivariable analysis, the only factor that was discovered to independently predict hospital mortality was energy intake achievement rate < 65% on the 10th ICU day (HR, 2.29; 95% CI, 1.12–4.69). We suggest that the potential mortality benefits from SBEN initiation are due to energy intake improvements in patients with very high disease severity. As such, if energy intake achievement is not improved substantially 3 days after SBEN initiation, supplementary PN or total PN should be considered to increase nutrition support.

This study has several limitations. First, the study design was a retrospective case-controlled study, in which two groups from a database were matched, rather than a prospective randomized controlled trial. Thus, heterogeneity may have existed between the two groups. Second, the study was conducted at a single ICU in a medical center, meaning that the results may not be generalizable. In practice, feeding protocols and patient populations may vary between ICUs. In our RICU, we followed a feeding protocol approved by the registered dietitian, who also provided nutrition risk evaluation and nutrition therapy recommendations in daily practice. For patients with an energy target achievement rate < 50% or a feeding volume < 750 mL/day, our protocol has provided the option since 2015 of consulting a gastroenterologist to evaluate the suitability of transpyloric tube insertion for SBEN on the seventh ICU day. Therefore, heterogeneity in ICU care and feeding protocols was minimal in the present study. Third, critically ill patients in ICU may require image studies, such as computed tomography and magnetic resonance imaging, invasive procedures, and gastrointestinal endoscopy, which can interrupt feeding protocols. Finally, the present results may not be generalizable to critically ill patients in pediatric, cardiac, neurosurgical, and surgical ICUs or even general ICUs because the current study was conducted only in RICU patients.

5. Conclusions

Replacing NGEN with SBEN on the seventh ICU day significantly improves energy delivery and may reduce hospital mortality risk in patients at high nutritional risk. The key factor determining survival in this population is an energy intake requirement rate > 65% within 3 days of SBEN initiation. For malnourished, critically ill patients at high nutritional risk (mNUTRIC score ≥ 5) who have been treated with all other available strategies to maximize EN tolerance, we suggest initiating SBEN on the seventh ICU day before PN initiation, and the clinician should follow up on the energy intake achievement rate (at least >65%) 3 days after SBEN initiation to determine the subsequent step of nutrition support therapy.

Author Contributions: Conceptualization, P.-K.F.; data curation, W.-N.W., C.-Y.W., and P.-K.F.; formal analysis, W.-N.W. and C.-Y.H.; funding acquisition, P.-K.F.; investigation, W.-N.W., C.-Y.H., and P.-K.F.; methodology, C.-Y.W., C.-Y.H., and P.-K.F.; software, C.-Y.H.; validation, C.-Y.W.; visualization, W.-N.W. and P.-K.F.; writing—original draft, P.-K.F.; writing—review and editing, W.-N.W., C.-Y.W., C.-Y.H., and P.-K.F. All authors read and approved the final manuscript.

Acknowledgments: This study was based in part on data from the Taichung Veterans General Hospital Research Database, which is managed by the Clinical Informatics Research & Development Center of Taichung Veterans General Hospital. This manuscript was edited by Wallace Academic Editing. An abstract of these findings has been submitted to the conference "Nutrition 2020" held by the American Society for Nutrition (ASN) on 30 January 2020. We thank Wei-Ning Wang for presenting the preliminary data in June 2020. The abstract has also been published in the journal of "Current Developments in Nutrition", Volume 4, Issue Supplement_2, June 2020, Page 1152 [34].

Abbreviations

The following abbreviations are used in this manuscript:

APACHE II	Acute Physiology and Chronic Health Evaluation II
ASPEN	American Society for Parenteral and Enteral Nutrition
CCI	Charlson Comorbidity Index
ESPEN	European Society for Clinical Nutrition and Metabolism
SBEN	Small bowel enteral nutrition
mNUTRIC	modified Nutrition Risk in Critically Ill
NGEN	Nasogastric tube enteral nutrition
PN	Parenteral nutrition
SCCM	Society of Critical Care Medicine
SOFA	Simplified Organ Failure Assessment

References

1. Weijs, P.J.M.; Mogensen, K.M.; Rawn, J.D.; Christopher, K.B. Protein Intake, Nutritional Status and Outcomes in ICU Survivors: A Single Center Cohort Study. *J. Clin. Med.* **2019**, *8*, 43. [CrossRef] [PubMed]
2. Mogensen, K.M.; Robinson, M.K.; Casey, J.D.; Gunasekera, N.S.; Moromizato, T.; Rawn, J.D.; Christopher, K.B. Nutritional Status and Mortality in the Critically Ill. *Crit. Care Med.* **2015**, *43*, 2605–2615. [CrossRef] [PubMed]
3. Kopp Lugli, A.; de Watteville, A.; Hollinger, A.; Goetz, N.; Heidegger, C. Medical Nutrition Therapy in Critically Ill Patients Treated on Intensive and Intermediate Care Units: A Literature Review. *J Clin. Med.* **2019**, *8*, 1395. [CrossRef] [PubMed]
4. Havens, J.M.; Columbus, A.B.; Seshadri, A.J.; Olufajo, O.A.; Mogensen, K.M.; Rawn, J.D.; Salim, A.; Christopher, K.B. Malnutrition at Intensive Care Unit Admission Predicts Mortality in Emergency General Surgery Patients. *J. Parenter. Enter. Nutr.* **2018**, *42*, 156–163. [CrossRef] [PubMed]
5. Singer, P.; Blaser, A.R.; Berger, M.M.; Alhazzani, W.; Calder, P.C.; Casaer, M.P.; Hiesmayr, M.; Mayer, K.; Montejo, J.C.; Pichard, C.; et al. ESPEN guideline on clinical nutrition in the intensive care unit. *Clin. Nutr.* **2019**, *38*, 48–79. [CrossRef]
6. Taylor, B.E.; McClave, S.A.; Martindale, R.G.; Warren, M.M.; Johnson, D.R.; Braunschweig, C.; McCarthy, M.S.; Davanos, E.; Rice, T.W.; Cresci, G.A.; et al. Guidelines for the Provision and Assessment of Nutrition Support Therapy in the Adult Critically Ill Patient: Society of Critical Care Medicine (SCCM) and American Society for Parenteral and Enteral Nutrition (A.S.P.E.N.). *Crit. Care Med.* **2016**, *44*, 390–438. [CrossRef]
7. McClave, S.A.; Taylor, B.E.; Martindale, R.G.; Warren, M.M.; Johnson, D.R.; Braunschweig, C.; McCarthy, M.S.; Davanos, E.; Rice, T.W.; Cresci, G.A.; et al. Guidelines for the Provision and Assessment of Nutrition Support Therapy in the Adult Critically Ill Patient: Society of Critical Care Medicine (SCCM) and American Society for Parenteral and Enteral Nutrition (A.S.P.E.N.). *J. Parenter. Enter. Nutr.* **2016**, *40*, 159–211. [CrossRef]
8. Wang, W.N.; Yang, M.F.; Wang, C.Y.; Hsu, C.Y.; Lee, B.J.; Fu, P.K. Optimal Time and Target for Evaluating Energy Delivery after Adjuvant Feeding with Small Bowel Enteral Nutrition in Critically Ill Patients at High Nutrition Risk. *Nutrients* **2019**, *11*, 645. [CrossRef]
9. Rattanachaiwong, S.; Zribi, B.; Kagan, I.; Theilla, M.; Heching, M.; Singer, P. Comparison of nutritional screening and diagnostic tools in diagnosis of severe malnutrition in critically ill patients. *Clin. Nutr.* **2020**, in press. [CrossRef]
10. De Vries, M.C.; Koekkoek, W.K.; Opdam, M.H.; van Blokland, D.; van Zanten, A.R. Nutritional assessment of critically ill patients: Validation of the modified NUTRIC score. *Eur. J. Clin. Nutr.* **2018**, *72*, 428–435. [CrossRef]
11. Sioson, M.S.; Martindale, R.; Abayadeera, A.; Abouchaleh, N.; Aditianingsih, D.; Bhurayanontachai, R.; Chiou, W.C.; Higashibeppu, N.; Mat Nor, M.B.; Osland, E.; et al. Nutrition therapy for critically ill patients across the Asia-Pacific and Middle East regions: A consensus statement. *Clin. Nutr. ESPEN* **2018**, *24*, 156–164. [CrossRef] [PubMed]
12. Arabi, Y.M.; Al-Dorzi, H.M.; Mehta, S.; Tamim, H.M.; Haddad, S.H.; Jones, G.; McIntyre, L.; Solaiman, O.; Sakkijha, M.H.; Sadat, M.; et al. Association of protein intake with the outcomes of critically ill patients: A post hoc analysis of the PermiT trial. *Am. J. Clin. Nutr.* **2018**, *108*, 988–996. [CrossRef] [PubMed]

13. Wang, C.Y.; Fu, P.K.; Huang, C.T.; Chen, C.H.; Lee, B.J.; Huang, Y.C. Targeted Energy Intake Is the Important Determinant of Clinical Outcomes in Medical Critically Ill Patients with High Nutrition Risk. *Nutrients* **2018**, *10*, 1731. [CrossRef]
14. Jung, Y.T.; Park, J.Y.; Jeon, J.; Kim, M.J.; Lee, S.H.; Lee, J.G. Association of Inadequate Caloric Supplementation with 30-Day Mortality in Critically Ill Postoperative Patients with High Modified NUTRIC Score. *Nutrients* **2018**, *10*, 1589. [CrossRef]
15. Wang, C.Y.; Huang, C.T.; Chen, C.H.; Chen, M.F.; Ching, S.L.; Huang, Y.C. Optimal Energy Delivery, Rather than the Implementation of a Feeding Protocol, May Benefit Clinical Outcomes in Critically Ill Patients. *Nutrients* **2017**, *9*, 527. [CrossRef] [PubMed]
16. Schuetz, P.; Stanga, Z. Nutritional Management and Outcomes in Malnourished Medical Inpatients in 2020: The Evidence Is Growing! *J. Clin. Med.* **2019**, *9*, 27. [CrossRef] [PubMed]
17. Allen, K.; Hoffman, L. Enteral Nutrition in the Mechanically Ventilated Patient. *Nutr. Clin. Pract.* **2019**, *34*, 540–557. [CrossRef]
18. Bendavid, I.; Zusman, O.; Kagan, I.; Theilla, M.; Cohen, J.; Singer, P. Early Administration of Protein in Critically Ill Patients: A Retrospective Cohort Study. *Nutrients* **2019**, *11*, 106. [CrossRef]
19. Davies, A.R.; Morrison, S.S.; Bailey, M.J.; Bellomo, R.; Cooper, D.J.; Doig, G.S.; Finfer, S.R.; Heyland, D.K. A multicenter, randomized controlled trial comparing early nasojejunal with nasogastric nutrition in critical illness. *Crit. Care Med.* **2012**, *40*, 2342–2348. [CrossRef]
20. Acosta-Escribano, J.; Fernandez-Vivas, M.; Grau Carmona, T.; Caturla-Such, J.; Garcia-Martinez, M.; Menendez-Mainer, A.; Solera-Suarez, M.; Sanchez-Paya, J. Gastric versus transpyloric feeding in severe traumatic brain injury: A prospective, randomized trial. *Intensive Care Med.* **2010**, *36*, 1532–1539. [CrossRef]
21. Hsu, C.W.; Sun, S.F.; Lin, S.L.; Kang, S.P.; Chu, K.A.; Lin, C.H.; Huang, H.H. Duodenal versus gastric feeding in medical intensive care unit patients: A prospective, randomized, clinical study. *Crit. Care Med.* **2009**, *37*, 1866–1872. [CrossRef] [PubMed]
22. White, H.; Sosnowski, K.; Tran, K.; Reeves, A.; Jones, M. A randomised controlled comparison of early post-pyloric versus early gastric feeding to meet nutritional targets in ventilated intensive care patients. *Crit. Care* **2009**, *13*, R187. [CrossRef] [PubMed]
23. Montejo, J.C.; Grau, T.; Acosta, J.; Ruiz-Santana, S.; Planas, M.; Garcia-De-Lorenzo, A.; Mesejo, A.; Cervera, M.; Sanchez-Alvarez, C.; Nunez-Ruiz, R.; et al. Multicenter, prospective, randomized, single-blind study comparing the efficacy and gastrointestinal complications of early jejunal feeding with early gastric feeding in critically ill patients. *Crit. Care Med.* **2002**, *30*, 796–800. [CrossRef] [PubMed]
24. Rahman, A.; Hasan, R.M.; Agarwala, R.; Martin, C.; Day, A.G.; Heyland, D.K. Identifying critically-ill patients who will benefit most from nutritional therapy: Further validation of the "modified NUTRIC" nutritional risk assessment tool. *Clin. Nutr.* **2016**, *35*, 158–162. [CrossRef] [PubMed]
25. Heidegger, C.P.; Berger, M.M.; Graf, S.; Zingg, W.; Darmon, P.; Costanza, M.C.; Thibault, R.; Pichard, C. Optimisation of energy provision with supplemental parenteral nutrition in critically ill patients: A randomised controlled clinical trial. *Lancet* **2013**, *381*, 385–393. [CrossRef]
26. Pradelli, L.; Graf, S.; Pichard, C.; Berger, M.M. Supplemental parenteral nutrition in intensive care patients: A cost saving strategy. *Clin. Nutr.* **2018**, *37*, 573–579. [CrossRef]
27. Gavri, C.; Kokkoris, S.; Vasileiadis, I.; Oeconomopoulou, A.C.; Kotanidou, A.; Nanas, S.; Routsi, C. Route of nutrition and risk of blood stream infections in critically ill patients; a comparative study. *Clin. Nutr. ESPEN* **2016**, *12*, e14–e19. [CrossRef]
28. Doig, G.S.; Simpson, F.; Sweetman, E.A.; Finfer, S.R.; Cooper, D.J.; Heighes, P.T.; Davies, A.R.; O'Leary, M.; Solano, T.; Peake, S. Early parenteral nutrition in critically ill patients with short-term relative contraindications to early enteral nutrition: A randomized controlled trial. *JAMA* **2013**, *309*, 2130–2138. [CrossRef]
29. Braunschweig, C.L.; Freels, S.; Sheean, P.M.; Peterson, S.J.; Perez, S.G.; McKeever, L.; Lateef, O.; Gurka, D.; Fantuzzi, G. Role of timing and dose of energy received in patients with acute lung injury on mortality in the Intensive Nutrition in Acute Lung Injury Trial (INTACT): A post hoc analysis. *Am. J. Clin. Nutr.* **2017**, *105*, 411–416. [CrossRef]
30. Mukhopadhyay, A.; Henry, J.; Ong, V.; Leong, C.S.; Teh, A.L.; van Dam, R.M.; Kowitlawakul, Y. Association of modified NUTRIC score with 28-day mortality in critically ill patients. *Clin. Nutr.* **2017**, *36*, 1143–1148. [CrossRef]

31. Arabi, Y.M.; Aldawood, A.S.; Al-Dorzi, H.M.; Tamim, H.M.; Haddad, S.H.; Jones, G.; McIntyre, L.; Solaiman, O.; Sakkijha, M.H.; Sadat, M.; et al. Permissive Underfeeding or Standard Enteral Feeding in High- and Low-Nutritional-Risk Critically Ill Adults. Post Hoc Analysis of the PermiT Trial. *Am. J. Respir. Crit. Care Med.* **2017**, *195*, 652–662. [CrossRef] [PubMed]
32. Compher, C.; Chittams, J.; Sammarco, T.; Nicolo, M.; Heyland, D.K. Greater Protein and Energy Intake May Be Associated With Improved Mortality in Higher Risk Critically Ill Patients: A Multicenter, Multinational Observational Study. *Crit. Care Med.* **2017**, *45*, 156–163. [CrossRef] [PubMed]
33. Alberda, C.; Gramlich, L.; Jones, N.; Jeejeebhoy, K.; Day, A.G.; Dhaliwal, R.; Heyland, D.K. The relationship between nutritional intake and clinical outcomes in critically ill patients: Results of an international multicenter observational study. *Intensive Care Med.* **2009**, *35*, 1728–1737. [CrossRef] [PubMed]
34. Wang, W.N.; Fu, P.K.; Hsu, C.Y. Comparison of Feeding Efficacy and Hospital Mortality Between Small Bowel and Nasogastric Tube Enteral Nutrition in Critical Illness at High Nutritional Risk. *Curr. Dev. Nutr.* **2020**, *4*, 1152. [CrossRef]

4

Association between Geriatric Nutritional Risk Index and Mortality in Older Trauma Patients in the Intensive Care Unit

Hang-Tsung Liu [1,†], Shao-Chun Wu [2,†], Ching-Hua Tsai [1], Chi Li [1], Sheng-En Chou [1], Wei-Ti Su [1], Shiun-Yuan Hsu [1] and Ching-Hua Hsieh [3,*]

1 Department of Trauma Surgery, Kaohsiung Chang Gung Memorial Hospital, Chang Gung University College of Medicine, Kaohsiung City 833, Taiwan; htl1688@yahoo.com.tw (H.-T.L.); tsai1737@cloud.cgmh.org.tw (C.-H.T.); foocollie7@gmail.com (C.L.); athenechou@gmail.com (S.-E.C.); s101132@adm.cgmh.org.tw (W.-T.S.); ah.lucy@hotmail.com (S.-Y.H.)

2 Department of Anesthesiology, Kaohsiung Chang Gung Memorial Hospital, Chang Gung University College of Medicine, Kaohsiung City 833, Taiwan; shaochunwu@gmail.com

3 Department of Plastic Surgery, Kaohsiung Chang Gung Memorial Hospital, Chang Gung University College of Medicine, Kaohsiung City 833, Taiwan

* Correspondence: m93chinghua@gmail.com

† These authors contributed equally to this work.

Abstract: The geriatric nutritional risk index (GNRI) is a simple and efficient tool to assess the nutritional status of patients with malignancies or after surgery. Because trauma patients constitute a specific population that generally acquires accidental and acute injury, this study aimed to identify the association between the GNRI at admission and mortality outcomes of older trauma patients in the intensive care unit (ICU). Methods: The study population included 700 older trauma patients admitted to the ICU between 1 January 2009 and 31 December 2019. The collected data included age, sex, body mass index (BMI), albumin level at admission, preexisting comorbidities, injury severity score (ISS), and in-hospital mortality. Multivariate logistic regression analysis was conducted to identify the independent effects of univariate predictive variables resulting in mortality in our study population. The study population was categorized into four nutritional risk groups: a major-risk group (GNRI < 82; n = 128), moderate-risk group (GNRI 82 to <92; n = 191), low-risk group (GNRI 92–98; n = 136), and no-risk group (GNRI > 98; n = 245). Results: There was no significant difference in sex predominance, age, and BMI between the mortality (n = 125) and survival (n = 575) groups. The GNRI was significantly lower in the mortality group than in the survival group (89.8 ± 12.9 vs. 94.2 ± 12.0, p < 0.001). Multivariate logistic regression analysis showed that the GNRI (odds ratio—OR, 0.97; 95% confidence interval (CI) 0.95–0.99; p = 0.001), preexisting end-stage renal disease (OR, 3.6; 95% CI, 1.70–7.67; p = 0.001), and ISS (OR, 1.1; 95% CI, 1.05–1.10; p < 0.001) were significant independent risk factors for mortality. Compared to the patients in group of GNRI > 98, those patients in group of GNRI < 82 presented a significantly higher mortality rate (26.6% vs. 13.1%; p < 0.001) and length of stay in hospital (26.5 days vs. 20.9 days; p = 0.016). Conclusions: This study demonstrated that GNRI is a significant independent risk factor and a promising simple screening tool to identify the subjects with malnutrition associated with higher risk for mortality in those ICU elderly trauma patients.

Keywords: trauma; intensive care unit; mortality; malnutrition; elderly; the geriatric nutritional risk index

1. Background

The prevalence of malnutrition in hospitalized patients ranges from 10% to 50%, depending on the study population and diagnosis criteria [1]. In patients aged >65 years, malnutrition appears to be a common problem [2], especially in older hospitalized patients [3]. However, malnutrition is generally unrecognized and not treated properly in hospitalized patients [4]. For the critically ill patients in the intensive care unit (ICU), their nutritional status deteriorates rapidly after admission due to stress-related severe catabolism and the effects of malnutrition are likely to be more magnified [5,6]. In a systemic review of 20 studies, malnutrition diagnosed by nutrition assessments was independently associated with increased in ICU length of stay (LOS), ICU readmission, incidence of infection, and in-hospital mortality rate [7]. Using appropriate nutrition screening and assessment tools will help identify effective strategies that reduce the negative impact of malnutrition [8,9]. Therefore, for those elderly patients admitted into the ICU, it is important to identify patients at risk of malnutrition early and to treat them adequately.

There are several methods for assessing the nutritional status, such as albumin level, body mass index (BMI), muscle circumference, prognostic nutritional index (based on the serum albumin level and peripheral blood lymphocyte count), and questionnaires. The serum albumin level can be modified by inflammatory processes, hydration, and hepatic or renal impairment [10]; therefore, serum albumin is considered a better marker of inflammation and severity of acute illness than nutritional status [11]. Furthermore, anthropometric parameters such as BMI, weight loss, muscle circumferences, and skinfold thicknesses do not reflect the actual nutritional status of patients when applied separately [12]. The nutritional risk index (NRI) is a screening method that was primarily developed to identify older patients with malnutrition [13]. It consists of serum albumin levels as well as body weight measurements. However, even under professional care, the usual body weight is often not documented for older patients [14]. To determine the usual body weight of older patients, the geriatric nutritional risk index (GNRI) was introduced in 2005 by Bouillanne et al. [15]—the formula included a combination of serum albumin levels and the ratio of body weight to ideal body weight. The GNRI formula replaces the usual body weight in the NRI formula with the ideal body weight, calculated using the Lorentz formula [15]. The ratio of body weight to ideal body weight used in the GNRI might reflect the degree of frailty and cachexia associated with a poor prognosis in older patients [16]. Thus, the GNRI, which combines the factors of albumin and body weight status, may predict nutrition-related risk better than the serum albumin level or BMI [15]. The GNRI has been found to be superior to the albumin level and BMI, when used separately, in predicting cardiovascular-related mortality [17]. On the other hand, The Subjective Global Assessment classifies patients using information on the history of illness and physical examination [18]. However, the tool is too complex and is not suitable for rapid screening purposes [19]. The Mini Nutritional Assessment (MNA) relies on the completeness of its questionnaire and thus cannot be used with older patients who have difficulty communicating, for example, intubated patients in the ICU. Because it requires only objective parameters that can be readily collected and does not depend on a caregiver or memory, the GNRI is clearly less time consuming than other questionnaire-based assessment procedures and requires minimal participation by patients [2,15], thus being suitable for older patients with critical illness in the ICU. The GNRI may also be useful for older patients with cognitive impairment or delirium [20]. In addition, the GNRI score was found to be superior to the Mini Nutritional Assessment-Short Form (MNA–SF) score for risk discrimination regarding the overall survival in cancer patients [21].Although the GNRI was developed using the data of patients who were admitted to a geriatric rehabilitation care unit [15], it was found to be a strong prognostic factor for certain malignancies [22,23] and a simple, objective, and quick method to determine the nutritional status of patients and long-term postoperative outcomes and the correlation between these elements [24–28]. Using this simple calculation, it is possible to evaluate the nutritional status of critically ill patients with acute respiratory distress syndrome in the ICU [29].

Considering that trauma patients constitute a specific population, as injuries generally occur accidentally and acutely, it is important to determine whether the GNRI can be used to link nutritional status and outcomes in trauma patients. Therefore, this study aimed to identify the association between GNRI at admission and mortality outcomes of older trauma patients in the ICU.

2. Methods

2.1. Ethics Statement

This study was approved by the Institutional Review Board (IRB) of Chang Gung Memorial Hospital (approval number 202001446B0). Because the study was designed for retrospective analysis of the registered database, the need for informed consent was waived according to IRB regulations.

2.2. Study Population and Data Collection

The medical records of 39,135 enrolled trauma patients registered between 1 January 2009 and 31 December 2019 were reviewed for this study (Figure 1). The enrolled patients experienced trauma from different injuries and were hospitalized for treatment. Of the 7136 patients who were admitted to the ICU, 1926 older trauma patients were aged ≥65 years. After excluding patients whose albumin data were not available and those with incomplete data (n = 1226), 700 older trauma patients were finally included in the study. The study population was categorized according to the original description provided by Bouillanne et al. [15] into four nutritional risk groups: a major-risk group (GNRI < 82; n = 128), moderate-risk group (GNRI 82 to <92; n = 191), low-risk group (GNRI 92–98; n = 136), and no-risk group (GNRI > 98; n = 245). Detailed information of the study population was extracted from the Trauma Registry System of the hospital [30–32]. The following data were collected: age, sex, body mass index (BMI), albumin level at admission, preexisting comorbidities (diabetes mellitus—DM, hypertension—HTN, coronary artery disease—CAD, congestive heart failure—CHF, cerebral vascular accident—CVA, end-stage renal disease—ESRD, and chronic obstructive pulmonary disease—COPD), injury severity score (ISS), and in-hospital mortality. The 1998 version of the Abbreviated Injury Scale (AIS) was used to record scores [33]. The AIS measures injury severity of a trauma patient with a numeric method for ranking anatomy-based specific injuries [1], with the severity of the anatomical injury assessed on a six-point ordinal scale ranging from minor (1), moderate (2), serious (3), severe (4), critical (5), to un-survivable injury (6) [34,35]. ISS, which represents the severity of injury in patients with multiple injuries and ranges from 1 to 75, was calculated using the sum of the squares of the three highest AIS scores in different body regions [36,37]. The GNRI was calculated using the albumin level and the ratio of body weight to ideal body weight as per the following formula: $-1.489 \times$ albumin (g/dL) + $41.7 \times$ (body weight/ideal body weight). The ideal body weight of men is (body height in cm $- 80) \times 0.7$, and that of women is (body height in cm $- 70) \times 0.6$.

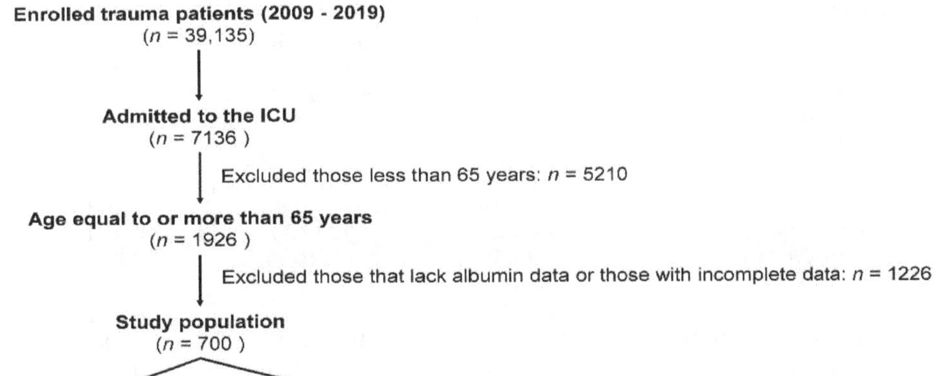
Enrolled trauma patients (2009 - 2019)
(n = 39,135)
Admitted to the ICU
(n = 7136)
Excluded those less than 65 years: n = 5210
Age equal to or more than 65 years
(n = 1926)
Excluded those that lack albumin data or those with incomplete data: n = 1226
Study population
(n = 700)
Death
(n = 125)
Survival
(n = 575)

Figure 1. Flow chart illustrating the inclusion of older trauma patients in the ICU and the allocation of these patients into the mortality group and survival group.

2.3. Statistical Analyses

In this study, all statistical analyses were performed using Window version 23.0 for SPSS (IBM Inc., Chicago, IL, USA). Two-sided Fisher's exact test or Pearson χ^2 test was used to compare categorical data. The normalization of the distributed data for continuous variables was assessed using the Kolmogorov–Smirnov test. Unpaired Student's t-test and the Mann–Whitney U test were used to analyze normally and non-normally distributed continuous data, respectively. The results are expressed as mean ± standard deviation, with ISS presented as median and interquartile range (IQR, Q1–Q3). Multivariate logistic regression analysis was conducted to identify the independent effects of univariate predictive variables leading to mortality in older patients with trauma. The odds ratios (ORs) of the risk factors associated with mortality and their 95% confidence intervals (CIs) were calculated with post hoc correction. p values < 0.05 were considered significant.

3. Results

3.1. Patient Demographics

As shown in Table 1, the study population was categorized into two groups: mortality (n = 125) and survival (n = 575). There was no significant difference in sex predominance, age, and BMI between the two groups. The albumin level and GNRI were significantly lower in the mortality group than in the survival group (albumin level: 3.0 ± 0.8 vs. 3.3 ± 0.6, p < 0.001; GNRI: 89.8 ± 12.9 vs. 94.2 ± 12.0, p < 0.001). There were no significant intergroup differences in the prevalence of preexisting comorbidities, except for a significantly lower rate of HTN (47.2% vs. 57.9%, p = 0.029) and higher rate of ESRD (10.4% vs. 4.2%, p = 0.005) in the mortality group than in the survival group. A significantly higher ISS was found in the group with fatal injuries than in the survival group (median—IQR: 25 [16–29] vs. 16 [13–25], p < 0.001). When stratified by ISS (1–15, 16–24, or ≥ 25), significantly fewer fatal patients had an ISS of 1–15 and 16–24 and more fatal patients had an ISS of ≥25 than survival patients. The patients in the mortality group had a shorter hospital LOS (19.7 days vs. 24.8 days, p = 0.006) than those in the survival group.

Table 1. Patient and injury characteristics of the mortality and survival groups of older trauma patients in the intensive care unit.

Variables	Death n = 125	Survival n = 575	p-Value
Gender			0.696
Male, n (%)	79 (63.2)	374 (65.0)	
Female, n (%)	46 (36.8)	201 (35.0)	
Age (years)	76.4 ± 7.5	75.7 ± 7.0	0.386
BMI	23.6 ± 4.5	23.4 ± 4.0	0.604
Albumin (g/dl)	3.0 ± 0.8	3.3 ± 0.6	<0.001
GNRI	89.8 ± 12.9	94.2 ± 12.0	<0.001
Co-morbidities			
DM, n (%)	39 (31.2)	165 (28.7)	0.577
HTN, n (%)	59 (47.2)	333 (57.9)	0.029
CAD, n (%)	22 (17.6)	83 (14.4)	0.369
CHF, n (%)	4 (3.2)	12 (2.1)	0.450
CVA, n (%)	12 (9.6)	58 (10.1)	0.869
ESRD, n (%)	13 (10.4)	24 (4.2)	0.005
COPD, n (%)	4 (3.2)	19 (3.3)	0.953
ISS, median (IQR)	25 (16–29)	16 (13–25)	<0.001
1–15, n (%)	12 (9.6)	158 (27.5)	<0.001
16–24, n (%)	44 (35.2)	267 (46.4)	0.022
≥25, n (%)	69 (55.2)	150 (26.1)	<0.001
LOS in hospital (days)	19.7 ± 20.9	24.8 ± 18.4	0.006

BMI = Body mass index; CAD = coronary artery disease; CHF = congestive heart failure; COPD = chronic obstructive pulmonary disease; CVA = cerebral vascular accident; DM = diabetes mellitus; ESRD = end-stage renal disease; GNRI =Geriatric Nutritional Risk Index; HTN = Hypertension; ISS = injury severity score; LOS = length of stay.

3.2. *Risk Factors for Mortality*

Univariate logistic regression analysis (Table 2) showed that the significant risk factors for mortality in older trauma patients in the ICU were the GNRI, preexisting HTN and ESRD, and ISS. Multivariate logistic regression analysis revealed that the GNRI (OR, 0.97; 95% CI, 0.95–0.99; $p = 0.001$), preexisting ESRD (OR, 3.6; 95% CI, 1.70–7.67; $p = 0.001$), and ISS (OR, 1.1; 95% CI, 1.05–1.10; $p < 0.001$) were significant independent risk factors for mortality. Gender (OR, 0.9; 95% CI, 0.57–1.33; $p = 0.511$), age (OR, 1.0; 95% CI, 0.99–1.05; $p = 0.129$), and preexisting HTN (OR, 0.7; 95% CI, 0.47–1.09; $p = 0.120$) was not recognized as a significant independent risk factor for mortality in older trauma patients in the ICU.

Table 2. Univariate and multivariate analysis to identify risk factors for mortality in older trauma patients in the intensive care unit.

Variables	Univariate Analysis		Multivariate Analysis	
	OR (95% CI)	*p*-Value	OR (95% CI)	*p*-Value
Gender	0.9 (0.62–1.38)	0.696	0.9 (0.57–1.33)	0.511
Age	1.0 (0.99–1.04)	0.385	1.0 (0.99–1.05)	0.129
GNRI	0.97 (0.95–0.99)	<0.001	0.97 (0.95–0.99)	0.001
HTN	0.7 (0.44–0.96)	0.029	0.7 (0.47–1.09)	0.120
ESRD	2.7 (1.32–5.39)	0.006	3.6 (1.70–7.67)	0.001
ISS	1.1 (1.05–1.10)	<0.001	1.1 (1.05–1.10)	<0.001

CI = confidence interval; ESRD = end-stage renal disease; GNRI = Geriatric Nutritional Risk Index; HTN = hypertension; ISS = injury severity score; OR = odds ratio.

3.3. *Comparison of Patients with Low and High GNRI*

As shown in Table 3, the patients in group of GNRI <82 were significantly older than the patients in group of GNRI >98. The patients in groups of GNRI <82, 82 to <92, and 92 to ≤98 presented a significantly lower BMI and level of albumin than the patients in group of GNRI >98. There were no significant intergroup differences in the prevalence of preexisting comorbidities, except HTN. There was no significant difference in the ISS among these groups of patients regardless of ISS stratification (1–15, 16–24, and ≥25). Compared to the patients in group of GNRI >98, those patients in group of GNRI < 82 presented a significantly higher mortality rate (26.6% vs. 13.1%; $p < 0.001$) and LOS in hospital (26.5 days vs. 20.9 days; $p = 0.012$). In contrast, no significant differences of mortality rate and LOS in hospital were found in those patients in groups of GNRI of 82 to <92 and of 92 to ≤98 than those patients in groups of GNRI >98.

Table 3. Patient characteristics and outcomes of the ICU elderly trauma patients with different risks of malnutrition according to GNRI.

GNRI: Variables	<82 *n* = 128	82 to <92 *n* = 191	92 to ≤98 *n* = 136	>98 *n* = 245	*p*-Value
Gender					0.862
Male, *n* (%)	86(67.2)	124(64.9)	89(65.4)	154(62.9)	
Female, *n* (%)	42(32.8)	67(35.1)	47(34.6)	91(37.1)	
Age (years)	78.2 ± 7.5 *	75.9 ± 7.5	76.1 ± 6.3	74.4 ± 6.7	<0.001
BMI	19.9 ± 2.7 *	21.7 ± 2.9 *	23.6 ± 2.9 *	26.5 ± 3.7	<0.001
Albumin (g/dl)	2.5 ± 0.6 *	3.0 ± 0.5 *	3.3 ± 0.5 *	3.8 ± 0.5	<0.001
Co-morbidities					
DM, *n* (%)	31(24.2)	51(26.7)	39(28.7)	83(33.9)	0.193
HTN, *n* (%)	57(44.5) *	99(51.8) *	79(58.1)	157(64.1)	0.002
CAD, *n* (%)	14(10.9)	30(15.7)	25(18.4)	36(14.7)	0.396
CHF, *n* (%)	3(2.3)	5(2.6)	5(3.7)	3(1.2)	0.474
CVA, *n* (%)	9(7.0)	19(9.9)	18(13.2)	24(9.8)	0.416
ESRD, *n* (%)	4(31.1)	12(6.3)	8(5.9)	13(5.3)	0.644
COPD, *n* (%)	6(4.7)	6(3.1)	5(3.7)	6(2.4)	0.703

Table 3. *Cont.*

GNRI: Variables	<82 $n = 128$	82 to <92 $n = 191$	92 to ≤98 $n = 136$	>98 $n = 245$	p-Value
ISS, median (IQR)	17(16–25)	17(16–25)	17(16–25)	16(13–25)	0.345
1–15, n (%)	31(24.2)	39(20.4)	28(20.6)	72(29.4)	0.110
16–24, n (%)	53(41.4)	92(48.2)	64(47.1)	102(41.6)	0.438
≥ 25, n (%)	44(34.4)	60(31.4)	44(32.4)	71(29.0)	0.742
Mortality, n (%)	34(26.6) *	37(19.4)	22(16.2)	32(13.1)	0.012
LOS in hospital (days)	26.5 ± 21.6 *	25.6 ± 18.7	24.4 ± 20.2	20.9 ± 16.7	0.020

BMI = Body mass index; CAD = coronary artery disease; CHF = congestive heart failure; CI = confidence interval; COPD = chronic obstructive pulmonary disease; CVA = cerebral vascular accident; DM = diabetes mellitus; ESRD = end-stage renal disease; GCS = Glasgow Coma Scale; HTN = hypertension; IQR = interquartile range; ISS = injury severity score; LOS = length of stay; OR= odds ratio. * indicate $p < 0.05$ when compared with those patients with GNRI > 98.

4. Discussion

In this study, multivariable logistic regression analysis identified the GNRI as an independent predictor of mortality in older trauma patients in the ICU. Although the odds ratio for mortality is small with the GNRI (OR 0.97; 95% CI, 0.95–0.99), the estimate is in accordance with the results showing that the GNRI was significantly lower in the mortality group than in the survival group and that the mortality rate was significantly higher in patients with low GNRI than in those with high GNRI. The GNRI has been validated by its correlation to indexes obtained from other nutritional scoring systems [10,11]. A strong association between the GNRI, mid-upper arm muscle circumference, arm muscle area, and handgrip strength in hospitalized patients [38] as well as with preoperative sarcopenia status in patients with cancer has been reported [39]. Malnourished patients are at a higher risk of developing postoperative complications, which in turn may affect their prognosis, leading to decreased survival rates [40,41].

In the original study by Bouillanne et al. [15], the GNRI scores were categorized into four nutrition-related risk groups (high-risk: GNRI < 82, moderate-risk: GNRI = 82 to <92, low-risk: GNRI = 92–98, and very low-risk: GNRI > 98), and the risk of infectious complications or mortality was significantly higher in the high-, moderate-, and low-risk groups than in the very low-risk group [7]. For older patients with sepsis, the odds of mortality for each GNRI group were reported to be 11.6-, 5.8-, and 2.3-fold times higher in the high-, moderate-, and low-risk groups, respectively, than in the very low-risk group [42]. In this study, the results demonstrated that the GNRI helps identify major risk-malnutrition elderly trauma patients in the ICU. Compared to the patients in group of GNRI > 98, those patients in group of GNRI < 82 presented a significantly higher mortality rate and LOS in hospital. Therefore, in the ICU, the group of elderly trauma patients with GNRI < 82 would require specific attention regarding their nutritional status. Some authors have proposed that a GNRI value of less than 87 is significantly associated with mortality in critically ill cancer patients [43]. While the GNRI measure is relevant for prognosis, the optimal GNRI cutoff values remain to be elucidated for older trauma patients with critical illnesses. Furthermore, preoperative nutritional interventions help patients cope with surgical stress and reduce the risk of postoperative complications [44]. Furthermore, high-risk GNRI patients can benefit from methods that aim to ameliorate the nutritional and functional status of cancer patients [45]. However, the effect of nutritional intervention in patients with high-risk GNRI remains to be validated.

Some of the limitations of this study are as follows: First, data of patients declared dead on arrival at the emergency room were not recorded in the registered database and only in-hospital mortality was evaluated. Second, selection bias may have been induced by the retrospective design of this study. Unknown conditions such as resuscitation, damage control, and surgical intervention could lead to bias. We assumed that the outcome of treatments was uniform across the studied population. Third, this study excluded many patients who had no albumin data or had incomplete data, and such a scenario may lead to selection bias. Fourth, the population included in this study was limited to that from a single urban trauma center in southern Taiwan; thus, these results may not be generalizable to other regions.

5. Conclusions

This study demonstrated that GNRI is a significant independent risk factor and a promising simple screening tool to identify the subjects with malnutrition associated with higher risk for mortality in those ICU elderly trauma patients.

Author Contributions: Conceptualization, C.-H.H.; Formal analysis, S.-Y.H.; Funding acquisition, H.-T.L.; Resources, C.-H.T. and C.L.; Software, W.-T.S.; Supervision, C.-H.H.; Validation, C.-H.H.; Writing—original draft, S.-C.W.; Writing—review & editing, H.-T.L. and S.-E.C. All authors have read and agreed to the published version of the manuscript.

Acknowledgments: We would like to appreciate the assistance with statistical analyses by Biostatistics Center, Kaohsiung Chang Gung Memorial Hospital.

References

1. Amaral, T.F.; Matos, L.C.; Teixeira, M.A.; Tavares, M.M.; Alvares, L.; Antunes, A. Undernutrition and associated factors among hospitalized patients. *Clin. Nutr.* **2010**, *29*, 580–585. [CrossRef] [PubMed]
2. Cereda, E.; Pedrolli, C. The Geriatric Nutritional Risk Index. *Curr. Opin. Clin. Nutr. Metab. Care* **2009**, *12*, 1–7. [CrossRef] [PubMed]
3. Gavazzi, G.; Krause, K.H. Ageing and infection. *Lancet Infect. Dis.* **2002**, *2*, 659–666. [CrossRef]
4. Barker, L.A.; Gout, B.S.; Crowe, T.C. Hospital malnutrition: Prevalence, identification and impact on patients and the healthcare system. *Int. J. Environ. Res. Public Health* **2011**, *8*, 514–527. [CrossRef]
5. Koekkoek, K.W.; van Zanten, A.R. Nutrition in the critically ill patient. *Curr. Opin. Anaesthesiol.* **2017**, *30*, 178–185. [CrossRef]
6. White, J.V.; Guenter, P.; Jensen, G.; Malone, A.; Schofield, M. Consensus statement of the Academy of Nutrition and Dietetics/American Society for Parenteral and Enteral Nutrition: Characteristics recommended for the identification and documentation of adult malnutrition (undernutrition). *J. Acad. Nutr. Diet.* **2012**, *112*, 730–738. [CrossRef]
7. Lew, C.C.H.; Yandell, R.; Fraser, R.J.L.; Chua, A.P.; Chong, M.F.F.; Miller, M. Association Between Malnutrition and Clinical Outcomes in the Intensive Care Unit: A Systematic Review [Formula: See text]. *JPEN J. Parenter. Enter. Nutr.* **2017**, *41*, 744–758. [CrossRef]
8. Vargas, N.; Tibullo, L.; Landi, E.; Carifi, G.; Pirone, A.; Pippo, A.; Alviggi, I.; Tizzano, R.; Salsano, E.; Di Grezia, F.; et al. Caring for critically ill oldest old patients: A clinical review. *Aging Clin. Exp. Res.* **2017**, *29*, 833–845. [CrossRef]
9. Rubinsky, M.D.; Clark, A.P. Early enteral nutrition in critically ill patients. *Dimens. Crit. Care Nurs. DCCN* **2012**, *31*, 267–274. [CrossRef]
10. Durán Alert, P.; Milà Villarroel, R.; Formiga, F.; Virgili Casas, N.; Vilarasau Farré, C. Assessing risk screening methods of malnutrition in geriatric patients: Mini Nutritional Assessment (MNA) versus Geriatric Nutritional Risk Index (GNRI). *Nutr. Hosp.* **2012**, *27*, 590–598. [CrossRef]
11. Cereda, E.; Pusani, C.; Limonta, D.; Vanotti, A. The ability of the Geriatric Nutritional Risk Index to assess the nutritional status and predict the outcome of home-care resident elderly: A comparison with the Mini Nutritional Assessment. *Br. J. Nutr.* **2009**, *102*, 563–570. [CrossRef] [PubMed]
12. Poziomyck, A.K.; Weston, A.C.; Lameu, E.B.; Cassol, O.S.; Coelho, L.J.; Moreira, L.F. Preoperative nutritional assessment and prognosis in patients with foregut tumors. *Nutr. Cancer* **2012**, *64*, 1174–1181. [CrossRef] [PubMed]
13. Buzby, G.P.; Knox, L.S.; Crosby, L.O.; Eisenberg, J.M.; Haakenson, C.M.; McNeal, G.E.; Page, C.P.; Peterson, O.L.; Reinhardt, G.F.; Williford, W.O. Study protocol: A randomized clinical trial of total parenteral nutrition in malnourished surgical patients. *Am. J. Clin. Nutr.* **1988**, *47*, 366–381. [CrossRef]

14. Labossiere, R.; Bernard, M.A. Nutritional considerations in institutionalized elders. *Curr. Opin. Clin. Nutr. Metab. Care* **2008**, *11*, 1–6. [CrossRef] [PubMed]
15. Bouillanne, O.; Morineau, G.; Dupont, C.; Coulombel, I.; Vincent, J.P.; Nicolis, I.; Benazeth, S.; Cynober, L.; Aussel, C. Geriatric Nutritional Risk Index: A new index for evaluating at-risk elderly medical patients. *Am. J. Clin. Nutr.* **2005**, *82*, 777–783. [CrossRef] [PubMed]
16. Fried, L.P.; Tangen, C.M.; Walston, J.; Newman, A.B.; Hirsch, C.; Gottdiener, J.; Seeman, T.; Tracy, R.; Kop, W.J.; Burke, G.; et al. Frailty in older adults: Evidence for a phenotype. *J. Gerontol. Ser. A Biol. Sci. Med. Sci.* **2001**, *56*, M146–M156. [CrossRef] [PubMed]
17. Takahashi, H.; Ito, Y.; Ishii, H.; Aoyama, T.; Kamoi, D.; Kasuga, H.; Yasuda, K.; Maruyama, S.; Matsuo, S.; Murohara, T.; et al. Geriatric nutritional risk index accurately predicts cardiovascular mortality in incident hemodialysis patients. *J. Cardiol.* **2014**, *64*, 32–36. [CrossRef]
18. Detsky, A.S.; McLaughlin, J.R.; Baker, J.P.; Johnston, N.; Whittaker, S.; Mendelson, R.A.; Jeejeebhoy, K.N. What is subjective global assessment of nutritional status? *JPEN J. Parenter. Enter. Nutr.* **1987**, *11*, 8–13. [CrossRef]
19. Kondrup, J.; Allison, S.P.; Elia, M.; Vellas, B.; Plauth, M. ESPEN guidelines for nutrition screening 2002. *Clin. Nutr.* **2003**, *22*, 415–421. [CrossRef]
20. Zhao, Y.; Xia, X.; Xie, D.; Liao, Y.; Wang, Y.; Chen, L.; Ge, N.; Yue, J. Geriatric Nutritional Risk Index can predict postoperative delirium and hospital length of stay in elderly patients undergoing non-cardiac surgery. *Geriatr. Gerontol. Int.* **2020**, *20*, 759–764. [CrossRef]
21. Gu, W.; Zhang, G.; Sun, L.; Ma, Q.; Cheng, Y.; Zhang, H.; Shi, G.; Zhu, Y.; Ye, D. Nutritional screening is strongly associated with overall survival in patients treated with targeted agents for metastatic renal cell carcinoma. *J. Cachexia Sarcopenia Muscle* **2015**, *6*, 222–230. [CrossRef] [PubMed]
22. Lidoriki, I.; Schizas, D.; Frountzas, M.; Machairas, N.; Prodromidou, A.; Kapelouzou, A.; Karavokyros, I.; Pikoulis, E.; Kales, S.N.; Liakakos, T. GNRI as a prognostic factor for outcomes in cancer patients: A systematic review of the literature. *Nutr. Cancer* **2020**, 1–13. [CrossRef] [PubMed]
23. Lv, G.Y.; An, L.; Sun, D.W. Geriatric nutritional risk index predicts adverse outcomes in human malignancy: A meta-analysis. *Dis. Markers* **2019**, *2019*, 4796598. [CrossRef] [PubMed]
24. Kushiyama, S.; Sakurai, K.; Kubo, N.; Tamamori, Y.; Nishii, T.; Tachimori, A.; Inoue, T.; Maeda, K. The preoperative geriatric nutritional risk index predicts postoperative complications in elderly patients with gastric cancer undergoing gastrectomy. *In Vivo* **2018**, *32*, 1667–1672. [CrossRef]
25. Lee, K.; Ahn, J.M.; Kang, D.Y.; Ko, E.; Kwon, O.; Lee, P.H.; Lee, S.W.; Kim, D.H.; Kim, H.J.; Kim, J.B.; et al. Nutritional status and risk of all-cause mortality in patients undergoing transcatheter aortic valve replacement assessment using the geriatric nutritional risk index and the controlling nutritional status score. *Clin. Res. Cardiol.* **2020**, *109*, 161–171. [CrossRef] [PubMed]
26. Mii, S.; Guntani, A.; Kawakubo, E.; Shimazoe, H.; Ishida, M. Impact of the geriatric nutritional risk index on the long-term outcomes of patients undergoing open bypass for intermittent claudication. *Circ. J.* **2019**, *83*, 1349–1355. [CrossRef] [PubMed]
27. Shibata, K.; Yamamoto, M.; Kano, S.; Koyama, Y.; Shimura, T.; Kagase, A.; Yamada, S.; Kobayashi, T.; Tada, N.; Naganuma, T.; et al. Importance of Geriatric Nutritional Risk Index assessment in patients undergoing transcatheter aortic valve replacement. *Am. Heart J.* **2018**, *202*, 68–75. [CrossRef]
28. Kubo, N.; Sakurai, K.; Tamura, T.; Toyokawa, T.; Tanaka, H.; Muguruma, K.; Yashiro, M.; Ohira, M. The impact of geriatric nutritional risk index on surgical outcomes after esophagectomy in patients with esophageal cancer. *Esophagus* **2019**, *16*, 147–154. [CrossRef]
29. Yoo, J.W.; Ju, S.; Lee, S.J.; Cho, Y.J.; Lee, J.D.; Kim, H.C. Geriatric nutritional risk index is associated with 30-day mortality in patients with acute respiratory distress syndrome. *Medicine* **2020**, *99*, e20671. [CrossRef]
30. Hsieh, C.H.; Hsu, S.Y.; Hsieh, H.Y.; Chen, Y.C. Differences between the sexes in motorcycle-related injuries and fatalities at a Taiwanese level I trauma center. *Biomed. J.* **2017**, *40*, 113–120. [CrossRef]
31. Hsieh, C.H.; Liu, H.T.; Hsu, S.Y.; Hsieh, H.Y.; Chen, Y.C. Motorcycle-related hospitalizations of the elderly. *Biomed. J.* **2017**, *40*, 121–128. [CrossRef] [PubMed]
32. Hsieh, C.H.; Chen, Y.C.; Hsu, S.Y.; Hsieh, H.Y.; Chien, P.C. Defining polytrauma by abbreviated injury scale >/= 3 for a least two body regions is insufficient in terms of short-term outcome: A cross-sectional study at a level I trauma center. *Biomed. J.* **2018**, *41*, 321–327. [CrossRef] [PubMed]

33. Loftis, K.L.; Price, J.; Gillich, P.J. Evolution of the Abbreviated Injury Scale: 1990–2015. *Traffic Inj. Prev.* **2018**, *19*, S109–S113. [CrossRef] [PubMed]
34. Committee on Medical Aspects of Automotive Safety. Rating the severity of tissue damage. I. The abbreviated scale. *JAMA* **1971**, *215*, 277–280. [CrossRef] [PubMed]
35. Hsu, S.Y.; Wu, S.C.; Rau, C.S.; Hsieh, T.M.; Liu, H.T.; Huang, C.Y.; Chou, S.E.; Su, W.T.; Hsieh, C.H. Impact of Adapting the Abbreviated Injury Scale (AIS)-2005 from AIS-1998 on injury severity scores and clinical outcome. *Int. J. Environ. Res. Public Health* **2019**, *16*, 5033. [CrossRef] [PubMed]
36. Aharonson-Daniel, L.; Giveon, A.; Stein, M.; Israel Trauma, G.; Peleg, K. Different AIS triplets: Different mortality predictions in identical ISS and NISS. *J. Trauma* **2006**, *61*, 711–717. [CrossRef]
37. Dong, X.R. Analysis of patients of multiple injuries with AIS-ISS and its clinical significance in the evaluation of the emergency managements. *Zhonghua Wai Ke Za Zhi* **1993**, *31*, 301–302.
38. Cereda, E.; Vanotti, A. The new Geriatric Nutritional Risk Index is a good predictor of muscle dysfunction in institutionalized older patients. *Clin. Nutr.* **2007**, *26*, 78–83. [CrossRef]
39. Han, J.Y.; Lee, K.H.; Kim, S.W.; Min, Y.J.; Cho, E.; Lee, Y.; Lee, S.H.; Kim, H.Y.; Lee, G.K.; Nam, B.H.; et al. A phase II study of poziotinib in patients with epidermal growth factor receptor (EGFR)-mutant lung adenocarcinoma who have acquired resistance to EGFR-tyrosine kinase inhibitors. *Cancer Res. Treat.* **2017**, *49*, 10–19. [CrossRef]
40. Artinyan, A.; Orcutt, S.T.; Anaya, D.A.; Richardson, P.; Chen, G.J.; Berger, D.H. Infectious postoperative complications decrease long-term survival in patients undergoing curative surgery for colorectal cancer: A study of 12,075 patients. *Ann. Surg.* **2015**, *261*, 497–505. [CrossRef]
41. Nathan, H.; Yin, H.; Wong, S.L. Postoperative complications and long-term survival after complex cancer resection. *Ann. Surg. Oncol.* **2017**, *24*, 638–644. [CrossRef] [PubMed]
42. Lee, J.S.; Choi, H.S.; Ko, Y.G.; Yun, D.H. Performance of the Geriatric Nutritional Risk Index in predicting 28-day hospital mortality in older adult patients with sepsis. *Clin. Nutr.* **2013**, *32*, 843–848. [CrossRef] [PubMed]
43. Fruchtenicht, A.V.; Poziomyck, A.K.; Kabke, G.B.; Loss, S.H.; Antoniazzi, J.L.; Steemburgo, T.; Moreira, L.F. Nutritional risk assessment in critically ill cancer patients: Systematic review. *Rev. Bras. Ter. Intensiva* **2015**, *27*, 274–283. [CrossRef] [PubMed]
44. Weimann, A.; Braga, M.; Carli, F.; Higashiguchi, T.; Hübner, M.; Klek, S.; Laviano, A.; Ljungqvist, O.; Lobo, D.N.; Martindale, R.; et al. ESPEN guideline: Clinical nutrition in surgery. *Clin. Nutr.* **2017**, *36*, 623–650. [CrossRef]
45. Caillet, P.; Liuu, E.; Raynaud Simon, A.; Bonnefoy, M.; Guerin, O.; Berrut, G.; Lesourd, B.; Jeandel, C.; Ferry, M.; Rolland, Y.; et al. Association between cachexia, chemotherapy and outcomes in older cancer patients: A systematic review. *Clin. Nutr.* **2017**, *36*, 1473–1482. [CrossRef]

5

Nutritional Laboratory Markers in Malnutrition

Ulrich Keller

FMH Endocrinology-Diabetology, Fichtlirain 33, CH-4105 Biel-Benken, Basel, Switzerland; ulrich.keller@unibas.ch

Abstract: Serum visceral proteins such as albumin and prealbumin have traditionally been used as markers of the nutritional status of patients. Prealbumin is nowadays often preferred over albumin due to its shorter half live, reflecting more rapid changes of the nutritional state. However, recent focus has been on an appropriate nutrition-focused physical examination and on the patient's history for diagnosing malnutrition, and the role of inflammation as a risk factor for malnutrition has been more and more recognized. Inflammatory signals are potent inhibitors of visceral protein synthesis, and the use of these proteins as biomarkers of the nutritional status has been debated since they are strongly influenced by inflammation and less so by protein energy stores. The current consensus is that laboratory markers could be used as a complement to a thorough physical examination. Other markers of the nutritional status such as urinary creatinine or 3-methylhistidine as indicators of muscle protein breakdown have not found widespread use. Serum IGF-1 is less influenced by inflammation and falls during malnutrition. However, its concentration changes are not sufficiently specific to be useful clinically as a marker of malnutrition, and serum IGF-1 has less been used in clinical trials. Nevertheless, biomarkers of malnutrition such as prealbumin may be of interest as easily measurable predictors of the prognosis for surgical outcomes and of mortality in severe illnesses.

Keywords: malnutrition; inflammation; nutritional assessment; biomarkers; albumin; prealbumin; IGF-1; elderly; prognostic marker

---

1. Introduction

Malnutrition has a substantial clinical and socioeconomic significance; it increases rates of complications in hospitalized patients and healthcare-associated costs. Its prevalence has been estimated in hospitals of Western countries to be 30–50% and in long-term care facilities up to 85% depending on the definition and the type of population studied [1–3].

One of the problems of diagnosing malnutrition is the lack of a unified definition and of standard methods for screening and diagnosis.

Malnutrition results from a mismatch of nutritional requirements with intake. In many malnourished patients, there is an associated disease-related inflammation, resulting in a complex interplay between the two. Inflammation influences both, requirements and intake. It promotes malnutrition and adverse outcomes by provoking anorexia and by altering metabolism with elevation of resting energy expenditure and by increasing muscle catabolism [4].

The appreciation that inflammation plays a major role in the pathophysiology of malnutrition is often lacking, and many clinicians assume that weight loss is the single most important criterion for a malnourished state. This has led to frequent underrecognition of the condition [5].

The purpose of this review is to review the published literature on the role of laboratory biomarkers as a tool to diagnose malnutrition, to assess nutritional risk and to monitor nutritional intervention.

2. Role of Biomarkers in Published Screening Tools to Assess the Risk of Malnutrition

About half of all published risk scores of malnutrition use serum laboratory markers such as visceral proteins, and others do not (Table 1).

Table 1. Anthropometric parameters and biomarkers in various nutritional assessment and screening tools (adapted from [3] with an update, in chronological order of publication.

Nutritional Assessment and Screening Tool	Anthropometric Parameters and History	Biomarkers
Prognostic Nutritional Index [6]	Triceps skin fold	Albumin, transferrin, skin sensitivity
Prognostic Inflammatory and Nutritional Index [7]	None	Albumin, prealbumin, C-reactive protein, α1-acid glycoprotein
Subjective Global Assessment (SGA) [8]	Weight history, diet history, primary diagnosis, stress level, physical symptoms (s.c. fat, muscle wasting, edema), functional capacity, gastrointestinal symptoms	None
Birmingham Nutrition Risk Score [9]	Weight loss, BMI, appetite, ability to eat, stress factor, (severity of diagnosis)	None
Nutrition Risk Classification [10]	Weight loss, percentage ideal body weight, dietary intake, gastrointestinal function	None
Mini Nutritional Assessment (MNA; [11]	Weight data, height, mid-arm circumference, calf circumference, diet history, appetite, feeding mode	Albumin, prealbumin, cholesterol, lymphocyte count
Malnutrition Screening Tool [12]	Appetite, unintentional weight loss	None
Simple Screening Tool [13]	Body mass index (BMI), percentage weight loss	Albumin
Full nutritional assessment [14]	BMI, information on unintended weight loss, triceps skinfold thickness, mid-arm muscle circumference	Serum albumin, prealbumin, and total lymphocyte count
Malnutrition Universal Screening Tool (MUST) [15]	BMI, change in weight, presence of acute disease	None
Nutritional Risk Screening (NRS) 2002 [1]	Weight loss, BMI, food intake, diagnosis (severity)	None
Short Nutrition Assessment Questionnaire [16]	Recent weight history, appetite, use of oral supplement or tube feeding	None
Controlling nutritional status (CONUT) [17]	None	Serum albumin, total cholesterol and total lymphocyte count
Maastricht Index [18]	Percentage ideal body weight	Albumin, prealbumin, lymphocyte count
Nutritional Risk Index [19]	Present and usual body weight	Albumin
Elderly Nutritional Indicators for Geriatric Malnutrition Assessment (ENIGMA) [20]	Nutritional history	Albumin, hemoglobin, total cholesterol and lymphocyte count

Results of these screening tests vary considerably, as shown in a Greek study in elderly subjects [2]. These authors found the highest validity coefficient for MUST but a lower specificity for NRS 2000 which has frequently been used.

A consensus committee of the European and US nutritional societies (ESPEN and ASPEN) proposed three sub-definitions of malnutrition. "Starvation-related malnutrition" is present when there is chronic starvation without inflammation; "chronic disease-related malnutrition" is defined as a condition when inflammation is chronic and of mild to moderate degree, and "acute disease or injury-related malnutrition" occurs when inflammation is acute and of severe degree [21]. The criteria for diagnosis of these sub-definitions were energy intake, weight loss, body fat, muscle mass, fluid accumulation and grip strength but no biomarkers [22]. Among ancillary parameters, serum visceral proteins were mentioned, but since they would rather reflect the state of inflammation it was proposed to use them with caution to diagnose malnutrition.

A meta-regression published recently [23] assessed the role of biomarkers in describing the severity of malnutrition according to established and validated nutritional assessment tools. A total of 111 studies (observational and cohort studies; randomized controlled trials were not available) were included, representing 52,911 participants from various clinical settings. The BMI ($p < 0.001$) and concentrations of albumin ($p < 0.001$), hemoglobin ($p < 0.001$), total cholesterol ($p < 0.001$), prealbumin ($p < 0.001$) and total protein ($p < 0.05$) among subjects at high risk of malnutrition assessed by MNA were significantly lower than those with low risk. Similar results were observed for malnutrition identified by SGA and NRS 2002. When patients with acute illnesses were included, the predictive value of albumin and prealbumin was distinctly reduced, confirming the conclusion that they are more markers of inflammation than of malnutrition. The authors concluded that BMI, hemoglobin, and total cholesterol were useful markers of malnutrition in older adults.

3. Serum Visceral Proteins as Biomarkers of the Nutritional Status

Visceral proteins are mostly synthesized in the liver. Poor protein and energy intake, impaired liver synthetic function as well as inflammatory status result in low circulating levels of visceral proteins. During inflammatory states and increased production of acute-phase proteins the liver reprioritizes protein synthesis, and lowers as a mirror visceral protein synthesis to a degree which correlates with the severity of the injury.

3.1. *Serum Albumin*

Albumin is the most abundant protein in human serum. It has been used for decades as an indicator of malnutrition in patients in clinically stable conditions (review and meta-analysis [24]). Serum albumin concentrations decrease with increasing age by approx. by 0.1 g/L per year; however, age itself is not a cause of distinct hypoalbuminemia.

There is a clear relationship between serum albumin concentrations and all-cause mortality in elderly subjects [25]. In patients with a hip fracture, albumin levels below 35 g/L were associated with higher rates of post-operative complications such as sepsis and higher overall mortality. Significant loss of muscle mass has been observed in elderly people with low albumin levels. Inflammatory states and in particular, high concentrations of the cytokines IL-6 and TNF-alpha, were two of the main factors causing low levels of serum albumin [24]. Systemic inflammation not only reduces albumin synthesis but increases its degradation and promotes its transcapillary leakage.

Other studies also found this protein to be a good predictor of surgical outcome [26,27]. Compared to nine other risk variables, serum albumin was the strongest predictor. These findings were confirmed in a later study [26], but whether hypoalbuminemia was due to undernutrition or advanced disease was not clarified in these trials.

When serum albumin as a biomarker for the differential diagnosis of unexplained weight loss (involuntary weight loss of more than 5 kg in the previous 6 months) was included in a study from Spain in 306 referred patients, a little more than one-third were ultimately diagnosed with a malignancy. Multivariate analysis found the strongest predictors of a neoplasm were age >80 years, white blood cell count > 12,000/mm^3 and serum albumin < 3.5 g/dL [28].

Albumin has been criticized as a player in nutritional assessment due to its lack of specificity and long half-life (approximately 20 days) [29]. Serum albumin concentrations not only decrease during decreased synthesis due to inflammatory cytokines as mentioned above or to hepatic insufficiency, they may also decrease following renal losses in nephrotic syndrome and to losses via the GI tract in protein-losing enteropathies [30].

3.2. *Serum Prealbumin*

Prealbumin, also named transthyretin, is a transport protein for thyroid hormone and is synthesized by the liver and partly catabolized by the kidneys. Serum prealbumin concentrations less than 10 mg/dL are associated with malnutrition [31].

The use of prealbumin has been advocated as a nutritional marker, particularly during refeeding and in the elderly [32]. The main advantage of prealbumin compared to albumin is its shorter half-life (two to three days) (Table 2), making it a more favorable marker of acute changes of the nutritional state. In addition, prealbumin was not influenced by intestinal protein losses in patients with protein-losing enteropathy [30].

Table 2. Characteristics of serum visceral proteins used as nutritional markers.

Protein	Molecular Weight	Half-Life	Reference Range
Albumin	65,000	20 days	3.30 to 4.80 g per dL
Transferrin	76,000	10 days	0.16 to 0.36 g per dL
Prealbumin	54,980	2 days	16 to 35 mg per dL
Retinol-binding protein	21,000	1/2 day	3–6 mg/dL

Table adapted from Spiekerman AM [33].

Prealbumin levels may be increased in the setting of renal dysfunction, corticosteroid therapy or dehydration, whereas they can be decreased during physiological stress, infection, liver dysfunction, and over-hydration [34].

An algorithm that uses prealbumin has recently been proposed as a practical guide to help the clinician to stratify general medical and intensive care patients by risk of complications and outcome [34]. Prealbumin screening should only performed when an acute inflammatory state (CRP > 15 mg/L) was excluded. A prealbumin level of < 0.11 g/L was associated with increased mortality and length of stay, and an increase by less than 0.04 g/L per week indicated failure of nutritional therapy.

An increase in the C-reactive protein/prealbumin ratio in medical intensive care unit patients has been associated with mortality [35], and a low C-reactive protein/prealbumin ratio in surgical patients predicted the successful closure of gastrointestinal fistulas [36]. Routine measurement of prealbumin has been advocated to be a useful nutritional and prognostic indicator in non-ICU patients without inflammation [34].

Several publications reported a role for prealbumin in predicting prognosis (mostly survival) in various clinical conditions such as gastric cancer [37], lung cancer [38] and cardiovascular diseases [39].

3.3. *Albumin and Prealbumin in Starved and Otherwise Healthy Malnourished Subjects*

A systematic review assessed the role of albumin and prealbumin in otherwise healthy subjects who were severely nutrient- deprived due to poor access to food or unwillingness to eat, mostly due to anorexia nervosa [40]. The study showed that serum albumin and prealbumin levels were maintained even in the presence of distinct weight loss, and they were lowered only during extreme starvation (BMI < 11 kg/m^2). The authors concluded that serum visceral proteins are not predictive of nutritional deprivation and should not be used to guide nutritional therapy in this group of patients.

3.4. *Transferrin*

This acute-phase reactant is a transport protein for iron. It has a relatively long half-life (approx. 10 days), and has also been used as a marker of the nutritional status [41] It is influenced by other factors including iron status, liver disease and inflammatory state. Like prealbumin, transferrin levels increase with renal failure [42]. Some authors found transferrin measurements useful for nutritional assessment [43], other did not [44].

During iron-deficiency the levels of transferrin are elevated whereas they are decreased in iron-overload states. Serum transferrin increased in parallel to prealbumin during nutritional intervention in critically ill children [45]. Serum levels decrease in the setting of severe malnutrition, but this marker has been found to be unreliable in the assessment of mild malnutrition and of fat-free mass in a group of elderly Italian patients [46].

3.5. Retinol-Binding Protein (RBP)

This is a low molecular weight protein with the physiological role to transport retinol from the liver to target organs. It represents the visceral protein with the shortest half-life (approx. 12 h) [33]. According to a review [47] it provides similar responses to energy intake to prealbumin, but it is more difficult to measure than the latter and it is influenced by the vitamin A status. For these reasons there RBP measurements have not found widespread application.

4. Laboratory Markers of Malnutrition Other Than Visceral Proteins

4.1. Urinary Creatinine

Creatinine is the end product of creatine which consists of 3 amino acids and is mainly present in muscle. Provided that renal function is intact its excretion reflects creatinine production which in turn is a mirror of skeletal muscle turnover. Each mmol of creatinine in urine is derived from 1.9 kg skeletal muscle [47]. The disadvantages are that it is slowly responding to changes of the nutritional status and that it depends on renal function and requires 24 h urine collections.

4.2. Urinary 3-Methylhistidine

3-methylhistidine is a component of muscle fibers and is not reutilized by the body. Its urinary excretion reflects the amount of fat-free mass and it can be used as a measure of the rate of muscle protein breakdown. It is less dependent on renal function than creatinine; it is often expressed per mmol of urinary creatinine [47]. Both assay of urinary creatinine and 3-methylhistidine have not found widespread use mainly due to the fact that urinary collections are often cumbersome, their excretion may increase after meat intake and they show a relatively poor sensitivity to monitor changes of body protein stores.

4.3. Serum Cholesterol

As can be seen in Table 1, some nutritional screening tools used total serum cholesterol as parameter of malnutrition. Serum cholesterol concentrations show a U-shaped relationship with mortality, and low levels have been associated with increased mortality [48]. However, sensitivity and specificity to monitor malnutrition are low.

4.4. Delayed Hypersensitivity and Blood Lymphocyte Count

The local inflammatory response to a s.c. injection of an antigen is impaired during severe malnutrition. At the same time, maturation of lymphocytes may be reduced in malnourished patients so that total circulating lymphocyte concentration falls to less than 1500/mm^3 (reference range 2000–3500) [47].

These abnormalities can be taken as supporting evidence for protein-energy malnutrition, however, they are not specific and insensitive, and concomitant diseases and a severe stress reaction may also have an effect. Both markers respond slowly to correction of the nutritional status. These reasons limit their use as diagnostic tools for malnutrition.

4.5. Serum Insulin-Like Growth Factor 1 (IGF-1)

IGF-1 (formerly called Somatomedin C) is a ubiquitous growth factor, and the circulating form is mainly produced by the liver. Pituitary growth hormone stimulates its release. Its serum half-life is short (approx. 24 h), and it is largely bound in plasma to binding proteins (mainly IGF BP 3). Fasting lowers plasma IGF-1 levels more than 4 fold and IGF-1 concentrations increases during nutritional repletion. A correlation between energy intake (and less so of protein intake) and plasma IGF-1 concentrations has been reported [49]. IGF-1 levels were a reliable index of protein-energy undernutrition in elderly patients in the recovery period after surgery for hip fracture; however, according to this trial, this marker was also influenced by inflammation [50]. In contrast, IGF-1 levels were not clearly influenced by inflammation in other groups of surgical patients [51,52]. IGF-1 concentrations are altered by liver disease, renal impairment and severe trauma such as burns [47]. Nevertheless, IGF-1 performed better during nutritional rehabilitation to monitor protein and energy status than albumin or transferrin [53]. Drawback of IGF-1 measurements is the fact that their serum concentrations are influenced by other factors such as the acute-phase response. More recently, there has been interest in free IGF-I which holds promise as a nutritional marker (review in [54]. In spite of the earlier positive reports, IFG-1 measurements have not been advocated in more recent publications.

4.6. Serum Leptin

Decreased serum leptin concentrations combined with elevated prothrombin time has been reported in malnourished hospitalized patients with end-stage liver disease [55].

4.7. Serum Nesfatin-1

Nesfatin-1 is an anorexigenic molecule and seems to play a role in appetite regulation and energy homeostasis. Serum nesfatin-1 concentrations have been shown to be increased in chronically malnourished but otherwise healthy children [56].

4.8. Serum Zinc

Zinc is the most abundant trace element in man beside iron; it is present in all body tissues and fluids and is an essential component of many enzymes. Zinc deficiency has been associated with impaired taste and smell, reduced immunity and increased risk of pneumonia [57]. In cases of severe zinc deficiency, skin lesions, anemia, diarrhea, anorexia, decreased lymphocyte function, impaired visual function and mental retardation may be observed. Several psychological functions were impaired in elderly subjects with zinc deficiency [58].

Zinc deficiency is due to low intake of zinc-containing foods such as meat and to decreased absorption caused by intestinal malabsorption [57]. According to a large sample of the TromsØ study, the risk of zinc deficiency was increased 3 fold in subjects at high risk of malnutrition, particularly in men [59]. Assessment of the zinc status carries the problems that only a small fraction of body zinc is circulating, and most serum zinc is bound to albumin. Therefore, albumin deficiency makes interpretation of serum zinc levels difficult. In spite of the widespread functions of zinc in the body and the potential importance replacing zinc in subjects with zinc deficiency, there is little high-quality evidence of the therapeutic benefit of zinc replacement in adult subjects. A randomized controlled trial in children with protein-energy malnutrition and zinc deficiency showed benefits of zinc replacement [60]. It is likely that zinc deficiency in subjects at risk of malnutrition remains often unrecognized.

4.9. Other Essential Micronutrients (Trace Elements and Vitamins)

Laboratory assessment of other trace elements such as iron is not specifically mentioned as part of current nutritional screening tools. This does not mean that in cases with clinical suspicion of micronutrient deficiency this should not be performed. The same can be stated for laboratory screening for vitamin deficiencies, in particular, those of vitamins A, B1, B6, B12, D, and folate.

5. Biomarkers of Nutritional Risk in Some Specific Clinical Conditions

5.1. Geriatric Patients

Dementia: Eating and swallowing problems increase the risk of malnutrition. According to a study from a memory clinic in the Netherlands, about 14% of community-dwelling subjects with newly diagnosed dementia were at risk of malnutrition [61]. These authors pointed out that it is important to detect malnutrition in dementia as early as possible.

In patients with dementia, the nutritional history may only be obtainable by asking family caregivers about appetite and weight change of patients. However, it is unknown whether nutritional information provided by family caregivers are reliable, and therefore biomarkers of malnutrition would be of particular interest.

A recent study compared biochemical blood markers among patients with Alzheimer's disease (AD), dementia with Lewy bodies (DLB), and frontotemporal lobar degeneration (FTLD) [62]. A total of 339 dementia outpatients and their family caregivers participated. Low serum albumin was 7.2 times more prevalent among patients with DLB and 10.1 times more prevalent among those with FTLD than among those with AD, with adjustment for age. The levels of biochemical markers were not significantly correlated with cognitive function. These authors proposed that a multidimensional approach including serological biomarkers such as albumin are needed to assess malnutrition in patients with dementia.

Sarcopenia in the elderly: A clinical investigation performed in elderly persons supported the view that prealbumin levels are useful surrogate indicators of lean body mass (LBM). Compared to serum albumin and RBP, prealbumin showed the highest positive correlation with LBM [46]. In order to improve its predictive potency for sarcopenia the reference values for prealbumin should be adapted to the corresponding age and sex [32]. Ingenbleek proposed that routine screening for protein malnutrition using prealbumin should be performed in elderly subjects [63].

5.2. Chronic Kidney Disease

A position paper from the International Society of Renal Nutrition and Metabolism (ISRNM) stated that serum biomarkers played a particular role in diagnosing malnutrition in patients with kidney failure [64]. Protein-energy wasting can be observed in chronic and in acute kidney disease, and protein-energy wasting is diagnosed according to this publication when low serum biomarkers (albumin, prealbumin, or cholesterol), reduced body mass and reduced muscle mass are present.

Serum prealbumin levels were positively correlated with body cell mass in pre-dialytic kidney patients [65]. Serum biomarkers were part of a new nutritional risk index for predicting mortality in Japanese hemodialysis patients [66]. Cox proportional hazard models indicated that in addition to low BMI, low albumin, low creatinine, and low serum cholesterol predicted independently and significantly mortality within one year.

6. Conclusions

The role played by serum biomarkers in diagnosing or monitoring malnutrition is controversial, particularly in more recent reports. This is explained by their relatively low specificity and by the fact that underlying diseases such as inflammation exert a major influence, particularly on serum visceral proteins. In addition, the role of biomarkers to guide nutritional therapy has not been studied in large randomized controlled trials. A recent randomized controlled multicenter trial in hospitalized patients with malnutrition might fill this gap in the near future [67]. Nevertheless, biomarkers such as prealbumin are valid prognostic indicators of disease outcome and of mortality in patients at risk of malnutrition.

Acknowledgments: The page charges for this article were covered by the Swiss Society for Clinical Nutrition.

References

1. Kondrup, J.; Rasmussen, H.H.; Hamberg, O.; Stanga, Z. Nutritional risk screening (NRS 2002): A new method based on an analysis of controlled clinical trials. *Clin. Nutr.* **2003**, *22*, 321–336. [CrossRef]

2. Poulia, K.-A.; Yannakoulia, M.; Karageorgou, D.; Gamaletsou, M.; Panagiotakos, D.B.; Sipsas, N.V.; Zampelas, A. Evaluation of the efficacy of six nutritional screening tools to predict malnutrition in the elderly. *Clin. Nutr.* **2012**, *31*, 378–385. [CrossRef] [PubMed]
3. Mueller, C.; Compher, C.; Ellen, D.M. ASPEN Clinical Guidelines. *J. Parenter. Enter. Nutr.* **2011**, *35*, 16–24. [CrossRef]
4. Jensen, G.L. Malnutrition and Inflammation—"Burning Down the House". *J. Parenter. Enter. Nutr.* **2015**, *39*, 56–62. [CrossRef] [PubMed]
5. Kirkland, L.L.; Kashiwagi, D.T.; Brantley, S.; Scheurer, D.; Varkey, P. Nutrition in the hospitalized patient. *J. Hosp. Med.* **2013**, *8*, 52–58. [CrossRef] [PubMed]
6. Buzby, G.P.; Mullen, J.L.; Matthews, D.C.; Hobbs, C.L.; Rosato, E.F. Prognostic nutritional index in gastrointestinal surgery. *Am. J. Surg.* **1980**, *139*, 160–167. [CrossRef]
7. Ingenbleek, Y.; Carpentier, Y.A. A prognostic inflammatory and nutritional index scoring critically ill patients. *Int. J. Vitam. Nutr. Res.* **1985**, *55*, 91–101.
8. Detsky, A.S.; Baker, J.P.; Johnston, N.; Whittaker, S.; Mendelson, R.A.; Jeejeebhoy, K.N. What is subjective global assessment of nutritional status? *J. Parenter. Enter. Nutr.* **1987**, *11*, 8–13. [CrossRef]
9. Reilly, H.M.; Martineau, J.K.; Moran, A.; Kennedy, H. Nutritional screening—Evaluation and implementation of a simple Nutrition Risk Score. *Clin. Nutr.* **1995**, *14*, 269–273. [CrossRef]
10. Kovacevich, D.S.; Boney, A.R.; Braunschweig, C.L.; Perez, A.; Stevens, M. Nutrition Risk Classification: A Reproducible and Valid Tool for Nurses. *Nutr. Clin. Pract.* **1997**, *12*, 20–25. [CrossRef]
11. Vellas, B.; Guigoz, Y.; Garry, P.J.; Nourhashemi, F.; Bennahum, D.; Lauque, S.; Albarede, J.L. The mini nutritional assessment (MNA) and its use in grading the nutritional state of elderly patients. *Nutrition* **1999**, *15*, 116–122. [CrossRef]
12. Ferguson, M.; Capra, S.; Bauer, J.; Banks, M. Development of a valid and reliable malnutrition screening tool for adult acute hospital patients. *Nutrition* **1999**, *15*, 458–464. [CrossRef]
13. Laporte, M.; Villalon, L.; Thibodeau, J.; Payette, H. Validity and reliability of simple nutrition screening tools adapted to the elderly population in healthcare facilities. *J. Nutr. Health Aging* **2001**, *5*, 292–294. [PubMed]
14. Thorsdottir, I.; Gunnarsdottir, I.; Eriksen, B. Screening Method Evaluated by Nutritional Status Measurements can be Used to Detect Malnourishment in Chronic Obstructive Pulmonary Disease. *J. Am. Diet. Assoc.* **2001**, *101*, 648–654. [CrossRef]
15. Elia, M. The 'MUST' Report. Nutritional Screening for Adults: A Multidisciplinary Responsibility. Development and Use of the 'Malnutrition Universal Screening Tool' (MUST) for Adults. 2003. Available online: https://eprints.soton.ac.uk/362499/ (accessed on 10 March 2019).
16. Kruizenga, H.M.; Van Tulder, M.W.; Seidell, J.C.; Thijs, A.; Ader, H.J.; Van Bokhorst-de van der Schueren, M.A. Effectiveness and cost-effectiveness of early screening and treatment of malnourished patients. *Am. J. Clin. Nutr.* **2005**, *82*, 1082–1089. [CrossRef]
17. De Ulíbarri, J.I.; González-Madroño, A.; De Villar, N.; González, P.; González, B.; Mancha, A.; Rodriguez, F.; Fernández, G. CONUT: A tool for controlling nutritional status. First validation in a hospital population. *Nutr. Hosp.* **2005**, *20*, 38–45.
18. Kuzu, M.A.; Terzioğlu, H.; Genç, V.; Erkek, A.B.; Özban, M.; Sonyürek, P.; Elhan, A.H.; Torun, N. Preoperative Nutritional Risk Assessment in Predicting Postoperative Outcome in Patients Undergoing Major Surgery. *World J. Surg.* **2006**, *30*, 378–390. [CrossRef]
19. The Veterans Affairs Total Parenteral Nutrition Cooperative Study Group. Perioperative Total Parenteral Nutrition in Surgical Patients. Available online: https://www.nejm.org/doi/10.1056/NEJM199108223250801?url_ver=Z39.88-2003&rfr_id=ori%3Arid%3Acrossref.org&rfr_dat=cr_pub%3Dwww.ncbi.nlm.nih.gov (accessed on 10 March 2019).
20. Ng, T.P.; Nyunt, M.S.Z.; Gao, Q.; Wee, S.L.; Yap, P.; Yap, K.B. Elderly Nutritional Indicators for Geriatric Malnutrition Assessment (ENIGMA): Development and validation of a nutritional prognostic index. *Clin. Nutr. ESPEN.* **2017**, *22*, 54–63. [CrossRef]
21. Jensen, G.L.; Mirtallo, J.; Compher, C.; Dhaliwal, R.; Forbes, A.; Grijalba, R.F.; Hardy, G.; Kondrup, J.; Labadarios, D.; Nyulasi, I.; et al. Adult Starvation and Disease-Related Malnutrition. *J. Parenter. Enter. Nutr.* **2010**, *34*, 156–159. [CrossRef]

22. White, J.V.; Guenter, P.; Jensen, G.; Malone, A.; Schofield, M. Consensus Statement: Academy of Nutrition and Dietetics and American Society for Parenteral and Enteral Nutrition. *J. Parenter. Enter. Nutr.* **2012**, *36*, 275–283. [CrossRef]
23. Zhang, Z.; Pereira, S.L.; Luo, M.; Matheson, E.M. Evaluation of Blood Biomarkers Associated with Risk of Malnutrition in Older Adults: A Systematic Review and Meta-Analysis. *Nutrients* **2017**, *9*, 829. [CrossRef]
24. Cabrerizo, S.; Cuadras, D.; Gomez-Busto, F.; Artaza-Artabe, I.; Marín-Ciancas, F.; Malafarina, V. Serum albumin and health in older people: Review and meta analysis. *Maturitas* **2015**, *81*, 17–27. [CrossRef]
25. Corti, M.-C.; Guralnik, J.M.; Salive, M.E.; Sorkin, J.D. Serum Albumin Level and Physical Disability as Predictors of Mortality in Older Persons. *JAMA* **1994**, *272*, 1036–1042. [CrossRef] [PubMed]
26. Kudsk, K.A.; Tolley, E.A.; DeWitt, R.C.; Janu, P.G.; Blackwell, A.P.; Yeary, S.; King, B.K. Preoperative albumin and surgical site identify surgical risk for major postoperative complications. *J. Parenter. Enter. Nutr.* **2003**, *27*, 1–9. [CrossRef]
27. Gibbs, J.; Cull, W.; Henderson, W.; Daley, J.; Hur, K.; Khuri, S.F. Preoperative Serum Albumin Level as a Predictor of Operative Mortality and Morbidity: Results from the National VA Surgical Risk Study. *Arch. Surg.* **1999**, *134*, 36–42. [CrossRef] [PubMed]
28. Hernández, J.L.; Riancho, J.A.; Matorras, P.; González-Macías, J. Clinical evaluation for cancer in patients with involuntary weight loss without specific symptoms. *Am. J. Med.* **2003**, *114*, 631–637. [CrossRef]
29. Levitt, D.G.; Levitt, M.D. Human serum albumin homeostasis: A new look at the roles of synthesis, catabolism, renal and gastrointestinal excretion, and the clinical value of serum albumin measurements. *Int. J. Gen. Med.* **2016**, *9*, 229–255. [CrossRef] [PubMed]
30. Takeda, H.; Ishihama, K.; Fukui, T.; Fujishima, S.; Orii, T.; Nakazawa, Y.; Shu, H.J.; Kawata, S. Significance of rapid turnover proteins in protein-losing gastroenteropathy. *Hepato-Gastroenterology* **2003**, *50*, 1963–1965.
31. Beck, F.K.; Rosenthal, T.C. Prealbumin: A Marker for Nutritional Evaluation. *Am. Fam. Physician* **2002**, *65*, 1575–1580. [PubMed]
32. Ingenbleek, Y. Plasma Transthyretin as a Biomarker of Sarcopenia in Elderly Subjects. *Nutrients* **2019**, *11*, 895. [CrossRef]
33. Spiekerman, A. Nutritional assessment (protein Nutriture). *Anal. Chem.* **1995**, *67*, 429–436. [CrossRef]
34. Dellière, S.; Cynober, L. Is transthyretin a good marker of nutritional status? *Clin. Nutr.* **2017**, *36*, 364–370. [CrossRef] [PubMed]
35. Li, L.; Dai, L.; Wang, X.; Wang, Y.; Zhou, L.; Chen, M.; Wang, H. Predictive value of the C-reactive protein-to-prealbumin ratio in medical ICU patients. *Biomark. Med.* **2017**, *11*, 329–337. [CrossRef]
36. Harriman, S.; Rodych, N.; Hayes, P.; Moser, M.A. The C-reactive protein-to-prealbumin ratio predicts fistula closure. *Am. J. Surg.* **2011**, *202*, 175–178. [CrossRef] [PubMed]
37. Shen, Q.; Liu, W.; Quan, H.; Pan, S.; Li, S.; Zhou, T.; Ouyang, Y.; Xiao, H. Prealbumin and lymphocyte-based prognostic score, a new tool for predicting long-term survival after curative resection of stage II/III gastric cancer. *Br. J. Nutr.* **2018**, *120*, 1359–1369. [CrossRef]
38. Shimura, T.; Shibata, M.; Inoue, T.; Owada-Ozaki, Y.; Yamaura, T.; Muto, S.; Hasegawa, T.; Shio, Y.; Suzuki, H. Prognostic impact of serum transthyretin in patients with non-small cell lung cancer. *Mol. Clin. Oncol.* **2019**, *10*, 597–604. [CrossRef]
39. Wang, W.; Wang, C.-S.; Ren, D.; Li, T.; Yao, H.-C.; Ma, S.-J. Low serum prealbumin levels on admission can independently predict in-hospital adverse cardiac events in patients with acute coronary syndrome. *Medicine* **2018**, *97*, e11740. [CrossRef] [PubMed]
40. Lee, J.L.; Oh, E.S.; Lee, R.W.; Finucane, T.E. Serum Albumin and Prealbumin in Calorically Restricted, Nondiseased Individuals: A Systematic Review. *Am. J. Med.* **2015**, *128*, 1203. [CrossRef]
41. Shetty, P.S.; Jung, R.T.; Watrasiewicz, K.E.; James, W.P. Rapid-turnover transport proteins: AN index of subclinical protein-energy malnutrition. *Lancet* **1979**, *314*, 230–232. [CrossRef]
42. Bharadwaj, S.; Ginoya, S.; Tandon, P.; Gohel, T.D.; Guirguis, J.; Vallabh, H.; Jevenn, A.; Hanouneh, I. Malnutrition: Laboratory markers vs nutritional assessment. *Gastroenterol. Rep.* **2016**, *4*, 272–280. [CrossRef] [PubMed]
43. Fletcher, J.P.; Little, J.M.; Guest, P.K. A Comparison of Serum Transferrin and Serum Prealbumin as Nutritional Parameters. *J. Parenter. Enter. Nutr.* **1987**, *11*, 144–147. [CrossRef]
44. Roza, A.M.; Tuitt, D.; Shizgal, H.M. Transferrin—A Poor Measure of Nutritional Status. *J. Parenter. Enter. Nutr.* **1984**, *8*, 523–528. [CrossRef]

45. Briassoulis, G.; Zavras, N.; Hatzis, T. Malnutrition, nutritional indices, and early enteral feeding in critically ill children. *Nutrition* **2001**, *17*, 548–557. [CrossRef]
46. Sergi, G.; Coin, A.; Enzi, G.; Volpato, S.; Inelmen, E.M.; Buttarello, M.; Peloso, M.; Mulone, S.; Marin, S.; Bonometto, P. Role of visceral proteins in detecting malnutrition in the elderly. *Eur. J. Clin. Nutr.* **2006**, *60*, 203–209. [CrossRef]
47. Shenkin, A.; Cederblad, G.; Elia, M.; Isaksson, B. Laboratory assessment of protein-energy status. *Clin. Chim. Acta.* **1996**, *253*, S5–S9. [CrossRef]
48. Neaton, J.D.; Blackburn, H.; Jacobs, D.; Kuller, L.; Lee, D.-J.; Sherwin, R.; Shih, J.; Stamler, J.; Wentworth, D. Serum Cholesterol Level and Mortality Findings for Men Screened in the Multiple Risk Factor Intervention Trial. *Arch. Intern. Med.* **1992**, *152*, 1490–1500. [CrossRef]
49. Isley, W.L.; Underwood, L.E.; Clemmons, D.R. Dietary components that regulate serum somatomedin-C concentrations in humans. *J. Clin. Investig.* **1983**, *71*, 175–182. [CrossRef]
50. Campillo, B.; Paillaud, E.; Bories, P.N.; Noel, M.; Porquet, D.; Le Parco, J.C. Serum levels of insulin-like growth factor-1 in the three months following surgery for a hip fracture in elderly: Relationship with nutritional status and inflammatory reaction. *Clin. Nutr.* **2000**, *19*, 349–354. [CrossRef]
51. López-Hellin, J.; Baena-Fustegueras, J.A.; Schwartz-Riera, S.; García-Arumí, E. Usefulness of short-lived proteins as nutritional indicators surgical patients. *Clin. Nutr.* **2002**, *21*, 119–125. [CrossRef]
52. Burgess, E.J. Insulin-Like Growth Factor 1: A Valid Nutritional Indicator during Parenteral Feeding of Patients Suffering an Acute Phase Response. *Ann. Clin. Biochem.* **1992**, *29*, 137–144. [CrossRef]
53. Unterman, T.G.; Vazquez, R.M.; Slas, A.J.; Martyn, P.A.; Phillips, L.S. Nutrition and somatomedin. XIII. Usefulness of somatomedin-C in nutritional assessment. *Am. J. Med.* **1985**, *78*, 228–234. [CrossRef]
54. Livingstone, C. Insulin-like growth factor-I (IGF-I) and clinical nutrition. *Clin. Sci.* **2013**, *125*, 265–280. [CrossRef]
55. Rachakonda, V.; Borhani, A.A.; Dunn, M.A.; Andrzejewski, M.; Martin, K.; Behari, J. Serum Leptin Is a Biomarker of Malnutrition in Decompensated Cirrhosis. *PLoS ONE* **2016**, *11*, e0159142. [CrossRef]
56. Acar, S.; Çatlı, G.; Küme, T.; Tuhan, H.; Gürsoy Çalan, Ö.; Demir, K.; Böber, E.; Abaci, A. Increased concentrations of serum nesfatin-1 levels in childhood with idiopathic chronic malnutrition. *Turk. J. Med. Sci.* **2018**, *48*, 378–385.
57. Tuerk, M.; Fazel, N. Zinc deficiency. *Curr. Opin. Gastroenterol.* **2009**, *25*, 136–143. [CrossRef]
58. Marcellini, F.; Giuli, C.; Papa, R.; Gagliardi, C.; Dedoussis, G.; Herbein, G.; Fulop, T.; Monti, D.; Rink, L.; Jajte, J.; et al. Zinc status, psychological and nutritional assessment in old people recruited in five European countries: Zincage study. *Biogerontology* **2006**, *7*, 339–345. [CrossRef]
59. Kvamme, J.-M.; Grønli, O.; Jacobsen, B.K.; Florholmen, J. Risk of malnutrition and zinc deficiency in community-living elderly men and women: The Tromsø Study. *Public Health Nutr.* **2015**, *18*, 1907–1913. [CrossRef]
60. Makonnen, B.; Venter, A.; Joubert, G. A Randomized Controlled Study of the Impact of Dietary Zinc Supplementation in the Management of Children with Protein–Energy Malnutrition in Lesotho. II: Special Investigations. *J. Trop. Pediatr.* **2003**, *49*, 353–360. [CrossRef]
61. Droogsma, E.; Van Asselt, D.Z.B.; Scholzel-Dorenbos, C.J.M.; Van Steijn, J.H.M.; Van Walderveen, P.E.; Van Der Hooft, C.S. Nutritional status of community-dwelling elderly with newly diagnosed Alzheimer's disease: Prevalence of malnutrition and the relation of various factors to nutritional status. *J. Nutr. Health Aging* **2013**, *17*, 606–610. [CrossRef]
62. Koyama, A.; Hashimoto, M.; Tanaka, H.; Fujise, N.; Matsushita, M.; Miyagawa, Y.; Hatada, Y.; Fukuhara, R.; Hasegawa, N.; Todani, S.; et al. Malnutrition in Alzheimer's Disease, Dementia with Lewy Bodies, and Frontotemporal Lobar Degeneration: Comparison Using Serum Albumin, Total Protein, and Hemoglobin Level. *PLoS ONE* **2016**, *11*, e0157053. [CrossRef]
63. Ingenbleek, Y. Why should plasma transthyretin become a routine screening tool in elderly persons? *J. Nutr. Health Aging* **2009**, *13*, 640–642. [CrossRef]
64. Fouque, D.; Kalantar-Zadeh, K.; Kopple, J.; Cano, N.; Chauveau, P.; Cuppari, L.; Franch, H.; Guarnieri, G.; Ikizler, T.A.; Kaysen, G.; et al. A proposed nomenclature and diagnostic criteria for protein–energy wasting in acute and chronic kidney disease. *Kidney Int.* **2008**, *73*, 391–398. [CrossRef]
65. Rymarz, A.; Bartoszewicz, Z.; Szamotulska, K.; Niemczyk, S. The Associations between Body Cell Mass and Nutritional and Inflammatory Markers in Patients with Chronic Kidney Disease and in Subjects Without Kidney Disease. *J. Ren. Nutr.* **2016**, *26*, 87–92. [CrossRef]

66. Kanda, E.; Kato, A.; Masakane, I.; Kanno, Y. A new nutritional risk index for predicting mortality in hemodialysis patients: Nationwide cohort study. *PLoS ONE* **2019**, *14*, e0214524. [CrossRef]
67. Schuetz, P.; Fehr, R.; Baechli, V.; Geiser, M.; Deiss, M.; Gomes, F.; Kutz, A.; Tribolet, P.; Bregenzer, T.; Braun, N.; et al. Individualised Nutritional Support in Medical Inpatients at Nutritional Risk: A Randomised Clinical Trial. *Lancet* **2019**. Available online: http://www.sciencedirect.com/science/article/pii/S0140673618327764 (accessed on 20 May 2019). [CrossRef]

6

Micronutrient Deficiencies in Medical and Surgical Inpatients

Mette M Berger *, Olivier Pantet, Antoine Schneider and Nawfel Ben-Hamouda

Service of Adult Intensive Care Medicine and Burns, Lausanne University Hospital (CHUV), BH 08.612, Rue du Bugnon 46, 1011 Lausanne, Switzerland
* Correspondence: Mette.Berger@chuv.ch

Abstract: Inpatients are threatened by global malnutrition, but also by specific micronutrient (i.e., trace element and vitamins) deficiencies that frequently are overseen in the differential diagnosis of major organ dysfunctions. Some of them are related to specific geographic risks (iodine, iron, selenium, zinc, vitamin A), while others are pathology related, and finally many are associated with specific feeding patterns, including low dose enteral feeding. Among the pathologies in which laboratory blood investigations should include a micronutrient outwork, anemia is in the front line, followed by obesity with bariatric surgery, chronic liver disease, kidney disease, inflammatory bowel disease, cardiomyopathies and heart failure. The micronutrients at the highest risk are iron, zinc, thiamine, vitamin B12 and vitamin C. Admission to hospital has been linked with an additional risk of malnutrition—feeding below 1500 kcal/day was frequent and has been associated with a structural additional risk of insufficient micronutrient intake to cover basal needs. Although not evidence based, systematic administration of liberal thiamine doses upon admission, and daily complementation of inpatients' food and enteral feeding solutions with multi-micronutrient tablets might be considered.

Keywords: iron; copper; selenium; zinc; thiamine; vitamin B12; obesity; inflammation; enteral nutrition

---

1. Introduction

Malnutrition includes a wide spectrum of conditions [1] that may affect energy, substrates and micronutrients (i.e., trace elements and vitamins) to variable degrees. Deficiency is defined as a lack, or shortage of a specific micronutrient that is essential for the proper growth and metabolism of a human: 11 trace elements and 13 vitamins qualify as essential in humans [2,3].

Disease related malnutrition has shown to be frequent upon admission [4]. The proportion of patients that have been admitted to hospital in a poor nutritional status varies between nearly zero in trauma and up to 50% in oncologic pathologies [5,6], and has an important impact on costs [6]. Malnutrition affects all ages from pediatric [7] to geriatric admissions [8]. Elderly subjects constituted an important, increasing part of our population with specific physiopathologic characteristics [9]. In developing countries, socio-economic factors will generate specific deficiencies [10], which will also be present in migrant populations [11]. Further, some pathologies threaten more, particularly the micronutrient status. Finally, the geographic place of living in the world, including some western countries and the local soil characteristics, will have their own impact [12,13]. Iodine and iron deficiencies are the most well-known. The below text will review some of these undermining deficiencies.

The definition of deficiency requires knowing the specific needs of diseased patients—this information is generally not available. Micronutrient requirements have been determined for the healthy population with age specificities [3]. They are called dietary reference intakes (DRI), a concept that has replaced the recommended daily allowance (RDA). There is minimal data that exists about the needs during disease. Therefore, the present review, which is based on searches in PubMed and the

Cochrane library, is focused on conditions in adults that have been best documented, such as elderly patients, and some selected conditions. The issue of refeeding syndrome in hospitalized patients is be given particular attention.

2. Undermining Micronutrients Deficiencies

The causes of deficiency can globally be divided into three: Low availability, reduction of intakes, and malabsorption. Some geographic soil and nutrition specificities have threatened the entire populations' micronutrient status. This knowledge is not new [2], and the below text provides a brief summary of their impact on acute diseases.

Micronutrient deficiencies have been called the hidden hunger [14], as they are determining and aggravating factors for one's health status and quality of life. The close relation between fetal malnutrition and the development of chronic non-communicable diseases later in life has been repeatedly confirmed [10,15]. Vitamin A (in developing countries), iodine, and iron deficiencies (worldwide) are the most important in terms of global public health [16]. The below deficiencies have affected patients before their hospital admission and should be integrated in the differential diagnosis of the acute condition.

2.1. Iodine

Deficiencies early in life impairs cognition and growth. Iodine status is also a key determinant of thyroid disorders in adults. Iodine deficiency disorders have affected 740 million people. A severe deficiency causes goiter and hypothyroidism because, despite an increase in thyroid activity to maximize iodine uptake and recycling, iodine concentrations are insufficient to enable synthesis of thyroid hormones [17].

2.2. Iron

Deficiencies are a public health problem worldwide [18]. In the year 2000, it was estimated that iron deficiency anemia affected two billion people, mostly women and children. Anemia concerns roughly a third of the world's population [19], but anemia represents the end stage of an iron deficiency [20] which is largely prevalent in all categories of society [21]. The diagnosis of this deficiency is complex in acute and chronic diseases presenting an inflammatory response that modulates blood iron concentrations [20,22]. Its efficient treatment has often been prevented by beliefs such as the risk of iron administration causing additional oxidative stress or favoring infection. These concerns have not been confirmed [23]. The exploration of the iron status (deficiency < 7.1 µg/L or 12.5 mmol/L) included determining the presence of inflammation reflected by C-reactive protein (CRP) > 10 mg/L [24]. In addition to hemoglobin, and erythrocyte morphology (microcytosis, hypochromia), the following have been required: Serum ferritin (<30 ng/L), transferrin saturation ($<15\%$), total iron-binding capacity (>13.1 µmol/L), soluble transferrin receptor (increased > 28.1 nmol/L) [20], and hepcidin (ranges men 0.6–23.3 nmol/L, women 0.4–19.7 nmol/L) [25].

With the availability of hepcidin as a marker of deficiency, the diagnosis should become easier [20,22,25]. Hepcidin is a hormone synthesized in the liver, secreted into the blood that systemically controls the rate of iron absorption as well as its mobilization from stores [26]. The synthesis of hepcidin is up-regulated by inflammatory cytokines (particularly interleukin-6), irrespective of the total level of iron in the body. This relationship most likely accounts for the development of anemia of chronic disease [27,28] (please see Section 3.7 for specificities in kidney diseases).

2.3. Selenium

Deficiencies have been an issue in Europe and in other parts of the world as the main source of human exposure is diet, which is related to the soil content [29]. Scientists have claimed that changes in climate and the organic carbon content of soil will lead to overall decreased soil Se concentrations, particularly in agricultural areas [30]. Europe and some parts of Australasia are particularly affected, while North America is spared by elevated soil content. Borderline Se status reduced endogenous antioxidant defenses via the reduction of the activity of the glutathione peroxidase (GPX) family of enzymes [31], which contributed to poor outcomes facing critical illness, and particularly sepsis [32]. In major trauma, the intravenous administration of selenium in combination with other micronutrients at 5 times DRI doses (see Table 1) resulted in normalization of plasma GPX3 activity and shortened hospital stays [33]. Nevertheless, the high dose single selenium trials (1000 μg/iv/day) in septic shock have been negative [34]. Therefore this strategy should not be considered, and has been advised against in the Surviving Sepsis Campaign 2017 recommendations [35].

Table 1. Micronutrient strategy in critically ill patients admitted to the Lausanne multidisciplinary ICU, according to disease and nutrition therapy.

Situation	Stress Profile in High Risk Patients in Organ Failure *	Parenteral Nutrition (and Combined Feeding)	Enteral Nutrition
Micro-Nutrients	1 vial multi-trace element (Addaven®, Fresenius Kabi, Oberdorf, Switzerland) + 5 mg Zinc + 1 vial multi-vitamin (Cernevit®, Baxter, Volketswil, Switzerland) + 500 mg vitamin C + 100 mg vitamin B1	Same as stress profile	Multi-micronutrient providing DRI needs (Supradyn®, Roche, Basel, Switzerland)
Duration Route	Diluted in 100 ml de NaCl 0.9% over 6 hours from admission for first 6 days during night shift	Daily with parenteral nutrition	Daily Mixed with enteral feeding

*: High risk conditions include shock (cardiogenic, septic, hypovolemic), pancreatitis, severe hepatopathy, major trauma, organ transplant, and malnutrition.

2.4. *Zinc*

Deficiencies were first identified in the 1960s [36], and have continued to plague multiple regions of the planet [37]. It has affected all ages, but particularly the elderly in western regions. Zinc deficiency affects cell-mediated immune dysfunction, susceptibility to infections, and increases oxidative stress. A randomized trial including 50 healthy elderly subjects tested the impact of a zinc-supplement (45 mg elemental Zn/day) orally for 12 months versus placebo [38]. First, the authors showed that compared to younger, healthy subjects, the elderly study subjects had lower plasma zinc, higher ex vivo generation of inflammatory cytokines and interleukin 10. The supplement resulted in a significant reduction of the incidence of infections and ex vivo generation of tumor necrosis factor alpha and plasma oxidative stress markers compared to the placebo group [38].

2.5. *Copper*

Deficiencies have also been shown to affect specific geographic areas—drinking water may or may not be rich in copper depending on the pipe composition. The deficiency is most frequently acquired [39], e.g., due to insufficient intakes in vulnerable populations, increased demands (pregnancy, lactation, wound healing), malabsorption (including high phytic content of vegetarian diets), increased losses (e.g., major burns, continuous renal replacement therapy), and from hereditary diseases [40,41].

2.6. *Vitamin A*

Deficiency is considered the world's most important cause of preventable blindness [42]. It affected 2.8 million children under five years of age. Tragically, the numbers have only grown over the last decades [20].

2.7. Vitamin D

Long known only for its role in calcium and bone homeostasis, and the development of osteoporosis, its deficiency seems to be a worldwide problem, and to particularly affect inpatients. The multiple effects of vitamin D are mediated by genomic and non-genomic effects, and include muscle function and metabolism, innate and adaptive immune system, lung epithelial function, cardiac function and numerous other functions as the specific nuclear vitamin D receptor are widely expressed throughout the body [43]. As shown in Table 1, low values can be found in nearly any severe condition. Many observational studies have consistently shown an association between low vitamin D levels and poor clinical outcomes. Nevertheless, high-quality evidence showing the benefits of vitamin D supplementation in inpatients is still lacking [44]. One of the largest studies (VITdAL-ICU) was analyzed retrospectively: 475 critically ill patients with 25(OH)D levels $\leq$ 20 ng/mL [45]. The deficiency was not associated with persistent critical illness, nor did supplementation with vitamin D3 mitigate the development of persistent critical illness. The actual evidence does not support general vitamin D screening and supplementation for the medical inpatient population in an acute care setting [44]. By contrast, screening of chronic kidney disease patients is probably rational (see Section 3.7).

3. Disease Specific Deficiency

The below Table 2 summarizes the most frequent deficits encountered in the different pathologies.

Table 2. Disease specific vitamins and in trace elements deficiencies.

Disease	Micronutrients at Risk
Alcoholism	Zn Vitamins A, D, E, K, B12, B9, B6, B1, B2, C
Anemia	Fe, Cu, Co Vitamins B12, B9
Cardiomyopathies/ Heart failure	Se, Fe Vitamin B1, D [?]
Inflammatory bowel diseases	Se, Zn Vitamins B12, A, D, E, K
Liver diseases	Se, Zn Vitamins B12, A, D, E
Obesity and Bariatric surgery	Cu, Zn, Fe Vitamins A, D, E, K, B1, B9, B12, C
Kidney diseases (chronic & acute)	Chronic: Vitamins K, D Acute: B1, Fe, Se, Zn, Cu

[?]: means uncertainty as to deficiency.

3.1. Alcoholism

Micronutrient deficiencies are commonly encountered in alcoholic patients, not only explained by a decrease of global dietary intake, but also because of maldigestion, malabsorption, impaired hepatic activation and an increased breakdown and excretion. The risk of developing micro and macronutrient deficiencies has been known to increase significantly when alcohol makes up more than 30 percent of total caloric intake [46].

All fat-soluble vitamins (A, D, E and K) are susceptible to be decreased [47], although vitamins A and K deficiencies are more common in the case of overt hepatic disease or chronic pancreatitis. Among water soluble vitamins, the vitamin B1 (thiamine) deficiency has been the most frequently described and feared [48], potentially leading to Wernicke's encephalopathy and its well-known triad (delirium, oculomotor abnormalities and ataxia). If left untreated, it can progress to the amnestic-confabulatory syndrome called Korsakoff. The therapeutic benefit of thiamin has been demonstrated in alcoholic patients even without severe Wernicke-Korsakoff encephalopathy [49]. In the emergency department, patients with acute alcohol intoxication have not all suffered thiamine deficiency [50,51]. A systematic review showed that thiamine and vitamin C were the most frequently identified deficiencies [51,52].

Nevertheless, considering the elevated prevalence of malnutrition in these patients, it is cautious and cheap, in case of hospital admission to provide 100–300 mg thiamine prior to any glucose IV infusion to prevent precipitating Wernicke's encephalopathy. Excessive alcohol consumption has also been linked to zinc and copper deficiency, which seems to be associated with a decreased quality of physical and mental life [53].

There has been one randomized trial testing the administration of 600 mg of benfotiamine in alcohol dependent patients—this thiamine analog was associated with a reduction of alcohol consumption, but no metabolic variables were tested [54]. In the absence of other randomized trials, most of the experts advocated the empiric administration to alcohol dependent patients of multivitamin cocktails, including in particular, thiamine (200–300 mg), folic acid, vitamin B6, and vitamin C upon admission.

3.2. *Anemia*

A third of the world's population is affected by anemia, and iron deficiency is involved in 50% of the cases [18]. The most common symptoms are paleness, fatigue, dyspnea and headache. Laboratory tests have shown low blood haemoglobin concentration (Hb < 130 g/L in men, <120 g/L in women and <110g/L in pregnancy) with microcytosis, hypochromia and serum ferritin below 30 μg/L. Iron deficiencies can be physiological (e.g., pregnancy), or pathological in case of blood loss (e.g., surgery, trauma, digestive tract bleeding), malabsorption (e.g., celiac disease, gastrectomy), chronic disease (cancer, chronic heart failure) or in some genetic disorders [19]. In the presence of iron-deficiency anemia, investigations to identify a cause of blood loss or malabsorption are required. Preventive iron supplementation should be prescribed in at-risk patients using the oral route, while treatment of in patients with a positive diagnosis [19], may require the intravenous route due to the frequent gastric intolerance and poor absorption of oral supplements.

Macrocytic anemia can be observed in vitamin B12 or/and vitamin B9 (folate) deficiencies. Vitamin B12 deficiencies occur in cases of severe malabsorption (bariatric surgery, gastrectomy, or autoimmune gastritis), in the abuse of nitrous oxide, and in cases of inherited metabolic disorders. Vitamin B12 supply is recommended after confirmed diagnosis. This treatment will be lifelong when the etiology of the deficiency is irreversible or unknown [55].

Copper deficiencies impair the activity of hephaestin, a copper-dependent ferroxidase responsible for transporting dietary iron from intestinal enterocytes into the circulatory system—its depression leads to iron deficiencies and low hemoglobin. Copper deficiency anemia has been treated with oral or intravenous copper supplementation [56]. Cobalt, a component of hydroxycobalamin, is considered one the most stimulator of erythrocyte production. In clinical practice, Cobalt administration is rare considering the high risk of toxicity of cobalt salts in humans [57].

3.3. *Cardiomyopathies and Heart Failure*

According to the European Society of Cardiology (ESC), cardiomyopathy (CM) is defined as a myocardial disorder in which the heart muscle is structurally and functionally abnormal, in the absence of coronary artery disease, hypertension, valvular disease and congenital heart disease [58]. CM can lead to heart failure (HF). Deficiencies in thiamine and selenium are nutritional factors that may be involved in the occurrence of such myocardial disorders [58,59] in malnutrition conditions, malabsorption, or exclusive parenteral nutrition (PN) [60–62]. Selenium deficiency cardiomyopathy is known as the Keshan disease in humans. It was initially described in China in 1935 in selenium-poor soils, with multiple case reports. In addition to the low plasma selenium levels, low glutathione peroxidase-1 activity has been reported in animals [63]. Some cases reported have been reversible by short-term oral or IV administration, and others have been fatal [60–63].

Thiamine plays a fundamental role in cellular metabolism, especially in the carbohydrate pathway. Severe and chronic thiamine deficiencies are known as Beriberi disease. The classic presentation includes neurologic features and encephalopathy. HF symptoms have been less frequent and have been associated to metabolic acidosis and hyperlactatemia (due to an inhibition of the pyruvate deshydrogenase) [64,65]. A fulminant form has also been described [64]. It has been shown that about 40% of the patients hospitalized for HF presented thiamine deficiencies [66]. Animal models have demonstrated that this deficiency causes cardiac disorders (cardiac hypertrophy, depressed cardiac contractility, and dysrhythmias) in the absence of beriberi. Finally, in human studies, the benefit of thiamine supplements in cases of chronic HF are unclear [66].

Iron deficiencies in HF are common (about 30–50%) in patients with chronic HF, independent of anemia, and have lead to skeletal muscle dysfunction. Recent ESC guidelines recommended screening for iron deficits in HF patients [28,59].

Recently, an association between vitamin D deficiency and HF has been suggested [67]. Vitamin D promoted cardioprotection in animals (anti-inflammatory, anti-apoptotic and anti-fibrotic mechanisms) [67].

3.4. *Inflammatory Bowel Disease*

Malnutrition is present in the vast majority of patients with inflammatory bowel disease (IBD), the deficiencies being more prevalent in Crohn's disease compared with ulcerative colitis and more important in active diseases [68]. Micronutrient deficiencies are essentially explained by the reduced dietary intake and the underlying malabsorption. They have been associated with prolonged hospitalization and higher mortality [69].

Fat-soluble vitamins are particularly prone to deficiency. A high prevalence of vitamin A and E deficiencies have been reported [70], but also of vitamin D, which has been suspected to play a role in the pathogenesis of IBD [71]. Vitamin K deficiencies are also frequent and correlated with disease activity [72].

Folate deficiencies are common in IBD and aggravated by treatment, such as sulfasalazine or methotrexate. Vitamin B12 has also been frequently observed, especially in Crohn's disease and after ileal resection of ≥30 cm [73]. Thiamin deficiency has also been reported, especially in IBD patients treated with parenteral nutrition [74].

Among trace elements, selenium deficiencies have been reported and may increase the severity of gut inflammation—the repletion data are conflicting [75]. Zinc deficiencies are also prevalent [76]. Iron deficiencies are very frequent and are the leading cause of anemia in patients with IBD. In the presence of inflammation, this diagnosis can be challenging and relies on the values of serum ferritin values.

3.5. *Liver Disease*

The liver plays a crucial role in maintaining systemic Zn homeostasis [77]. Chronic liver disease, such as chronic hepatitis, liver cirrhosis, or fatty liver, impairs Zn metabolism, and has resulted in Zn deficiency, which in turn has caused multiple metabolic abnormalities, including insulin resistance, hepatic steatosis and hepatic encephalopathy. Zn deficiency may also favor carcinogenesis of hepatocellular carcinoma (HCC). In chronic liver disease, low levels of selenium [78] have been generally observed. In comparison, copper levels have often been elevated [79]. It is argued that doses required to achieve an effect in chronic hepatitis are far beyond DRI with 150–200 mg/day [80].

In cases of liver disease secondary to alcoholism, please see 3.1 (same picture). Group B vitamin deficiencies, especially thiamine, are common in cirrhosis [81]. Unlike observations for alcoholic patients without liver disease, vitamin B12 levels have been frequently elevated in viral hepatitis, cirrhosis and hepatocellular carcinoma (HCC) [82]. This increase has been explained by the cytolysis of hepatocytes, and vitamin B12 being mainly stored in the liver.

Fat-soluble vitamin deficiencies have been observed in cases of alcoholism, but also in cholestasis with malabsorption and bile salt deficiency [83]. Levels of vitamins A, D and E should therefore be routinely checked as well as prothrombin time. However, prolonged prothrombin time does not purely reflect vitamin K deficiencies, but also reduced levels of coagulation factor V. Importantly, vitamin D has pleiotropic effects for liver disease, including anti-inflammatory, immune-modulatory and anti-fibrotic properties in addition to its classical skeletal effects. This may impact on disease progression [84], especially in HCC and non-alcoholic steatohepatitis, although any benefit from its repletion has not been formally proven by prospective studies [85].

3.6. Obesity & Bariatric Surgery

In patients with grade III obesity (body mass index ≥ 40 kg·m^{-2} or ≥ 35 kg·m^{-2} with comorbid conditions), bariatric surgery has become common. In 2013, over 450,000 bariatric surgeries were performed worldwide. Roux-en-Y gastric bypass, adjustable gastric band, and sleeve gastrectomy were the most frequent procedures [86,87]. Micronutrient deficiencies were observed before (in obese patients, vitamin C deficiency in about 40% and zinc deficiency is up to 50%) and after the surgery. Due to fat malabsorption and maldigestion, all fat-soluble vitamins are at risk. The bypass of the duodenum and proximal jejunum lead to thiamine deficiencies [86], leading to a risk of clinical Wernicke's encephalopathy [88]. Vitamin B9 is approximately 10%. Vitamin B12 deficiencies have been widely described in the literature because of their neurologic complications, especially an acquired myelopathy with paresthesias, ataxia and muscle weakness [89]. It is recalled that the intrinsic factor produced in the stomach is needed for ileal absorption of vitamin B12. The severity of a vitamin B6 deficiencies vary from peripheral neuropathy to seizures [89]. The common trace elements deficiencies after bariatric surgery include copper (absorbed in the stomach and the duodenum), iron (absorbed in the duodenum), and zinc (absorbed in the jejunum). The prevalence of copper deficiency has been reported to be as high as 90% post- surgery (70% for zinc). Further, systematic supplements of micronutrients are recommended after bariatric surgery by the American Society for Parenteral and Enteral Nutrition (ASPEN) [86] and the American Society for Metabolic and Bariatric Surgery clinical practice guidelines (ASMBS) [90].

3.7. Kidney Disease

Kidney disease, whether chronic (CKD) or acute, affects micronutrient homeostasis and might lead to either deficiency or toxic excess. Indeed, a decreased glomerular filtration rate might lead to accumulation of molecules normally excreted by the kidney such as selenium. On the other hand, renal replacement therapy when applied might lead to uncompensated losses of other micronutrients (copper). Finally, the loss of renal activation might lead to decreased biological activity (vitamin D). Unfortunately, the authors knowledge remains limited [91].

Anemia is commonly observed in CKD. Beyond the lack of erythropoietin, which is now clearly established and easily administered, it might also be associated with alterations in iron metabolism and inflammation. Oral corrections of iron deficiencies in pre-dialysis CKD patients have been shown to be an efficient option in a recent randomized trial [92]. The role of hepcidin, a key regulator of circulating iron level in CKD associated anemia is increasingly recognized. Indeed, the condition has been associated with elevated hepcidin serum levels as it is typically excreted by the kidney [93]. This leads to reduced iron availability and anemia. Its measurement and potential anti-hepcidin therapies could help managing anemia in CKD [27,94].

Subclinical vitamin K deficiencies have been shown to be clinically relevant as requirements have increased due to the vitamin K-dependent proteins required to inhibit calcification [95]. This vitamin governs the gamma-carboxylation of matrix Gla protein for inhibiting vascular calcification, and the vitamin D binding protein receptor is related to vitamin K gene expression [96]. Deficiency may favor vascular calcification.

Chronic dialysis is typically associated with elevated oxidative stress leading to low levels of zinc, selenium and GPX. A French team showed three decades ago that weekly administration of selenium with zinc was able to restore GPX activity and reduced thiobarbituric acid reactants (TBARs) plasma concentrations [97]. In a large cohort of 1278 patients on incident hemodialysis, it was observed that lower selenium and zinc concentrations were strongly and independently associated with death and all-cause hospitalization [98]. Trimestrial monitoring of selenium and zinc may thus be justified, with repletion in case of low values.

In acute kidney failure requiring continuous renal replacement therapy, other micronutrients such as thiamine and copper will be lost in the effluent fluid [39,40,99]. Copper losses causing low blood levels can be associated with severe arrhythmias and wound healing complications. Very low plasma levels (<8 mmol/L) might require active intravenous repletion with doses 6–10 mg/day, i.e., 5–10 times the usual DRI [40].

3.8. Migrant Populations

Being a migrant is not a disease, but a difficult social condition frequently associated with malnutrition for multiple reasons ranging from insufficient food intake, to exposure to unusual food or unbalanced diet due to incapacity to find the traditional foods. Migrants represent a growing category of inpatients. Micronutrients of concern have shown to be retinol, vitamin D, magnesium, potassium, copper, and selenium [11], in addition to iron.

3.9. Laboratory Investigations

Laboratory investigations of micronutrient deficiencies have often not been systematic except for 2 conditions: (1) Anemia outwork, which generally included determination of blood Vitamin B6, B12, iron, ferritin and transferrin; (2) screening before and the follow-up after bariatric surgery included thiamine, vitamin B12, folic acid, iron, zinc, copper, calcium and the liposoluble vitamins D, A, E and K were recommended [90]. In other conditions, the diagnosis lacked standardization. A pragmatic approach upon admission or during hospitalization could be to draw an additional blood sample for further diagnostic outwork, and to empirically administer multi-micronutrients without delay.

Inflammation causes a redistribution of micronutrients between the various compartments and generally reduces circulating levels. The intensity of inflammation has been reflected by CRP levels [24]. The example of vitamin D has been emblematic. While a CRP > 80 mg/L has been associated with a reduction of its blood concentration by 40% below reference ranges [24], CRP has never been mentioned in the vitamin D trials. CRP should belong to any micronutrients outwork as low levels do not necessarily indicate a deficiency.

4. Micronutrient Unavailability as Cause of Deficiency

4.1. Nutritional Sources

Hospital related malnutrition is a well know entity that is observed worldwide and is related to being bedridden [100]. A large proportion of patients only consume a third or half of the proposed meals [4]. In our hospital, a standard daily serving provides 1700–1800 kcal. If only half is consumed, the daily micronutrients cannot be covered.

The sickest patients are fed with enteral nutrition. Due to regulatory constraints, the industry must respect micronutrient recommendations intended for the general healthy population, the previously mentioned DRI. The concentrations of the products are calculated for feeding doses varying between 1500 and 2500 kcal/day. However, worldwide it has been shown that many patients receive no more than 1000 kcal/day by this route [101]. In addition, the most recent nutrition guidelines for critical care patients recommended ramping up the feeding over several days [102]. The consequences might be an even further reduction of nutrition delivery. By design, the enteral feeding solutions will not be able to cover needs as long as quantities below 1500 kcal per day are provided. Table 3 shows the detailed micronutrient provision for 1000 kcal/day provided by the 10 most frequently used enteral feeding solutions provided by 4 international companies on the Swiss market. While intakes below DRI of fluor and iodine may be less important during an acute phase, low intakes of iron and of the B vitamin group are a concern considering their essential role in energy (ATP synthesis) and carbohydrate metabolism. Moreover, as absorption is unreliable and as needs might be higher, several micronutrients such as vitamin C are just in the reference range, which may be insufficient.

Table 3. Energy, protein and micronutrient data for 1000 kcal for a selection of frequent products available on the Swiss market compared to the dietary reference intakes (DRI). The values which are below the DRI appear in red and bold characters; in violet-bold, those for which DRI is just covered.

	Abbott	**Abbott**	**Nestlé**	**Nestlé**	**Nestlé**	**Fresenius K**	**Fresenius K**	**Fresenius K**	**Nutricia**	**Nutricia**	
Values for 1000 kcal	**Promote Fibres Plus**	**Jevity Plus**	**NovaSource GI Advance**	**Isosource Energy**	**Peptamen Intense**	**Fresubin 2 kcal HP**	**Fresubin HP Energy**	**Fresubin Intensive**	**Nutrison Protein + Mulitf**	**Nutrison**	**DRI Adults**
Energy density kcal/ml	1.3	1.2	1.55	1.57	1.0	2.0	1.5	1.2	1.3	1.0	
Proteins g/1000 kcal	62.5	46.3	61.9	38.9	93.0	50.0	50.0	83.3	49.2	40.0	
Fer (Fe) mg	**12.3**	**15.0**	**11.0**	**10.2**	**16.0**	**13.5**	**8.7**	**16.7**	**15.6**	**16.0**	18
Zinc (Zn) mg	13.1	11.7	11.6	9.6	13	12	**8.0**	12.5	11.7	12	8
Cuivre (Cu) mg	1.5	1.7	1.5	1.5	1.8	1.5	**0.7**	1.7	1.8	1.8	0.9
Manganèse (Mn) mg	3.1	3.5	2.3	2.3	1.4	2.5	2.0	4.2	3.2	3.3	1.8
Fluor	**0.0**	**0.0**	**1.0**	**1.3**	**1.6**	**1.5**	**0.7**	**1.7**	**1.0**	**1.0**	3
Iode (I) µg	**123**	**125**	**142**	**146**	**120**	**134**	**89**	183	**102**	**130**	150
Molybdène (Mo) µg	92	108	116	115	170	100	67	117	102	100	45
Chrome (Cr) µg	54	67	97	96	60	67	45	92	65	67	20
Selenium (Se) µg	65	63	65	64	80	67	**45**	88	**55**	**57**	55
A (RE) µg	1154	**700**	1097	1083	**650**	925	**613**	1500	**797**	820	750
D µg	**6.9**	**8.3**	14.2	14	14	**10**	**8.7**	17	**13.3**	**10**	10
E (α-TE) mg	18.2	20	17.4	16.6	**14**	**13.5**	**8.7**	25	**12.5**	**13**	15
K µg	**54**	**67**	**71**	**76**	**44**	**67**	**45**	**75**	**52**	**53**	90
C mg	154	100	123	102	80	**67**	**45**	183	102	100	75
B1 mg	1.5	1.6	1.6	1.5	**1.0**	1.5	**0.7**	1.7	1.5	1.5	1.1
B2 Riboflavin mg	2.2	1.8	1.7	1.7	1.3	2.0	1.3	1.7	1.6	1.6	1.1
B3 Niacin mg	21.5	18.3	20.0	17.2	30	**16**	**11**	20	18	18	14
B5 Pantothenic acid mg	7.7	8.3	**5.2**	5.5	**4.5**	**4.5**	3.3	7.5	**5.2**	**5.3**	5
B6 Pyridoxin mg	2.2	2.2	1.8	1.8	1.7	**1.5**	**0.8**	2.5	**1.6**	**1.7**	1.5
B12 Cyancobalamin µg	4.6	2.9	3.8	3.7	2.9	**2.5**	**2.0**	4.2	**2.0**	**2.1**	2.4
B9 Folic acid µg	**231**	**250**	**290**	**287**	**300**	**267**	**180**	**263**	**258**	**270**	400
B8 Biotin µg	46	43	45	45	**30**	50	**33**	57	**39**	40	30
Choline mg	**462**	500	**368**	**382**	670	**0**	178	**0**	**359**	**370**	425

Regarding these low micronutrient doses, it might be justified to deliver standard multivitamin and trace element products daily providing DRI doses to the majority of inpatients. This strategy has been applied for many years in the Lausanne university hospital's ICU, as critically ill patients do have higher needs. In the sickest patients, multi-micronutrients cocktails have been delivered IV for the first 5 days [33], resulting in a shortening of the hospital stay, particularly in major trauma patients.

4.2. Geriatric Population

The qualification, elderly, encompasses patients aged 60 to over 100 years. While the younger seniors often are fit until the seventies, some physiological changes already occur that become exacerbated with growing age. The elderly often present with anorexia which is considered a complex geriatric syndrome and a risk factor for frailty [9]. These changes are associated with lower weight, and lower energy expenditure. The body undergoes specific changes—the gastric mucosa tends to atrophy, reducing vitamin B12 absorption. Indeed, the decline in vitamin B12 is independent of nutrition but caused by a decline of both the intestinal uptake and the renal reabsorption system for vitamin B12 [103]. The elderly also require higher doses of vitamin B6 and D to maintain health, which has been integrated into DRI recommendations for older subjects. Deficiencies can be overcome by supplementation, as shown by a large randomized controlled trial including 652 geriatric patients—daily oral nutrition supplements enriched with proteins, hydroxy-methyl-butyrate, vitamin D and other micronutrients reduced mortality [104].

4.3. Partial or Complete Starving upon Hospital Admission and Refeeding

The incidence and importance of the refeeding has often been underestimated [105]. The absence of a uniform definition participates in its underestimation [105]. Refeeding syndrome consists of metabolic changes that occur on the reintroduction of food or simply a glucose infusion. A few days of feeding grossly below needs will be sufficient to create the metabolic crisis which is characterized by sudden shifts in the electrolytes that are needed for energy and substrate (mainly glucose) metabolism. The NutritionDay survey, an initiative that analysed the relation between nutritional intakes and outcomes of a wide range of institutionalized and hospitalized patients worldwide, has shown that more than half of the patients admitted to hospital were eating less than half of their normal food intake before admission [106]. This places the majority of hospitalized patients at risk of a refeeding syndrome.

Some categories of patients, such as chronic, alcohol consumers, which are largely prevalent in western countries, being present in nearly 30% of hospital admissions, are at higher risk of thiamine deficiencies—these patients are at particularly high risk of refeeding syndrome and its worst neurologic complication, the Wernicke encephalopathy. A recent review of the literature confirmed the importance of administering intravenous thiamine to these patients in order to prevent severe sequelae [107]. The recommended doses ranged from 50–100 mg/day to 250–500 mg 3 times a day. The IV route was recommended due to the frequent presence of gastritis in these patients, which reduced absorption.

4.4. Economic Considerations

A Canadian prospective cohort study showed that approximately 40% of the 956 patients admitted to hospital were moderately to severely malnourished. These patients had longer hospital stays, and as a result, cost more than the well-nourished patients [108]. A European narrative review showed that malnutrition increased the length of hospital stays by 2.4 to 7.2 days [5]. Malnutrition led to an additional individual cost ranging between 1640 € and 5829 €.

Clinical evidences are lacking for empirical multi-micronutrient supplements. The cost of malnutrition attributable to micronutrient deficiencies have not been assessed in adult inpatients and several studies have failed to demonstrate significant beneficial effects of various micronutrient supplements in the general population [109]. Nevertheless, there are data suggesting a benefit, at least in the sickest patients [33,110].

However, data exists for children. A study focusing on estimates of disability-adjusted life years and their monetization showed that short-term economic costs of micronutrient malnutrition in India amounted to 0.8% to 2.5% of the gross domestic product [14]. The health and cost consequences of iodine, iron, vitamin A, and zinc deficiencies were assessed in Pakistani children: Societal costs amounted to 1.44% of gross domestic product and 4.45% of disability-adjusted life-years in Pakistan in 2013, which hindered the country's development [111].

When deciding about an empirical administration of micronutrients, the analytical costs of deficiency diagnosis must be considered. The European Society for Clinical Nutrition and Metabolism (ESPEN) monitoring recommendations indicate that some vitamin and trace element analysis (inductively coupled plasma mass spectrometry: ICP-MS) are expensive [112]. They are actually more expensive than the empirical administration. A semi-automatic weekly determination of blood selenium levels in our ICU resulted in major costs that could be contained by the decision to let blood sampling be prescribed only by the ICU nutritionists and dieticians in patients at risk [113].

A multi-micronutrient tablet costs 0.80 € (the IV dose in Table 1 costs 25 €), which is negligible compared to the cost of one day in hospital, or worse, in the ICU. This prescription is likely to be beneficial if the administration is standardized, and limited to the first week of hospitalization, and to patients on enteral feeding.

5. Conclusions

Micronutrient deficiencies and borderline status are more frequent than generally acknowledged. The most important potential acute deficiency that may compromise outcome is thiamine deficiency. Other deficiencies will impact on immune defenses and anabolic capacity. Therefore, an empirical and cheap complementation strategy, based on daily oral multi-micronutrient products providing DRI, may be justified for hospital inpatients for one week. It is important to state that the evidence from trials is still missing.

Author Contributions: Conceptualization M.M.B.; Search methodology M.M.B., N.B.-H., O.P.; validation, M.M.B., O.P., A.S. and N.B.-H.; writing—original draft preparation, M.M.B., O.P., N.B.-H.; writing—review and editing, N.B.-H., O.P., A.S., and M.M.B.

Abbreviations

DRI	Dietary Reference Intakes
CKD	Chronic kidney disease
CM	cardiomyopathy
CRP	C-reactive protein
ESC	European Society of Cardiology
ESPEN	European Society for Clinical Nutrition and Metabolism
GPX	Glutathione peroxidase
HF	Heat failure
IBD	inflammatory bowel disease
IV	Intravenous
RDA	recommended daily allowance

References

1. Cederholm, T.; Jensen, G.L.; Correia, M.I.T.D.; Gonzalez, M.C.; Fukushima, R.; Higashiguchi, T.; Baptista, G.; Barazzoni, R.; Blaauw, R.; Coats, A.; et al. GLIM criteria for the diagnosis of malnutrition—A consensus report from the global clinical nutrition community. *Clin. Nutr.* **2019**, *38*, 1–9. [CrossRef] [PubMed]

2. Allen, L.; de Benoist, B.; Dary, O.; Hurrel, R. Guidelines on food fortification with micronutrients. In *World Health Organization (WHO) Food and Agricultural Organization (FAO) of the United Nations*; WHO: Geneva, Switzerland, 2006; pp. 1–376. Available online: http://www.who.int/nutrition/publications/guide_food_fortification_micronutrients.pdf (accessed on 25 June 2019).
3. Trumbo, P.; Yates, A.; Schlicker, S.; Poos, M. Dietary reference intakes: Vitamin A, vitamin K, arsenic, boron, chromium, copper, iodine, iron, manganese, molybdenum, nickel, silicon, vanadium, and zinc. *J. Am. Diet. Assoc.* **2001**, *101*, 294–301. [CrossRef]
4. Schuetz, P.; Fehr, R.; Baechli, V.; Geiser, M.; Deiss, M.; Gomes, F.; Kutz, A.; Tribolet, P.; Bregenzer, T.; Braun, N.; et al. Individualised nutritional support in medical inpatients at nutritional risk: A randomised clinical trial. *Lancet* **2019**, *393*, 2312–2321. [CrossRef]
5. Khalatbari-Soltani, S.; Marques-Vidal, P. The economic cost of hospital malnutrition in Europe; a narrative review. *Clin. Nutr. ESPEN* **2015**, *10*, e89–e94. [CrossRef] [PubMed]
6. Norman, K.; Pichard, C.; Lochs, H.; Pirlich, M. Prognostic impact of disease-related malnutrition. *Clin. Nutr.* **2008**, *27*, 5–15. [CrossRef] [PubMed]
7. Pawellek, I.; Dokoupil, K.; Koletzko, B. Prevalence of malnutrition in paediatric hospital patients. *Clin. Nutr.* **2008**, *27*, 72–76. [CrossRef] [PubMed]
8. Orlandoni, P.; Venturini, C.; Jukic Peladic, N.; Costantini, A.; Di Rosa, M.; Cola, C.; Giorgini, N.; Basile, R.; Fagnani, D.; Sparvoli, D.; et al. Malnutrition upon Hospital Admission in Geriatric Patients: Why Assess It? *Front. Nutr.* **2017**, *4*, 50. [CrossRef]
9. Sanford, A.M. Anorexia of aging and its role for frailty. *Curr. Opin. Clin. Nutr. Metab. Care* **2017**, *20*, 54–60. [CrossRef]
10. World Health Organisation. In *Nutrition for Health and Development: A Global Agenda for Combating Malnutrition*; Docemunt WHO/NHD/00.6; WHO: Geneva, Switzerland, 2000.
11. Castaneda-Gameros, D.; Redwood, S.; Thompson, J. Nutrient Intake and Factors Influencing Eating Behaviors in Older Migrant Women Living in the United Kingdom. *Ecol. Food Nutr.* **2018**, *57*, 50–68. [CrossRef]
12. Black, R. Global distribution and disease burden related to micronutrient deficiencies. *Nestle Nutr. Inst. Workshop Ser.* **2014**, *78*, 21–28. [CrossRef]
13. White, J.; Zasoski, R. Mapping soil micronutrients. *Field Crop. Res.* **1999**, *60*, 11–26. [CrossRef]
14. Stein, A.; Qaim, M. The human and economic cost of hidden hunger. *Food Nutr. Bull.* **2007**, *28*, 125–134. [CrossRef] [PubMed]
15. Diaz, J.; de las Cagigas, A.; Rodriguez, R. Micronutrient deficiencies in developing and affluent countries. *Eur. J. Clin. Nutr.* **2003**, *57* (Suppl. 1), S70–S72. [CrossRef]
16. World Health Orgniasation. Micronutrients. Available online: https://www.who.int/nutrition/topics/micronutrients/en/ (accessed on 25 April 2019).
17. Zimmermann, M.B.; Boelaert, K. Iodine deficiency and thyroid disorders. *Lancet Diabetes Endocrinol.* **2015**, *3*, 286–295. [CrossRef]
18. Stoltzfus, R. Defining iron-deficiency anemia in public health terms: A time for reflection. *J. Nutr.* **2001**, *131*, 565S–567S. [CrossRef] [PubMed]
19. Lopez, A.; Cacoub, P.; Macdougall, I.; Peyrin-Biroulet, L. Iron deficiency anaemia. *Lancet* **2016**, *367*, 907–917. [CrossRef]
20. Camaschella, C. Iron deficiency. *Blood* **2019**, *133*, 30–39. [CrossRef] [PubMed]
21. Schuepbach, R.; Bestmann, L.; Bechir, M.; Fehr, J.; Bachli, E. High prevalence of Iron deficiency among educated hospital employees in Switzerland. *Int. J. Biomed. Sci. IJBS* **2011**, *7*, 150–157.
22. Heming, N.; Montravers, P.; Lasocki, S. Iron deficiency in critically ill patients: Highlighting the role of hepcidin. *Crit. Care* **2011**, *15*, 210. [CrossRef]
23. Lasocki, S.; Piednoir, P.; Couffignal, C.; Rineau, E.; Dufour, G.; Lefebvre, T.; Puy, H.; Duval, X.; Driss, F.; Schilte, C. Does IV Iron Induce Plasma Oxidative Stress in Critically Ill Patients? A comparison with healthy volunteers. *Crit. Care Med.* **2016**, *44*, 521–530. [CrossRef]
24. Duncan, A.; Talwar, D.; McMillan, D.; Stefanowicz, F.; O'Reilly, D. Quantitative data on the magnitude of the systemic inflammatory response and its effect on micronutrient status based on plasma measurements. *Am. J. Clin. Nutr.* **2012**, *95*, 64–71. [CrossRef] [PubMed]

25. Galesloot, T.E.; Vermeulen, S.H.; Geurts-Moespot, A.J.; Klaver, S.M.; Kroot, J.; van Tienoven, D.; Wetzels, J.F.; Kiemeney, L.; Sweep, F.C.; den Heijer, M.; et al. Serum hepcidin: Reference ranges and biochemical correlates in the general population. *Blood* **2011**, *117*, e218–e225. [CrossRef] [PubMed]
26. Johnson-Wimbley, T.D.; Graham, D.Y. Diagnosis and management of iron deficiency anemia in the 21st century. *Ther. Adv. Gastroenterol.* **2011**, *4*, 177–184. [CrossRef] [PubMed]
27. Ueda, N.; Takasawa, K. Impact of Inflammation on Ferritin, Hepcidin and the Management of Iron Deficiency Anemia in Chronic Kidney Disease. *Nutrients* **2018**, *10*, 1173. [CrossRef] [PubMed]
28. Cohen-Solal, A.; Leclercq, C.; Deray, G.; Lasocki, S.; Zambrowski, J.; Mebazaa, A.; de Groote, P.; Damy, T.; Galinier, M. Iron deficiency: An emerging therapeutic target in heart failure. *Heart* **2014**, *100*, 1414–1420. [CrossRef]
29. Vinceti, M.; Filippini, T.; Wise, L.A. Environmental Selenium and human health: An update. *Curr. Environ. Health Rep.* **2018**, *5*, 464–485. [CrossRef] [PubMed]
30. Jones, G.D.; Droz, B.; Greve, P.; Gottschalk, P.; Poffet, D.; McGrath, S.P.; Seneviratne, S.I.; Smith, P.; Winkel, L.H. Selenium deficiency risk predicted to increase under future climate change. *Proc. Natl. Acad. Sci. USA* **2017**, *114*, 2848–2853. [CrossRef]
31. Rayman, M.P. Selenium and human health. *Lancet* **2012**, *379*, 1256–1268. [CrossRef]
32. Alhazzani, W.; Jacobi, J.; Sindi, A.; Hartog, C.; Reinhart, K.; Kokkoris, S.; Gerlach, H.; Andrews, P.; Drabek, T.; Manzanares, W.; et al. The effect of selenium therapy on mortality in patients with sepsis syndrome: A systematic review and meta-analysis of randomized controlled trials. *Crit. Care Med.* **2013**, *41*, 1555–1564. [CrossRef]
33. Berger, M.M.; Soguel, L.; Shenkin, A.; Revelly, J.P.; Pinget, C.; Baines, M.; Chiolero, R.L. Influence of early antioxidant supplements on clinical evolution and organ function in critically ill cardiac surgery, major trauma and subarachnoid hemorrhage patients. *Crit. Care* **2008**, *12*, R101. [CrossRef]
34. Bloos, F.; Trips, E.; Nierhaus, A.; Briegel, J.; Heyland, D.K.; Jaschinski, U.; Moerer, O.; Weyland, A.; Marx, G.; Grundling, M.; et al. Effect of sodium selenite administration and procalcitonin-guided therapy on mortality in patients with severe sepsis or septic shock: A randomized clinical trial. *JAMA Intern. Med.* **2016**, *176*, 1266–1276. [CrossRef] [PubMed]
35. Rhodes, A.; Evans, L.E.; Alhazzani, W.; Levy, M.M.; Antonelli, M.; Ferrer, R.; Kumar, A.; Sevransky, J.E.; Sprung, C.L.; Nunnally, M.E.; et al. Surviving Sepsis Campaign: International Guidelines for Management of Sepsis and Septic Shock: 2016. *Intensive Care Med.* **2017**, *43*, 304–377. [CrossRef] [PubMed]
36. Prasad, A.S. Zinc deficiency. *BMJ* **2003**, *326*, 409–410. [CrossRef] [PubMed]
37. Prasad, A.S. Impact of the discovery of human zinc deficiency on health. *J. Trace Elem. Med. Biol.* **2014**, *28*, 357–363. [CrossRef] [PubMed]
38. Prasad, A.S.; Beck, F.W.; Bao, B.; Fitzgerald, J.T.; Snell, D.C.; Steinberg, J.D.; Cardozo, L.I. Zinc supplementation decreases incidence of infections in the elderly: Effect of zinc on generation of cytokines and oxidative stress. *Am. J. Clin. Nutr.* **2007**, *85*, 837–844. [CrossRef] [PubMed]
39. Altarelli, M.; Ben-Hamouda, N.; Schneider, A.; Berger, M.M. Copper Deficiency—Causes, Manifestations, and Treatment. *Nutr. Clin. Prac.* **2019**. [CrossRef] [PubMed]
40. Ben-Hamouda, N.; Charrière, M.; Voirol, P.; Berger, M.M. Massive copper and selenium losses cause life-threatening deficiencies during prolonged continuous renal replacement. *Nutrition* **2017**, *34*, 71–75. [CrossRef] [PubMed]
41. Wapnir, R.A. Copper absorption and bioavailability. *Am. J. Clin. Nutr.* **1998**, *67*, 1054S–1060S. [CrossRef] [PubMed]
42. World Health Organization. The Global Burden of Disease: 2004 Update. 1. Cost of Illness. 2. World Health—Statistics. 3. Mortality—Trends. Available online: http://www.who.int/healthinfo/global_burden_disease/GBD_report_2004update_full.pdf (accessed on 30 August 2012).
43. Amrein, K.; Papinutti, A.; Mathew, E.; Vila, G.; Parekh, D. Vitamin D and critical illness: What endocrinology can learn from intensive care and vice versa. *Endocr. Connect.* **2018**, *7*, R304–R315. [CrossRef] [PubMed]
44. Gradel, L.; Merker, M.; Mueller, B.; Schuetz, P. Screening and Treatment of Vitamin D Deficiency on Hospital Admission: Is There a Benefit for Medical Inpatients? *Am. J. Med.* **2016**, *129*, 116.e111–116.e134. [CrossRef] [PubMed]

45. Viglianti, E.M.; Zajic, P.; Iwashyna, T.J.; Amrein, K. Neither vitamin D levels nor supplementation are associated with the development of persistent critical illness: A retrospective cohort analysis. *Crit. Care Resusc.* **2019**, *21*, 39–44. [PubMed]
46. Lieber, C.S. Alcohol: Its metabolism and interaction with nutrients. *Annu. Rev. Nutr.* **2000**, *20*, 395–430. [CrossRef] [PubMed]
47. Leo, M.A.; Lieber, C.S. Alcohol, vitamin A, and beta-carotene: Adverse interactions, including hepatotoxicity and carcinogenicity. *Am. J. Clin. Nutr.* **1999**, *69*, 1071–1085. [CrossRef] [PubMed]
48. Leevy, C.M. Thiamin deficiency and alcoholism. *Ann. N. Y. Acad. Sci.* **1982**, *378*, 316–326. [CrossRef] [PubMed]
49. Ambrose, M.L.; Bowden, S.C.; Whelan, G. Thiamin treatment and working memory function of alcohol-dependent people: Preliminary findings. *Alcohol. Clin. Exp. Res.* **2001**, *25*, 112–116. [CrossRef] [PubMed]
50. Li, S.F.; Jacob, J.; Feng, J.; Kulkarni, M. Vitamin deficiencies in acutely intoxicated patients in the ED. *Am. J. Emerg. Med.* **2008**, *26*, 792–795. [CrossRef]
51. Lee, H.J.; Shin, J.; Hong, K.; Jung, J.H. Vitamin C deficiency of Korean homeless vatients visiting to Emergency Department with acute alcohol intoxication. *J. Korean Med Sci.* **2015**, *30*, 1874–1880. [CrossRef]
52. Ijaz, S.; Jackson, J.; Thorley, H.; Porter, K.; Fleming, C.; Richards, A.; Bonner, A.; Savovic, J. Nutritional deficiencies in homeless persons with problematic drinking: A systematic review. *Int. J. Equity Health* **2017**, *16*, 71. [CrossRef]
53. Ordak, M.; Bulska, E.; Jablonka-Salach, K.; Luciuk, A.; Maj-Zurawska, M.; Matsumoto, H.; Nasierowski, T.; Wojnar, M.; Matras, J.; Muszynska, E.; et al. Effect of Disturbances of Zinc and Copper on the Physical and Mental Health Status of Patients with Alcohol Dependence. *Biol. Trace Elem. Res.* **2018**, *183*, 9–15. [CrossRef]
54. Manzardo, A.M.; He, J.; Poje, A.; Penick, E.C.; Campbell, J.; Butler, M.G. Double-blind, randomized placebo-controlled clinical trial of benfotiamine for severe alcohol dependence. *Drug Alcohol. Depend.* **2013**, *133*, 562–570. [CrossRef]
55. Green, R. Vitamin B12 deficiency from the perspective of a practicing hematologist. *Blood* **2017**, *129*, 2603–2611. [CrossRef] [PubMed]
56. Myint, Z.W.; Oo, T.H.; Thein, K.Z.; Tun, A.M.; Saeed, H. Copper deficiency anemia: Review article. *Ann. Hematol.* **2018**, *97*, 1527–1534. [CrossRef] [PubMed]
57. Oliveira, D.C.; Nogueira-Pedro, A.; Santos, E.W.; Hastreiter, A.; Silva, G.B.; Borelli, P.; Fock, R.A. A review of select minerals influencing the haematopoietic process. *Nutr. Res. Rev.* **2018**, *31*, 267–280. [CrossRef] [PubMed]
58. Elliott, P.; Andersson, B.; Arbustini, E.; Bilinska, Z.; Cecchi, F.; Charron, P.; Dubourg, O.; Kuhl, U.; Maisch, B.; McKenna, W.J.; et al. Classification of the cardiomyopathies: A position statement from the European Society Of Cardiology Working Group on Myocardial and Pericardial Diseases. *Eur. Heart J.* **2008**, *29*, 270–276. [CrossRef] [PubMed]
59. Ponikowski, P.; Voors, A.A.; Anker, S.D.; Bueno, H.; Cleland, J.G.F.; Coats, A.J.S.; Falk, V.; Gonzalez-Juanatey, J.R.; Harjola, V.P.; Jankowska, E.A.; et al. 2016 ESC Guidelines for the diagnosis and treatment of acute and chronic heart failure: The Task Force for the diagnosis and treatment of acute and chronic heart failure of the European Society of Cardiology (ESC)Developed with the special contribution of the Heart Failure Association (HFA) of the ESC. *Eur. Heart J.* **2016**, *37*, 2129–2200. [CrossRef] [PubMed]
60. Levy, J.B.; Jones, H.W.; Gordon, A.C. Selenium deficiency, reversible cardiomyopathy and short-term intravenous feeding. *Postgrad. Med. J.* **1994**, *70*, 235–236. [CrossRef] [PubMed]
61. Fleming, C.R.; Lie, J.T.; McCall, J.T.; O'Brien, J.F.; Baillie, E.E.; Thistle, J.L. Selenium deficiency and fatal cardiomyopathy in a patient on home parenteral nutrition. *Gastroenterology* **1982**, *83*, 689–693.
62. Burke, M.P.; Opeskin, K. Fulminant heart failure due to selenium deficiency cardiomyopathy (Keshan disease). *Med. Sci. Law* **2002**, *42*, 10–13. [CrossRef]
63. Oropeza-Moe, M.; Wisloff, H.; Bernhoft, A. Selenium deficiency associated porcine and human cardiomyopathies. *J. Trace Elem. Med. Biol.* **2015**, *31*, 148–156. [CrossRef]
64. Dabar, G.; Harmouche, C.; Habr, B.; Riachi, M.; Jaber, B. Shoshin Beriberi in Critically-Ill patients: Case series. *Nutr. J.* **2015**, *14*, 51. [CrossRef]
65. Ben-Hamouda, N.; Haesler, L.; Liaudet, L. Hyperlactatemia and lactic acidosis in the critically ill patient. *Rev. Med. Suisse* **2013**, *9*, 2335–2340. [PubMed]

66. Smithline, H.A. Thiamine for the treatment of acute decompensated heart failure. *Am. J. Emerg. Med.* **2007**, *25*, 124–126. [CrossRef] [PubMed]
67. Rai, V.; Agrawal, D.K. Role of Vitamin D in Cardiovascular Diseases. *Endocrinol. Metab. Clin. N. Am.* **2017**, *46*, 1039–1059. [CrossRef] [PubMed]
68. Kalantari, H.; Barekat, S.M.; Maracy, M.R.; Azadbakht, L.; Shahshahan, Z. Nutritional status in patients with ulcerative colitis in Isfahan, Iran. *Adv. Biomed. Res.* **2014**, *3*, 58. [CrossRef] [PubMed]
69. O'Sullivan, M. Symposium on The challenge of translating nutrition research into public health nutrition. Session 3: Joint Nutrition Society and Irish Nutrition and Dietetic Institute Symposium on 'Nutrition and autoimmune disease'. Nutrition in Crohn's disease. *Proc. Nutr. Soc.* **2009**, *68*, 127–134. [CrossRef] [PubMed]
70. Hashemi, J.; Asadi, J.; Amiriani, T.; Besharat, S.; Roshandel, G.R.; Joshaghani, H.R. Serum vitamins A and E deficiencies in patients with inflammatory bowel disease. *Saudi Med. J.* **2013**, *34*, 432–434. [PubMed]
71. Torki, M.; Gholamrezaei, A.; Mirbagher, L.; Danesh, M.; Kheiri, S.; Emami, M.H. Vitamin D Deficiency Associated with Disease Activity in Patients with Inflammatory Bowel Diseases. *Dig. Dis. Sci.* **2015**, *60*, 3085–3091. [CrossRef] [PubMed]
72. Nowak, J.K.; Grzybowska-Chlebowczyk, U.; Landowski, P.; Szaflarska-Poplawska, A.; Klincewicz, B.; Adamczak, D.; Banasiewicz, T.; Plawski, A.; Walkowiak, J. Prevalence and correlates of vitamin K deficiency in children with inflammatory bowel disease. *Sci. Rep.* **2014**, *4*, 4768. [CrossRef]
73. Bermejo, F.; Algaba, A.; Guerra, I.; Chaparro, M.; De-La-Poza, G.; Valer, P.; Piqueras, B.; Bermejo, A.; Garcia-Alonso, J.; Perez, M.J.; et al. Should we monitor vitamin B12 and folate levels in Crohn's disease patients? *Scand. J. Gastroenterol.* **2013**, *48*, 1272–1277. [CrossRef]
74. Larnaout, A.; El-Euch, G.; Kchir, N.; Filali, A.; Hamida, M.B.; Hentati, F. Wernicke's encephalopathy in a patient with Crohn's disease: A pathological study. *J. Neurol.* **2001**, *248*, 57–60. [CrossRef]
75. Hiller, F.; Oldorff, L.; Besselt, K.; Kipp, A.P. Differential acute effects of selenomethionine and sodium selenite on the severity of colitis. *Nutrients* **2015**, *7*, 2687–2706. [CrossRef] [PubMed]
76. Saod, W.M.; Darwish, N.T.; Zaidan, T.A.; Alfalujie, A.W.A. Trace Elements in Sera of Patients with Hepatitis B: Determination and Analysis. In Proceedings of the Advanced nanotechnology in engineering and medical sciences (ANEMS) – International conference 2017, Langkawi, Malaysia, 20–21 November 2017.
77. Vagianos, K.; Bector, S.; McConnell, J.; Bernstein, C.N. Nutrition assessment of patients with inflammatory bowel disease. *JPEN J. Parenter. Enter. Nutr.* **2007**, *31*, 311–319. [CrossRef] [PubMed]
78. Himoto, T.; Masaki, T. Associations between Zinc Deficiency and Metabolic Abnormalities in Patients with Chronic Liver Disease. *Nutrients* **2018**, *10*, 88. [CrossRef] [PubMed]
79. Agarwal, A.; Avarebeel, S.; Choudhary, N.S.; Goudar, M.; Tejaswini, C.J. Correlation of Trace Elements in Patients of Chronic Liver Disease with Respect to Child- Turcotte- Pugh Scoring System. *J. Clin. Diagn. Res.* **2017**, *11*, OC25–OC28. [CrossRef] [PubMed]
80. Murakami, Y.; Koyabu, T.; Kawashima, A.; Kakibuchi, N.; Kawakami, T.; Takaguchi, K.; Kita, K.; Okita, M. Zinc supplementation prevents the increase of transaminase in chronic hepatitis C patients during combination therapy with pegylated interferon alpha-2b and ribavirin. *J. Nutr. Sci. Vitaminol. (Tokyo)* **2007**, *53*, 213–218. [CrossRef] [PubMed]
81. Schenker, S.; Halff, G.A. Nutritional therapy in alcoholic liver disease. *Semin. Liver Dis.* **1993**, *13*, 196–209. [CrossRef] [PubMed]
82. Ermens, A.A.; Vlasveld, L.T.; Lindemans, J. Significance of elevated cobalamin (vitamin B12) levels in blood. *Clin. Biochem.* **2003**, *36*, 585–590. [CrossRef] [PubMed]
83. Lindor, K.D. Management of osteopenia of liver disease with special emphasis on primary biliary cirrhosis. *Semin. Liver Dis.* **1993**, *13*, 367–373. [CrossRef]
84. Konstantakis, C.; Tselekouni, P.; Kalafateli, M.; Triantos, C. Vitamin D deficiency in patients with liver cirrhosis. *Ann. Gastroenterol.* **2016**, *29*, 297–306. [CrossRef]
85. Kitson, M.T.; Roberts, S.K. D-livering the message: The importance of vitamin D status in chronic liver disease. *J. Hepatol.* **2012**, *57*, 897–909. [CrossRef]
86. Patel, J.J.; Mundi, M.S.; Hurt, R.T.; Wolfe, B.; Martindale, R.G. Micronutrient Deficiencies After Bariatric Surgery: An Emphasis on Vitamins and Trace Minerals [Formula: See text]. *Nutr. Clin. Pract.* **2017**, *32*, 471–480. [CrossRef] [PubMed]
87. Roust, L.R.; DiBaise, J.K. Nutrient deficiencies prior to bariatric surgery. *Curr. Opin. Clin. Nutr. Metab. Care* **2017**, *20*, 138–144. [CrossRef] [PubMed]

88. Singh, S.; Kumar, A. Wernicke encephalopathy after obesity surgery: A systematic review. *Neurology* **2007**, *68*, 807–811. [CrossRef] [PubMed]
89. Koffman, B.M.; Greenfield, L.J.; Ali, I.I.; Pirzada, N.A. Neurologic complications after surgery for obesity. *Muscle Nerve* **2006**, *33*, 166–176. [CrossRef] [PubMed]
90. Parrott, J.; Frank, L.; Rabena, R.; Craggs-Dino, L.; Isom, K.; Greiman, L. American Society for Metabolic and Bariatric Surgery Integrated Health Nutritional Guidelines for the Surgical Weight Loss Patient 2016 Update: Micronutrient. *Surg. Obes. Relat. Dis.* **2017**, *13*, 727–741. [CrossRef] [PubMed]
91. Jankowska, M.; Rutkowski, B.; Debska-Slizien, A. Vitamins and Microelement Bioavailability in Different Stages of Chronic Kidney Disease. *Nutrients* **2017**, *9*, 282. [CrossRef] [PubMed]
92. Jensen, G.; Goransson, L.; Fernstrom, A.; Furuland, H.; Christensen, J. Treatment of iron deficiency in patients with chronic kidney disease: A prospective observational study of iron isomaltoside (NIMO Scandinavia). *Clin. Nephrol.* **2019**, *91*, 246–253. [CrossRef]
93. Valenti, L.; Messa, P.; Pelusi, S.; Campostrini, N.; Girelli, D. Hepcidin levels in chronic hemodialysis patients: A critical evaluation. *Clin. Chem. Lab. Med.* **2014**, *52*, 613–619. [CrossRef]
94. Santos-Silva, A.; Ribeiro, S.; Reis, F.; Belo, L. Hepcidin in chronic kidney disease anemia. *Vitam. Horm.* **2019**, *110*, 243–264. [CrossRef]
95. Cozzolino, M.; Mangano, M.; Galassi, A.; Ciceri, P.; Messa, P.; Nigwekar, S. Vitamin K in Chronic Kidney Disease. *Nutrients* **2019**, *11*, 168. [CrossRef]
96. Hou, Y.C.; Lu, C.L.; Zheng, C.M.; Chen, R.M.; Lin, Y.F.; Liu, W.C.; Yen, T.H.; Chen, R.; Lu, K.C. Emerging Role of Vitamins D and K in Modulating Uremic Vascular Calcification: The aspect of passive calcification. *Nutrients* **2019**, *11*, 152. [CrossRef] [PubMed]
97. Richard, M.; Ducros, V.; Foret, M.; Arnaud, J.; Coudray, C.; Fusselier, M.; Favier, A. Reversal of selenium and zinc deficiencies in chronic hemodialysis patients by intravenous sodium selenite and zinc gluconate supplementation—Time-course of glutathione peroxidase repletion and lipid peroxidation decrease. *Biol. Trace Elem. Res.* **1993**, *39*, 149–159. [CrossRef] [PubMed]
98. Tonelli, M.; Wiebe, N.; Bello, A.; Field, C.J.; Gill, J.S.; Hemmelgarn, B.R.; Holmes, D.T.; Jindal, K.; Klarenbach, S.W.; Manns, B.J.; et al. Concentrations of Trace Elements and Clinical Outcomes in Hemodialysis Patients: A prospective cohort study. *Clin. J. Am. Soc. Nephrol.* **2018**, *13*, 907–915. [CrossRef] [PubMed]
99. Berger, M.M.; Shenkin, A.; Bollmann, M.D.; Revelly, J.P.; Cayeux, M.C.; Schaller, M.D.; Tappy, L.; Chioléro, R. Trace element balances during continuous venovenous hemodiafiltration (CVVHD). *Kardiovasc. Med.* **2003**, *6* (Suppl. 5), 81S.
100. Schindler, K.; Themessl-Huber, M.; Hiesmayr, M.J.; Kosak, S.; Lainscak, M.; Laviano, A.; Ljungqvist, O.; Mouhieddine, M.; Schneider, S.; de van der Schueren, M.; et al. To eat or not to eat? Indicators for reduced food intake in 91,245 patients hospitalized on nutritionDays 2006–2014 in 56 countries worldwide: A descriptive analysis. *Am. J. Clin. Nutr.* **2016**, *104*, 1393–1402. [CrossRef] [PubMed]
101. Alberda, C.; Gramlich, L.; Jones, N.; Jeejeebhoy, K.; Day, A.G.; Dhaliwal, R.; Heyland, D.K. The relationship between nutritional intake and clinical outcomes in critically ill patients: Results of an international multicenter observational study. *Intensive Care Med.* **2009**, *35*, 1728–1737. [CrossRef] [PubMed]
102. Singer, P.; Reintam-Blaser, A.; Berger, M.M.; Alhazzani, W.; Calder, P.C.; Casaer, M.; Hiesmayr, M.J.; Mayer, K.; Montejo, J.M.; Pichard, C.; et al. ESPEN Guidelines: Nutrition in the ICU. *Clin. Nutr.* **2019**, *38*, 48–79. [CrossRef] [PubMed]
103. Pannerec, A.; Migliavacca, E.; De Castro, A.; Michaud, J.; Karaz, S.; Goulet, L.; Rezzi, S.; Ng, T.; Bosco, N.; Larbi, A.; et al. Vitamin B12 deficiency and impaired expression of amnionless during aging. *J. Cachexia Sarcopenia Muscle* **2018**, *9*, 41–52. [CrossRef]
104. Deutz, N.E.; Matheson, E.M.; Matarese, L.E.; Luo, M.; Baggs, G.E.; Nelson, J.L.; Hegazi, R.A.; Tappenden, K.A.; Ziegler, T.R.; Group, Nourish Study. Readmission and mortality in malnourished, older, hospitalized adults treated with a specialized oral nutritional supplement: A randomized clinical trial. *Clin. Nutr.* **2016**, *35*, 18–26. [CrossRef]
105. Friedli, N.; Stanga, Z.; Sobotka, L.; Culkin, A.; Kondrup, J.; Laviano, A.; Mueller, B.; Schuetz, P. Revisiting the refeeding syndrome: Results of a systematic review. *Nutrition* **2017**, *35*, 151–160. [CrossRef]
106. Sauer, A.; Goates, S.; Malone, A.; Mogensen, K.; Gewirtz, G.; Sulz, I.; Moick, S.; Laviano, A.; Hiesmayr, M. Prevalence of Malnutrition Risk and the Impact of Nutrition Risk on Hospital Outcomes: Results From nutritionDay in the U.S. *JPEN. J. Parenter. Enter. Nutr.* **2019**. [CrossRef] [PubMed]

107. Pruckner, N.; Baumgartner, J.; Hinterbuchinger, B.; Glahn, A.; Vyssoki, S.; Vyssoki, B. Thiamine Substitution in Alcohol Use Disorder: A Narrative Review of Medical Guidelines. *Eur. Addict. Res.* **2019**, *25*, 103–110. [CrossRef] [PubMed]
108. Curtis, L.; Bernier, P.; Jeejeebhoy, K.; Allard, J.; Duerksen, D.; Gramlich, L.; Laporte, M.; Keller, H. Costs of hospital malnutrition. *Clin. Nutr.* **2017**, *36*, 1391–1396. [CrossRef] [PubMed]
109. Hercberg, S.; Galan, P.; Preziosi, P.; Bertrais, S.; Mennen, L.; Malvy, D.; Roussel, A.; Favier, A.; Briancon, S. The SU.VI.MAX Study: A randomized, placebo-controlled trial of the health effects of antioxidant vitamins and minerals. *Arch. Intern. Med.* **2004**, *164*, 2335–2342. [CrossRef]
110. Visser, J.; Labadarios, D.; Blaauw, R. Micronutrient supplementation for critically ill adults: A systematic review and meta-analysis. *Nutrition* **2011**, *27*, 745–758. [CrossRef]
111. Wieser, S.; Brunner, B.; Tzogiou, C.; Plessow, R.; Zimmermann, M.B.; Farebrother, J.; Soofi, S.; Bhatti, Z.; Ahmed, I.; Bhutta, Z.A. Societal costs of micronutrient deficiencies in 6- to 59-month-old children in Pakistan. *Food Nutr. Bull.* **2017**, *38*, 485–500. [CrossRef]
112. Berger, M.M.; Reintam-Blaser, A.; Calder, P.C.; Casaer, M.; Hiesmayr, M.; Mayer, K.; Montejo, J.C.; Pichard, P.; Preiser, J.; van Zanten, A.; et al. Monitoring nutrition in the ICU. *Clin. Nutr.* **2019**, *38*, 584–593. [CrossRef]
113. Gagnon, G.; Voirol, P.; Soguel, L.; Boulat, O.; Berger, M.M. Trace element monitoring in the ICU: Quality and economic impact of a change in sampling practice. *Clin. Nutr.* **2014**, *34*, 422–427. [CrossRef]

7

Protein Intake, Nutritional Status and Outcomes in ICU Survivors: A Single Center Cohort Study

Peter J.M. Weijs [1,2], Kris M. Mogensen [3], James D. Rawn [4] and Kenneth B. Christopher [5,*]

1 Department of Nutrition and Dietetics, Amsterdam University Medical Centers, VU University, 1081 HV Amsterdam, The Netherlands; p.weijs@vumc.nl
2 Faculty of Sports and Nutrition, Amsterdam University of Applied Sciences, 1067 SM Amsterdam, The Netherlands
3 Department of Nutrition, Brigham and Women's Hospital, Boston, MA 02115, USA; kmogensen@bwh.harvard.edu
4 Department of Surgery, Brigham and Women's Hospital, Boston, MA 02115, USA; jrawn@bwh.harvard.edu
5 The Nathan E. Hellman Memorial Laboratory, Division of Renal Medicine, Brigham and Women's Hospital, Boston, MA 02115, USA
* Correspondence: kbchristopher@bwh.harvard.edu

Abstract: Background: We hypothesized that protein delivery during hospitalization in patients who survived critical care would be associated with outcomes following hospital discharge. Methods: We studied 801 patients, age $\geq$ 18 years, who received critical care between 2004 and 2012 and survived hospitalization. All patients underwent a registered dietitian formal assessment within 48 h of ICU admission. The exposure of interest, grams of protein per kilogram body weight delivered per day, was determined from all oral, enteral and parenteral sources for up to 28 days. Adjusted odds ratios for all cause 90-day post-discharge mortality were estimated by mixed- effects logistic regression models. Results: The 90-day post-discharge mortality was 13.9%. The mean nutrition delivery days recorded was 15. In a mixed-effect logistic regression model adjusted for age, gender, race, Deyo-Charlson comorbidity index, acute organ failures, sepsis and percent energy needs met, the 90-day post-discharge mortality rate was 17% (95% CI: 6–26) lower for each 1 g/kg increase in daily protein delivery (OR = 0.83 (95% CI 0.74–0.94; p = 0.002)). Conclusions: Adult medical ICU patients with improvements in daily protein intake during hospitalization who survive hospitalization have decreased odds of mortality in the 3 months following hospital discharge.

Keywords: protein; malnutrition; critical care; mortality; outcomes; hospital readmission; ICU Survivors

---

1. Introduction

A hallmark of critical illness is muscle wasting related to a dramatic increase in muscle protein catabolism in the setting of inflammation [1]. Catabolic critical illness results in a protracted and dramatic loss of nitrogen and reduces exogenous amino acid deposition into endogenous proteins [2]. Nutritionally compromised hospitalized patients commonly present with sarcopenia [3]. Inflammation related endogenous skeletal muscle protein catabolism that can quickly progress to severe muscle atrophy [4]. In the critically ill, muscle mass loss and decreased strength are common complications [5].

Protein intake recommended for healthy adults is 0.8 g/kg per day. While the most common recommended protein intake in the critically ill is 1.5 g/kg per day [6,7], up to 1.5–2.5 g protein/kg per day may be most advantageous [7,8]. ICU patients commonly receive less than even the lowest guideline recommendation regarding adequate protein intake [7,9–11]. Recent trials [12–15] demonstrate that "calorie-supplemented, protein-deficient nutrition" [4] does not improve clinical outcomes. Early energy provision of 70–80% of measured energy expenditure appears to be associated with improved outcome [16,17]. Although the correct amount of protein to provide critically ill patients is unknown, higher than 1.2 g/kg is associated with reduced mortality in non-septic non-energy overfed ICU patients [16]. A recent large observational study suggests achieving ≥80% of prescribed protein intake in the ICU is associated with decreased mortality [18].

Although short term survival is studied in the critically ill regarding protein delivery [18], post-hospital discharge outcomes in such ICU survivors relative to protein intake and nutrition status is not known. In patients who survive critical illness, pre-existing malnutrition may be a risk factor for adverse events following hospital discharge [19]. As ICU patients with low protein delivery [18] and with malnutrition [20] have elevated in-hospital mortality, we studied the association between increases in daily protein delivery in malnourished critically ill patients would be associated with lower 90-day mortality following hospital discharge. We hypothesized that in hospital survivors who received critical care, those with higher daily protein delivery would have a lower risk of post discharge mortality and this effect would be magnified in patients with pre-existing malnutrition.

2. Materials and Methods

2.1. Data Sources

We obtained administrative and laboratory data from critically ill medical patients admitted to the Brigham and Women's Hospital (BWH), an academic medical center in Boston with 777 beds. Patient data was collected by the Research Patient Data Registry (RPDR) a clinical data warehouse for patient records at BWH that has been utilized and validated in other studies [20]. The Partners Human Research Committee Institutional Review Board granted approval for the study. Between 2004 and 2012 there were 801 unique patients ≥18 years, assigned the CPT code 99291 (critical care, first 30–74 min) [21] who had nutrition risk assessed, protein intake measured, and survived to hospital discharge.

2.2. Exposure of Interest and Comorbidities

All medical ICU patients at BWH are screened by a registered dietitian (RD). Patients at risk for malnutrition are then evaluated by an RD with a structured objective assessment. The exposure of interest, grams of protein per kilogram body weight delivered per day, was determined by an RD from all oral, enteral and parenteral sources for up to 28 days. We included all nutrition data collected by an RD in the ten days prior to ICU admission to two days following an ICU discharge. The determination of nutrition status is described in detail previously [20,22]. The RD determines the diagnosis of malnutrition based on literature [23,24], clinical judgment, and on data related to inadequate nutrient intake, muscle wasting, subcutaneous fat wasting and unintended weight loss [22]. As in our prior study, we categorized nutrition diagnoses a priori into four groups of increasing severity: malnutrition absent, at risk for malnutrition, non-specific malnutrition, or any protein-energy malnutrition [22]. Patients that meet criteria for non-specific malnutrition have risk factors for malnutrition (insufficient intake of energy, protein, and micronutrients) in addition to metabolic stress and/or obvious signs of malnutrition (muscle and/or subcutaneous fat wasting) without supporting biochemical or anthropometric data. Patients that meet criteria for protein-energy malnutrition have a combination of disease-related weight loss, obvious muscle wasting, peripheral edema, inadequate energy or protein intake and are considered underweight by percent ideal body weight [25]. Patients with absence of malnutrition are diagnosed by an RD as well-nourished and not at risk for malnutrition.Race was self-determined or determined by the patient's family or healthcare proxy. The Deyo-Charlson comorbidity index was determined using validated ICD-9 coding algorithms [26]. To define sepsis we used the presence of the ICD-9 codes 038, 785.52, 995.91, or 995.92 in the three days before ICU admission to the 7 days after ICU admission [27]. The vasopressors/inotropes covariate is the prescription of any vasopressor or inotrope in the three days prior to ICU admission to the seven days after ICU admission [20].

The number of acute organ failures was a combination of ICD-9-CM and CPT codes relating to acute organ dysfunction assigned from three days prior to ICU admission day to the 30 days after [28,29]. Intubation was defined as the presence of ICD-9 codes mechanical ventilation (96.7×) following hospital admission [30]. Acute kidney injury is the RIFLE class Injury or Failure taking place in the three days prior to ICU admission and the seven days after ICU admission [31]. Chronic kidney disease is <60 mL/min glomerular filtration rate calculated from the Modification of Diet in Renal Disease (MDRD) equation using pre-hospital or hospital admission creatinine as baseline [32]. Changes from the expected hospital length of stay (LOS) are determined by subtracting the actual LOS from the geometric mean LOS for each Diagnostic Related Grouping (DRG) a classification system for hospital cases [33]. The geometric mean LOS is the United States national mean LOS for each DRG per the Centers for Medicare & Medicaid Services [34].

2.3. End Points

Our primary outcome was all cause 90-day post-discharge mortality. Mortality status for the study cohort was obtained from the United States Social Security Administration Death Master File. Mortality determination via the Death Master File is validated in our administrative database [21]. The entire cohort had mortality status present for the year following hospital discharge. The censoring date was 15 March 2012. All patients in the cohort had at least 90-day follow-up after hospital discharge or expired before the 90-days post-hospitalization.

2.4. Power Calculations and Statistical Analysis

90-day post-discharge mortality rate was 9.6% in our prior study nutrition in critical illness [35]. From these data, we assumed that 90-day post-discharge mortality would be 6.0% greater in patients with <1.0 g/kg/day protein delivery compared to those with >1.0 g/kg/day protein delivery. With a power of 80% and an alpha error level of 5%, the sample size required for the 90-day post-discharge mortality outcome was 393 patients with >1.0 g/kg/day protein delivery and 393 patients with <1.0 g/kg/day protein delivery.

We described categorical covariates via frequency distribution, and compared variables in outcome groups with chi-square testing. We compared continuous variables across outcome groups using one-way analysis of variance (ANOVA) or the Kruskal–Wallis test. We utilized mixed-effect logistic regression models [36,37] which contain both fixed and random-effects for analysis of the association between g/kg/day protein delivery and 90-day post-discharge mortality by use of the command xtmelogit [38] in STATA 14.1 MP (College Station, TX, USA). The dates of protein delivery of individual patients were used as the random effect. We assessed the following covariates for confounding: age, gender, race, Deyo-Charlson comorbidity index, energy delivery, nutrition status, acute organ failure, sepsis, metastatic malignancy, acute kidney injury and chronic kidney disease. We selected the final model confounders by analyzing the maximum model and then conducting backward elimination of covariates with a $p > 0.10$. The final model had an independent covariance structure of the random effects; a fixed effect for age, gender, race, Deyo-Charlson comorbidity index, energy delivery, nutrition status, acute organ failure and sepsis; and gaussian-distributed random intercepts and slopes. We then used mixed-effect linear regression to analyze the association between the change in daily protein delivery and hospital LOS where random effects accounted for the dates of protein delivery within individual patients. Data visualization was performed utilizing the DistillerSR Forest Plot Generator (Evidence Partners, Ottawa, ON, Canada). p-values presented are two-tailed with $p < 0.05$ considered to be significant. We utilized STATA 14.1MP (College Station, TX, USA) for all analyses.

3. Results

Patient characteristics were stratified according to 90-day post-discharge mortality (Table 1). In our cohort the mean (SD) age was 62.3 (16.6) years, 55.3% were male and 78.9% were white. The majority of patients were assessed by an RD within 24 hours of ICU admission (median [IQR] time between ICU admission and RD assessment was 0 [1, 1] days). The mean number of recorded nutrition delivery days was 15. A total of 8735 days with protein intake were determined. The mean peak protein daily delivery was 0.32 g protein/kg. Figure 1 shows protein delivery over time in the cohort.

The mean (SD) length of hospital stay was 22.1 (15.2) days. The 30-, 90- and 365-day post-discharge mortality rates were 7.1%, 13.9%, and 24.5%, respectively. Age, race, Deyo-Charlson comorbidity index, malnutrition, the acute organ failure score and chronic kidney disease are significantly associated with 90-day post-discharge mortality (Table 1).

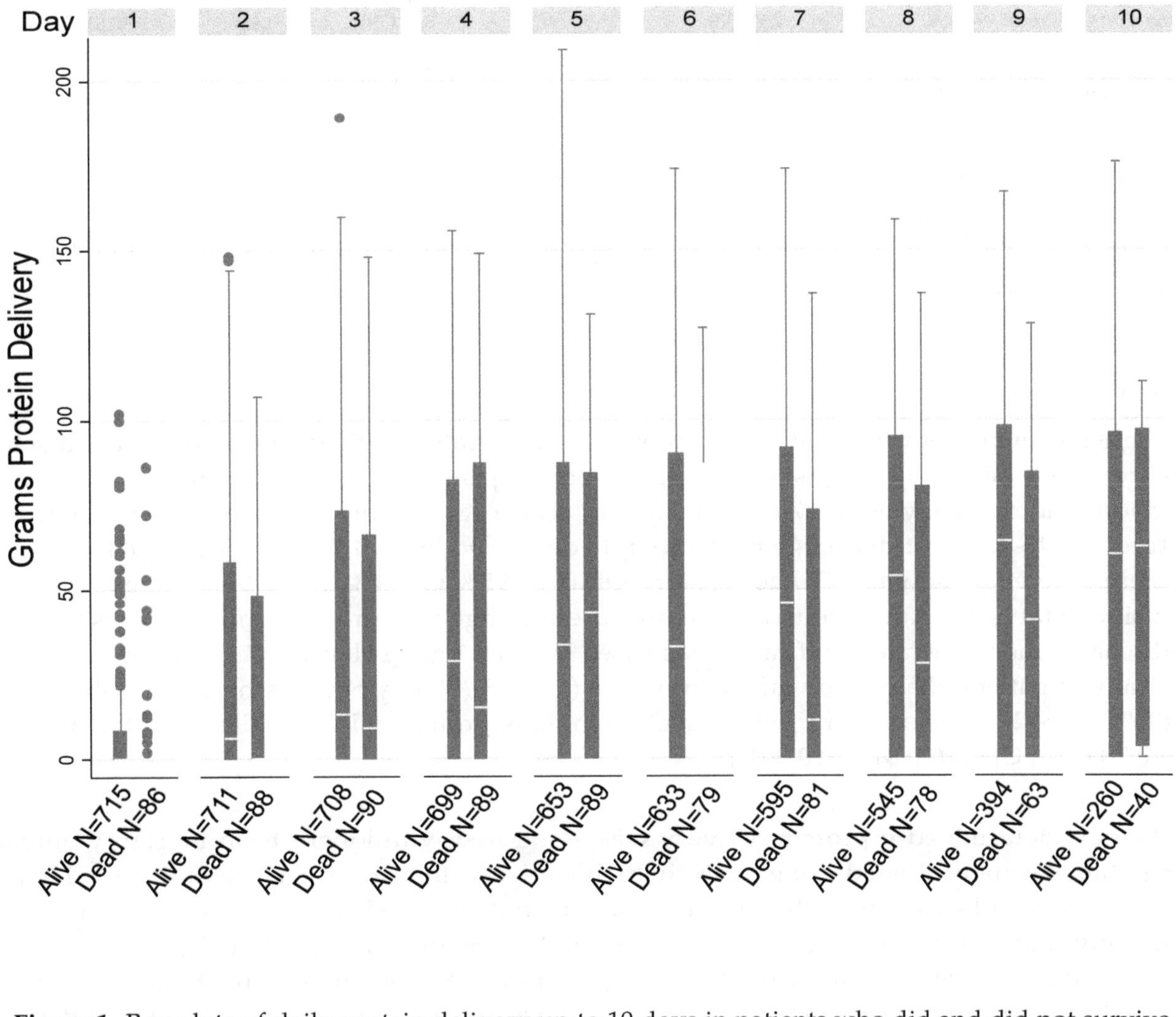

Figure 1. Box plots of daily protein delivery up to 10 days in patients who did and did not survive to 90-day post-discharge mortality, showing the median (white line), the third quartile (Q3) and first quartile (Q1) range of the data and data outliers (observations outside the 9–91 percentile range).

Table 1. Clinical and demographic characteristics of the study cohort ($n = 801$).

Characteristics	Alive at 90-Days Post-Discharge	Expired by 90-Days Post-Discharge	Total	p-Value	Unadjusted OR (95%CI) for 90-Day Post-Discharge Mortality
	690	111	801		
Age-Mean ± SD	61.1 ± 16.7	69.8 ± 14	62.3 ± 16.6	<0.001 *	1.04 (1.02, 1.05)
Male Gender-No. (%)	384 (56)	58 (52)	442 (55)	0.50	0.87 (0.58, 1.30)
Non-White Race-No. (%)	154 (22)	15 (14)	169 (21)	0.035	0.54 (0.31, 0.96)
Deyo-Charlson Index-No. (%)				0.003	
0	182 (26.38)	15 (13.39)	197 (24.56)		1.00 (Referent)
1–2	440 (63.77)	75 (66.96)	515 (64.21)		2.07 (1.16, 3.70)
≥3	68 (9.86)	22 (19.64)	90 (11.22)		3.93 (1.92, 8.01)
Acute Organ Failures-No. (%)				0.030	
0	86 (12)	16 (14)	102 (13)		1.00 (Referent)
1	217 (31)	29 (26)	246 (31)		0.72 (0.37, 1.39)
2	192 (28)	26 (23)	218 (27)		0.73 (0.37, 1.43)
3	136 (20)	20 (18)	156 (19)		0.79 (0.39, 1.61)
≥4	59 (9)	20 (18)	79 (10)		1.82 (0.87, 3.80)
Sepsis-No. (%)	138 (20)	28 (25)	166 (21)	0.21	1.35 (0.85, 2.15)
Intubation-No. (%)	400 (58)	60 (54)	460 (57)	0.44	0.85 (0.57, 1.28)
Acute Organ Failure Score-Mean ± SD	10.2 ± 4.4	11.4 ± 4.6	10.4 ± 4.5	0.0082 *	1.06 (1.02, 1.11)
Vasopressors/Inotropes-No. (%)	264 (38)	51 (46)	315 (39)	0.12	1.37 (0.92, 2.05)
Metastatic Malignancy-No. (%)	296 (43)	58 (52)	354 (44)	0.066	1.46 (0.97, 2.18)
Acute Kidney Injury-No. (%) †	55 (10)	6 (7)	61 (10)	0.381	0.68 (0.28, 1.63)
Chronic Kidney Disease-No. (%) ††	169 (31)	42 (49)	211 (33)	0.001	1.23 (1.06, 1.41)
Malnutrition-No. (%)				0.035	
At Risk for Malnutrition	291 (43)	33 (30)	324 (41)		1.00 (Referent)
Non-Specific Malnutrition	343 (51)	65 (60)	408 (52)		1.67 (1.07, 2.61)
Protein-Energy Malnutrition	45 (7)	11 (10)	56 (7)		2.16 (1.02, 4.57)

Data presented as n (%) unless otherwise indicated. p values determined by chi-square unless designated by (*) then p value determined by ANOVA. † Data available to determine Acute Kidney Injury in 638 patients. †† Data available to determine Chronic Kidney Disease was present in 638 patients.

Primary Outcome

Higher protein delivery in ICU survivors was associated with lower 90-day post-discharge mortality. In our mixed-effect logistic regression model adjusted for age, gender, race, Deyo-Charlson comorbidity index, energy delivery, nutrition status, acute organ failure, sepsis and the random-effects structure, the 90-day post-discharge mortality rate decreased by 18% for each 1 g/kg/day elevation in protein delivery following ICU admission (OR 0.82, 95% CI 0.73–0.92). Following stratification for nutrition status, the same multivariable mixed-effect logistic regression model shows the 90-day post-discharge mortality rate significantly decreased for each 1 g/kg elevation in daily protein delivery. Specifically, in patients diagnosed with malnutrition ($n = 473$), 90-day post-discharge mortality rate was 30% (95% CI: 6–26) less for each 1 g/kg elevation in daily protein delivery following ICU admission (OR = 0.70 (95% CI 0.61–0.81; $p < 0.001$)).

We next determined if protein delivery was associated with longer term mortality outcomes. When patients were evaluated using a multivariable mixed-effect logistic regression model with the same covariates and structure as the primary outcome model, 180-day post-discharge mortality was significantly reduced for each 1 g/kg elevation in daily protein delivery (OR 0.74, 95% CI 0.67–0.83; $p < 0.001$). When patients were evaluated using the multivariable mixed-effect logistic regression model with the same covariates and structure as the primary outcome model, the 365- and 720-day post-discharge mortality rate was significantly reduced for each 1 g/kg elevation in daily protein delivery (OR 0.76, 95% CI 0.69–0.83; $p < 0.001$), (OR 0.77, 95% CI 0.71–0.84; $p < 0.001$) respectively (Table 2, Figure 2). All estimates are for each 1 g/kg/day increase in protein delivery.

Table 2. Associations between Protein Delivery and post-hospital mortality outcomes.

Outcome	OR	95% CI	p-Value	Association for Each 1 g/kg/Day Increase in Protein Delivery
90-day post-discharge Mortality				
Full Cohort (n = 801)	0.83	0.74–0.94	0.002	17% decrease odds of death
Malnutrition (n = 473)	0.70	0.61–0.81	<0.001	30% decrease odds of death
180-day post-discharge Mortality				
Full Cohort (n = 801)	0.74	0.67–0.83	<0.001	26% decrease odds of death
365-day post-discharge Mortality				
Full Cohort (n = 801)	0.76	0.69–0.83	<0.001	24% decrease odds of death
720-day post-discharge Mortality				
Full Cohort (n = 801)	0.77	0.71–0.84	<0.001	23% decrease odds of death

All estimates were produced via a mixed-effect logistic regression model adjusted for age, gender, race, Deyo-Charlson comorbidity index, energy delivery, nutrition status, acute organ failure, sepsis and the random-effects structure.

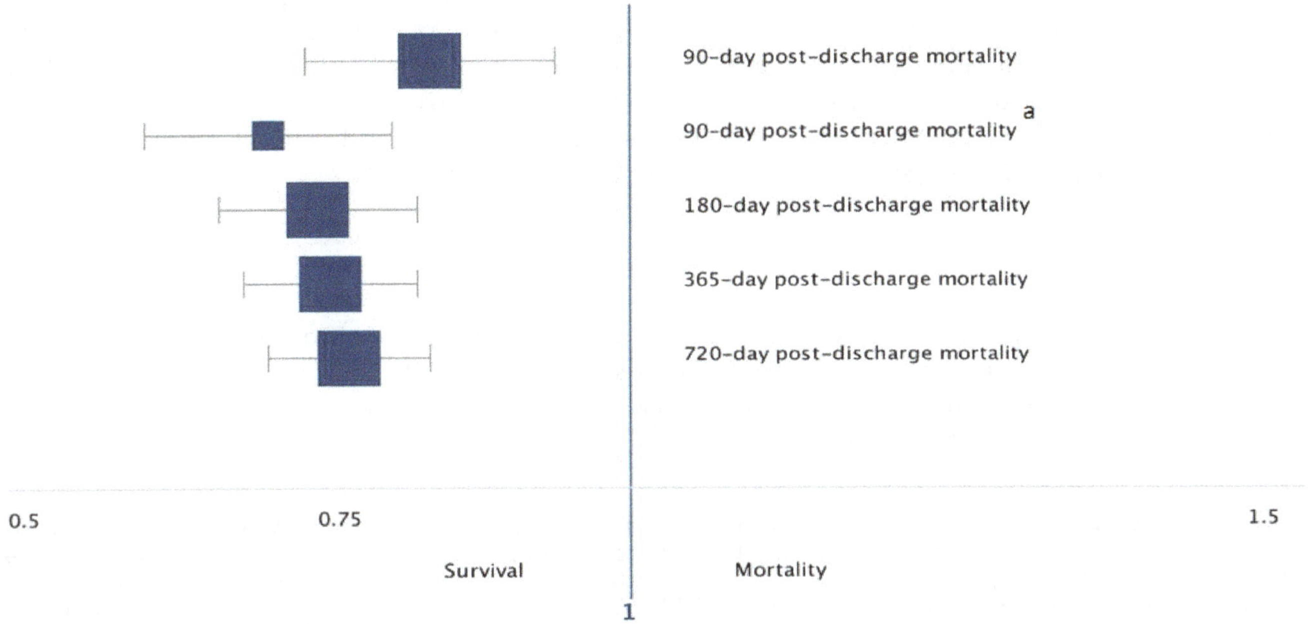

Figure 2. Forest plot of post-discharge mortality associated for each 1 g/kg/day increase in protein delivery in our study cohort. Odds ratios with corresponding 95% CIs shown of the individual outcomes under study. [a] Restricted to patients diagnosed with Malnutrition.

Finally we examined the association between protein delivery and hospital length of stay. In a mixed-effect linear regression model adjusted for age, gender, race, Deyo-Charlson comorbidity index, energy delivery, nutrition status, acute organ failure, sepsis and the random-effects structure, the actual hospital length of stay (LOS) was reduced by 0.87 days (95% CI −1.7 to −0.10) compared with the average LOS for the DRG for each 1 g/kg/day increase in protein delivery ($p = 0.028$).

4. Discussion

In our study, we examined the association between protein delivery in critical illness survivors and post-hospital discharge outcomes. We demonstrate that improvement in daily protein delivery is associated with a significant decrease in the odds of post-discharge hospital mortality. We also show that patients with improved daily protein delivery have decreased hospital length of stay.

Long-term morbidity and mortality are substantial problems in ICU survivors [39]. Adverse events following discharge from an ICU admission are known to include comorbidity, illness severity and organ failures [40]. In critical illness survivors, the risk factors for outside hospital adverse events are not well known. Our results show an association between higher daily protein delivery during hospitalization and improved post-discharge mortality in critical illness survivors. While our observational study cannot be interpreted as causal, the protein delivery-post-discharge outcome association has biologic plausibility.

Our study may have limitations due to its observational design. Causality is limited and as such our observations should be considered hypothesis generating. As protein intake in our cohort is only collected in patients considered to be at least at risk for malnutrition, ascertainment bias may be present. Unmeasured variables may influence outcomes following hospitalization independent of protein delivery, which can result in bias. We are unable to adjust for gut failure which associated with lower nutrition tolerance, lower protein intake and contributes to adverse outcomes [41]. Though ICD-9 code assignment data is collected from individual provider encounters, determination of covariates via ICD-9 codes may not completely capture the true incidence or prevalence. Finally, residual confounding may remain despite multivariable adjustment which may contribute to observed estimates.

Our study has several strengths. We utilize mixed-effects models to incorporate multiple measures and sources of protein intake over a total of 8735 days which allow for more complete information to be captured in parameter estimations. Mixed-effects models are ideal for such longitudinal data because each patient may have an unequal number of repeated measures. Additionally, a highly trained RD utilized weight loss history, clinical assessment, anthropometric metrics and protein intake to make an in person assessment of nutritional risk and daily protein delivery. Finally, the Master Death File is shown to capture post discharge mortality in our cohort accurately [21].

5. Conclusions

Our data show that in critically ill patients who survive hospitalization, higher daily protein delivery during hospitalization is associated with decreased mortality following hospital discharge. Increasing protein delivery following the acute phase of illness may be a strategy to assist with critical illness recovery and longer term outcomes.

Author Contributions: Conceptualization, P.J.M.W. and K.B.C.; Methodology, P.J.M.W. and K.B.C.; Software, K.B.C.; Validation, K.B.C.; Formal Analysis, K.B.C.; Investigation, P.J.M.W., K.M.M., and K.B.C.; Resources, K.M.M., J.D.R., and K.B.C.; Data Curation, J.D.R., and K.B.C.; Writing—Original Draft Preparation, P.J.M.W., K.M.M., and K.B.C.; Writing—Review & Editing, P.J.M.W., K.M.M., J.D.R., and K.B.C.; Supervision, K.B.C.; Project Administration, K.B.C.; Funding Acquisition, K.B.C.

Acknowledgments: This manuscript is dedicated to the memory of our dear friend and colleague Nathan Edward Hellman. The authors thank Shawn Murphy and Henry Chueh and the Partners Health Care Research Patient Data Registry group for facilitating use of their database.

References

1. Gabay, C.; Kushner, I. Acute-phase proteins and other systemic responses to inflammation. *N. Engl. J. Med.* **1999**, *340*, 448–454. [CrossRef] [PubMed]
2. Hoffer, L.J.; Bistrian, B.R. Nutrition in critical illness: A current conundrum. *F1000Research* **2016**, *5*, 2531. [CrossRef] [PubMed]
3. Cerri, A.P.; Bellelli, G.; Mazzone, A.; Pittella, F.; Landi, F.; Zambon, A.; Annoni, G. Sarcopenia and malnutrition in acutely ill hospitalized elderly: Prevalence and outcomes. *Clin. Nutr.* **2015**, *34*, 745–751. [CrossRef] [PubMed]
4. Hoffer, L.J. Protein requirement in critical illness. *Appl. Physiol. Nutr. Metab.* **2016**, *41*, 573–576. [CrossRef] [PubMed]

5. Batt, J.; dos Santos, C.C.; Cameron, J.I.; Herridge, M.S. Intensive care unit-acquired weakness: Clinical phenotypes and molecular mechanisms. *Am. J. Respir. Crit. Care Med.* **2013**, *187*, 238–246. [CrossRef] [PubMed]
6. Ziegler, T.R. Parenteral nutrition in the critically ill patient. *N. Engl. J. Med.* **2009**, *361*, 1088–1097. [CrossRef] [PubMed]
7. Hoffer, L.J.; Bistrian, B.R. Why critically ill patients are protein deprived. *JPEN J. Parenter. Enter. Nutr.* **2013**, *37*, 300–309. [CrossRef]
8. Hoffer, L.J.; Bistrian, B.R. What is the best nutritional support for critically ill patients? *Hepatobiliary Surg. Nutr.* **2014**, *3*, 172–174. [CrossRef]
9. Heyland, D.K. Should We PERMIT Systematic Underfeeding in All Intensive Care Unit Patients? Integrating the Results of the PERMIT Study in Our Clinical Practice Guidelines. *JPEN J. Parenter. Enter. Nutr.* **2016**, *40*, 156–158. [CrossRef]
10. Alberda, C.; Gramlich, L.; Jones, N.; Jeejeebhoy, K.; Day, A.G.; Dhaliwal, R.; Heyland, D.K. The relationship between nutritional intake and clinical outcomes in critically ill patients: Results of an international multicenter observational study. *Intensive Care Med* **2009**, *35*, 1728–1737. [CrossRef]
11. Heyland, D.K.; Dhaliwal, R.; Wang, M.; Day, A.G. The prevalence of iatrogenic underfeeding in the nutritionally 'at-risk' critically ill patient: Results of an international, multicenter, prospective study. *Clin. Nutr.* **2015**, *34*, 659–666. [CrossRef] [PubMed]
12. Doig, G.S.; Simpson, F.; Sweetman, E.A.; Finfer, S.R.; Cooper, D.J.; Heighes, P.T.; Davies, A.R.; O'Leary, M.; Solano, T.; Peake, S.; et al. Early parenteral nutrition in critically ill patients with short-term relative contraindications to early enteral nutrition: A randomized controlled trial. *JAMA* **2013**, *309*, 2130–2138. [CrossRef] [PubMed]
13. Casaer, M.P.; Mesotten, D.; Hermans, G.; Wouters, P.J.; Schetz, M.; Meyfroidt, G.; Van Cromphaut, S.; Ingels, C.; Meersseman, P.; Muller, J.; et al. Early versus late parenteral nutrition in critically ill adults. *N. Engl. J. Med.* **2011**, *365*, 506–517. [CrossRef] [PubMed]
14. Heidegger, C.P.; Berger, M.M.; Graf, S.; Zingg, W.; Darmon, P.; Costanza, M.C.; Thibault, R.; Pichard, C. Optimisation of energy provision with supplemental parenteral nutrition in critically ill patients: A randomised controlled clinical trial. *Lancet* **2013**, *381*, 385–393. [CrossRef]
15. Singer, P.; Anbar, R.; Cohen, J.; Shapiro, H.; Shalita-Chesner, M.; Lev, S.; Grozovski, E.; Theilla, M.; Frishman, S.; Madar, Z. The tight calorie control study (TICACOS): A prospective, randomized, controlled pilot study of nutritional support in critically ill patients. *Intensive Care Med.* **2011**, *37*, 601–609. [CrossRef] [PubMed]
16. Weijs, P.J.; Looijaard, W.G.; Beishuizen, A.; Girbes, A.R.; Oudemans-van Straaten, H.M. Early high protein intake is associated with low mortality and energy overfeeding with high mortality in non-septic mechanically ventilated critically ill patients. *Crit. Care* **2014**, *18*, 701. [CrossRef]
17. Zusman, O.; Theilla, M.; Cohen, J.; Kagan, I.; Bendavid, I.; Singer, P. Resting energy expenditure, calorie and protein consumption in critically ill patients: A retrospective cohort study. *Crit. Care* **2016**, *20*, 367. [CrossRef]
18. Nicolo, M.; Heyland, D.K.; Chittams, J.; Sammarco, T.; Compher, C. Clinical Outcomes Related to Protein Delivery in a Critically Ill Population: A Multicenter, Multinational Observation Study. *JPEN J. Parenter. Enter. Nutr.* **2016**, *40*, 45–51. [CrossRef]
19. Weijs, P.J.; Looijaard, W.G.; Dekker, I.M.; Stapel, S.N.; Girbes, A.R.; Oudemans-van Straaten, H.M.; Beishuizen, A. Low skeletal muscle area is a risk factor for mortality in mechanically ventilated critically ill patients. *Crit. Care* **2014**, *18*, R12. [CrossRef]
20. Mogensen, K.M.; Robinson, M.K.; Casey, J.D.; Gunasekera, N.S.; Moromizato, T.; Rawn, J.D.; Christopher, K.B. Nutritional Status and Mortality in the Critically Ill. *Crit. Care Med.* **2015**, *43*, 2605–2615. [CrossRef]
21. Zager, S.; Mendu, M.L.; Chang, D.; Bazick, H.S.; Braun, A.B.; Gibbons, F.K.; Christopher, K.B. Neighborhood poverty rate and mortality in patients receiving critical care in the academic medical center setting. *Chest* **2011**, *139*, 1368–1379. [CrossRef] [PubMed]
22. Robinson, M.K.; Mogensen, K.M.; Casey, J.D.; McKane, C.K.; Moromizato, T.; Rawn, J.D.; Christopher, K.B. The relationship among obesity, nutritional status, and mortality in the critically ill*. *Crit. Care Med.* **2015**, *43*, 87–100. [CrossRef] [PubMed]
23. Swails, W.S.; Samour, P.Q.; Babineau, T.J.; Bistrian, B.R. A proposed revision of current ICD-9-CM malnutrition code definitions. *J. Am. Diet. Assoc.* **1996**, *96*, 370–373. [CrossRef]

24. Blackburn, G.L.; Bistrian, B.R.; Maini, B.S.; Schlamm, H.T.; Smith, M.F. Nutritional and metabolic assessment of the hospitalized patient. *JPEN J. Parenter. Enter. Nutr.* **1977**, *1*, 11–22. [CrossRef] [PubMed]
25. Simopoulos, A.P. Obesity and body weight standards. *Annu. Rev. Public Health* **1986**, *7*, 481–492. [CrossRef] [PubMed]
26. Quan, H.; Sundararajan, V.; Halfon, P.; Fong, A.; Burnand, B.; Luthi, J.C.; Saunders, L.D.; Beck, C.A.; Feasby, T.E.; Ghali, W.A. Coding algorithms for defining comorbidities in ICD-9-CM and ICD-10 administrative data. *Med. Care* **2005**, *43*, 1130–1139. [CrossRef]
27. Liu, V.; Escobar, G.J.; Greene, J.D.; Soule, J.; Whippy, A.; Angus, D.C.; Iwashyna, T.J. Hospital deaths in patients with sepsis from 2 independent cohorts. *JAMA* **2014**, *312*, 90–92. [CrossRef]
28. Martin, G.S.; Mannino, D.M.; Eaton, S.; Moss, M. The epidemiology of sepsis in the United States from 1979 through 2000. *N. Engl. J. Med.* **2003**, *348*, 1546–1554. [CrossRef]
29. McMahon, G.M.; Mendu, M.L.; Gibbons, F.K.; Christopher, K.B. Association between hyperkalemia at critical care initiation and mortality. *Intensive Care Med.* **2012**, *38*, 1834–1842. [CrossRef]
30. Thickett, D.R.; Moromizato, T.; Litonjua, A.A.; Amrein, K.; Quraishi, S.A.; Lee-Sarwar, K.A.; Mogensen, K.M.; Purtle, S.W.; Gibbons, F.K.; Camargo, C.A., Jr.; et al. Association between prehospital vitamin D status and incident acute respiratory failure in critically ill patients: A retrospective cohort study. *BMJ Open Respir. Res.* **2015**, *2*, e000074. [CrossRef]
31. Braun, A.B.; Litonjua, A.A.; Moromizato, T.; Gibbons, F.K.; Giovannucci, E.; Christopher, K.B. Association of low serum 25-hydroxyvitamin D levels and acute kidney injury in the critically ill*. *Crit. Care Med.* **2012**, *40*, 3170–3179. [CrossRef] [PubMed]
32. Levey, A.S.; Bosch, J.P.; Lewis, J.B.; Greene, T.; Rogers, N.; Roth, D. A more accurate method to estimate glomerular filtration rate from serum creatinine: A new prediction equation. Modification of Diet in Renal Disease Study Group. *Ann. Intern. Med.* **1999**, *130*, 461–470. [CrossRef] [PubMed]
33. Rapoport, J.; Gehlbach, S.; Lemeshow, S.; Teres, D. Resource utilization among intensive care patients. Managed care vs traditional insurance. *Arch. Intern. Med.* **1992**, *152*, 2207–2212. [CrossRef] [PubMed]
34. Amrein, K.; Litonjua, A.A.; Moromizato, T.; Quraishi, S.A.; Gibbons, F.K.; Pieber, T.R.; Camargo, C.A., Jr.; Giovannucci, E.; Christopher, K.B. Increases in pre-hospitalization serum 25(OH)D concentrations are associated with improved 30-day mortality after hospital admission: A cohort study. *Clin. Nutr.* **2016**, *35*, 514–521. [CrossRef] [PubMed]
35. Mogensen, K.M.; Horkan, C.M.; Purtle, S.W.; Moromizato, T.; Rawn, J.D.; Robinson, M.K.; Christopher, K.B. Malnutrition, Critical Illness Survivors, and Postdischarge Outcomes: A Cohort Study. *JPEN J. Parenter. Enter. Nutr.* **2017**, *42*, 557–565. [CrossRef] [PubMed]
36. Hedeker, D. A mixed-effects multinomial logistic regression model. *Stat. Med.* **2003**, *22*, 1433–1446. [CrossRef]
37. Hartzel, J.; Agresti, A.; Caffo, B. Multinomial logit random effects models. *Stat. Model.* **2001**, *1*, 81–102. [CrossRef]
38. Nicholson, B.D.; Shinkins, B.; Pathiraja, I.; Roberts, N.W.; James, T.J.; Mallett, S.; Perera, R.; Primrose, J.N.; Mant, D. Blood CEA levels for detecting recurrent colorectal cancer. *Cochrane Database Syst. Rev.* **2015**, CD011134. [CrossRef]
39. Desai, S.V.; Law, T.J.; Needham, D.M. Long-term complications of critical care. *Crit. Care Med.* **2011**, *39*, 371–379. [CrossRef]
40. Horkan, C.M.; Purtle, S.W.; Mendu, M.L.; Moromizato, T.; Gibbons, F.K.; Christopher, K.B. The association of acute kidney injury in the critically ill and postdischarge outcomes: A cohort study. *Crit. Care Med.* **2015**, *43*, 354–364. [CrossRef]
41. Puleo, F.; Arvanitakis, M.; Van Gossum, A.; Preiser, J.C. Gut failure in the ICU. *Semin. Respir. Crit. Care Med.* **2011**, *32*, 626–638. [CrossRef] [PubMed]

8

Nutritional Challenges in Patients with Advanced Liver Cirrhosis

Jessica Stirnimann [1] and Guido Stirnimann [2,*]

1 Division of Diabetology, Endocrinology, Nutritional Medicine and Metabolism, University Hospital Inselspital and University of Bern, 3010 Bern, Switzerland; jessica.stirnimann@insel.ch

2 University Clinic for Visceral Surgery and Medicine, University Hospital Inselspital and University of Bern, 3010 Bern, Switzerland

* Correspondence: guido.stirnimann@dbmr.unibe.ch or guido.stirnimann@insel.ch

Abstract: Patients with advanced liver cirrhosis are at risk of malnutrition and nutrition-associated complications. Significant ascites, a frequent finding in these patients, has an especially negative impact on oral nutrition. A negative caloric and protein balance can further deteriorate the already impaired synthetic function of the cirrhotic liver. An important factor in this situation is the diminished capacity of glycogen production and storage in the cirrhotic liver and, consequently, a reduced tolerability for fasting episodes. These episodes are frequently observed in hospitalized patients, e.g., while waiting for investigations, interventions or surgery. A comprehensive work-up of patients with advanced liver cirrhosis should include not only a thorough assessment regarding nutritional deficits, but also a muscularity analysis to identify patients with sarcopenia. The overall nutritional treatment goal is to cover caloric deficits and assure a sufficiently high protein intake. Furthermore, vitamin and micronutrient deficiencies should be identified and corrective measures implemented where required. Ideally, optimal nutrition management can not only prevent the progression of malnutrition and sarcopenia in patients with advanced liver cirrhosis, but positively influence the evolution of the liver disease.

Keywords: cirrhosis; ascites; sarcopenia; sarcopenic obesity; nutrition; vitamins; micronutrients

---

1. Introduction

Liver cirrhosis is a common end stage of several liver diseases. The most prevalent aetiologies are chronic hepatitis B virus (HBV) and hepatitis C virus (HCV) infection, alcoholism, and nonalcoholic steatohepatitis [1]. As, with the introduction of direct acting antiviral therapy, HCV and HCV-related complications are rapidly declining, nonalcoholic steatohepatitis is now a growing burden of cirrhosis.

In patients with advanced liver cirrhosis, malnutrition and sarcopenia are not only related to alterations in the nutritional behavior, but also to changes in the GI-tract, the liver and the muscle. An increased protein loss, via the GI-tract, the kidneys or frequent paracenteses, can further aggravate the situation.

Patients with chronic advanced liver disease suffer from increased fatigue, nausea, bloating, and anorexia, which can result in a reduced food intake. In the presence of clinically relevant ascites, mechanical effects may further compromise nutrition by compression of the stomach, resulting in early satiety [2]. Inadequate appetite regulation and energy expenditure may be related to an elevation in bound leptin in patients with cirrhosis. Whereas free leptin correlates with fat mass in cirrhotic patients as well as in healthy controls, bound leptin was positively correlated with energy expenditure in patients with cirrhosis [3]. Increased serum concentrations of bound leptin could be associated with wasting in patients with liver cirrhosis, as has been shown in patients with symptomatic human immunodeficiency virus [4]. Furthermore, leptin is also a known contributor to fibrinogenesis in chronic liver disease [5]. Small bowel transit time is correlated with the severity of liver disease, and patients with decompensated cirrhosis or spontaneous bacterial peritonitis in the context of ascites have a slower transit time [6].

In patients with alcoholic cirrhosis, anorexia and irregular unbalanced nutrition uptake are common, and energy supply may be achieved through the consumption of alcohol rather than by a balanced food intake [7]. A low socioeconomic status is an additional risk factor for poor nutrition [2].

Dietary restrictions, e.g., an untasty, sodium-reduced diet, inadequate protein supply, or taste alterations, may further compromise the nutrition of patients with cirrhosis [2].

For the assessment of malnutrition and sarcopenia different tools, comprising clinical and laboratory parameters, physical assessments, image analysis and anthropometric measurements, are available. Clinical bedside assessments are easy to perform and inexpensive, but may lack precision in patients with advanced cirrhosis, especially if significant ascites is present. In contrast, muscularity analysis on cross-sectional images is precise but technically demanding and may require special software tools and trained personnel.

2. Comprehensive Assessment of Patients with Advanced Liver Cirrhosis

2.1. Malnutrition

To assess the nutritional status of patients, the subjective global assessment (SGA) is a well-established and widely used bedside tool. Patients are assigned to one of the three different risk categories: A (well nourished), B (mildly/moderately malnourished), and C (severely malnourished), based on five items that can be derived from the patient's history and three items that are based on clinical examinations. SGA is an independent predictor of outcome in liver transplant recipients [8,9]. However, especially in decompensated patients with ascites or peripheral fluid accumulation, the performance of SGA is limited [10].

2.2. Liver Function

Unfortunately, a simple test to assess the main dimensions of liver function (synthetic function, metabolic capacity and excretion function) does not exist. In the context of malnutrition, the synthetic function of the liver is of special interest. Albumin levels are frequently tested in patients with liver disease, and albumin is part of the widely used Child–Pugh–Turcotte (CPT) score to determine the stage of liver disease [11]. However, albumin levels do not solely reflect endogenous albumin production, but may also be low due to infection/inflammation, or an increased albumin loss or high in the case of albumin substitution, for instance, in patients that frequently require large volume paracenteses. In recent years, functional aspects, like the binding of lipopolisaccharides or other bacterial products and qualitative alterations (oxidation and glycation) of albumin, have been investigated in more detail. However, to date, it is not clear what the impact of these findings is [12].

Prealbumin (transthyretin) is an alternative parameter to assess the synthetic function in patients with liver cirrhosis. Prealbumin plasma levels decrease progressively from CPT stage A to C and correlate with galactose elimination capacity, a test to assess functional liver capacity [13]. A major advantage of this parameter compared to albumin is the fact that it is not influenced by exogenous albumin administration, a frequent treatment in patients with decompensated liver cirrhosis. The addition of prealbumin to the Model for End-stage Liver Disease (MELD) score improved outcome prediction in patients with decompensated liver cirrhosis [14], and prealbumin was a predictive factor regarding postoperative liver insufficiency and survival in CPT A patients with hepatocellular carcinoma-related surgery [15–17]. In clinical practice, prealbumin is an inexpensive and easy to determine functional liver parameter that helps to assess the synthetic liver function in cirrhotic patients. However, compared to albumin, the available evidence is limited in patients with liver cirrhosis.

Prothrombin time (PT) is the second parameter reflecting synthetic liver function that is an integral part of the CPT score (all coagulation factors, with the exception of factor VIII, are produced in the liver). However, production of coagulation factors may be preserved even in advanced cirrhosis and patients may still present with a normal or only slightly decreased PT in this situation. In contrast, patients with acute liver failure frequently have markedly decreased PT values.

2.3. Sarcopenia

Although sarcopenia is usually a visual diagnosis in malnourished patients with cirrhosis, diagnosis may be more challenging in obese patients, e.g., in patients with non-alcoholic fatty liver disease (NAFLD). To obtain an objective measure of sarcopenia, a quantitative analysis of the patient's muscularity should be performed.

The most-validated method to date is the muscle assessment on cross-sectional CT or MR images. Several methods have been proposed, e.g., area of the psoas muscle at the level of the 4th lumbar vertebra without and with normalization by height [18,19], the skeletal muscles index at the level of the 3rd lumbar vertebra (SMI) [19,20], or transversal psoas thickness at the level of the umbilicus [21]. Importantly, by using the SMI with the gender specific cut-offs (42 cm^2/m^2 for women and 50 cm^2/m^2 for men), muscle wasting was not limited to underweight patients, but could be detected in cirrhotic patients with a normal or even elevated BMI [20]. Regarding mortality risk in patients with cirrhosis, the skeletal muscle index (SMI) seems to be superior to the psoas index, especially in men with cirrhosis [22].

Special attention is required for patients with advanced liver cirrhosis who have a BMI >25 kg/m^2. Sarcopenia in obese patients is frequently overlooked, since it is less expected than in underweight or normal-weight patients with malnutrition. It is important to note that sarcopenic obesity, as well as myosteatosis, characterized by an increased proportion of muscular fat, are independent risk factors regarding long-term mortality [23].

Apart from simple measurements, like psoas muscle diameter, the assessment of cross-sectional image analysis is technically demanding and may require special image analysis software and trained personnel. Therefore, image analysis is mainly used in the context of clinical research projects.

In clinical practice, bio impedance analysis (BIA), dual-energy X-ray absorptiometry (DEXA) and anthropometric measurements are easier to perform. However, DEXA and BIA results may be altered in patients with significant ascites and general fluid overload, limiting their use in decompensated patients [24]. Restricting DEXA to the upper limb lean mass, and therefore excluding the body parts that are most prone to fluid overload, resulted in a good sarcopenia-related prediction of mortality in men with advanced cirrhosis [25]. Mid-arm muscle circumference (MAMC) measurement is easy to perform, but its relevance in clinical practice is limited [26].

Unfortunately, the most frequently used scores in patients with cirrhosis, CPT and MELD score [27], do not contain specific information about the nutritional status of a given patient. Therefore, new scores have been developed and evaluated, with a focus on outcome, in patients awaiting liver transplantation. The MELD-psoas score includes transversal psoas muscle thickness normalized by height at the level of the umbilicus. This score was significantly associated with mortality, especially in patients with refractory ascites [21].

The addition of the skeletal muscle index (SMI), as a measure of sarcopenia, to the MELD score resulted in an improved prediction of mortality in patients with cirrhosis [20,28]. Especially in low MELD patients on a liver transplant list, the inclusion of sarcopenia resulted in a better association with mortality [21].

2.4. Deficiencies of Vitamins and Micronutrients

2.4.1. Vitamin D

Vitamin D is synthesized in the skin from 7-dehydrocholesterol. An alternative source is food-derived vitamin D that is absorbed in the gastrointestinal tract with the help of bile acids. Vitamin D subsequently undergoes two hydroxylation steps, 25-hydroxylation in the liver and 1α-hydroxylation in the kidney. Whereas vitamin D is considered biologically inactive, 25-hydroxy(OH)-vitamin D is the main circulating metabolite. Conversion to 1,25-dihydroxy-vitamin D in the kidney increases the affinity for the vitamin D receptor (VDR).

The main purpose of vitamin D is the regulation of mineral and bone homeostasis. However, several other functions in different tissues (kidney, intestine, skin, immune cells and non-parenchymal hepatic cells) are known, too [29].

Vitamin D deficiency is common in liver cirrhosis. Whereas liver function correlates with vitamin D deficiency, aetiology of the liver disease seems to be of minor importance [30,31]. Decreased vitamin D levels are associated with an unfavorable outcome in patients with chronic advanced liver disease. The relative risk for hepatic decompensation and for mortality was 6.37 (95% confidence interval (CI) 1.75–23.2) and 4.31 (95% CI 1.38–13.5), respectively, for patients in the lowest OH-vitamin D level group, compared to patients in the highest OH-vitamin D level group [31].

2.4.2. Vitamin A

The liver is the organ where most (>90%) of the body vitamin A is stored. Plasma contains only a fraction (1%) of the total amount of vitamin A. While normal and high vitamin A concentrations do not show a linear correlation with liver vitamin A reserves, low retinol plasma levels do correlate [32]. In patients with chronic liver disease, vitamin A levels are frequently reduced, and the concentration progressively decreases with the progression of liver disease. Importantly, patients with hepatocellular carcinoma have the lowest levels, independent of the stage of liver disease [33]. While, in patients with CPT A cirrhosis, severe deficiency was absent, 52.8% of Child–Pugh C patients presented with a severe vitamin A deficiency (<0.35 μmol/L) [34]. It is important to note that chronic high dose supplementation over a period of several years has been associated with relevant liver damage [35].

2.4.3. Zinc

Zinc deficiency is a common finding in patients with advanced chronic liver disease. Reasons for low zinc levels are inadequate dietary intake and an increased zinc loss in the urine that is related to severe muscle catabolism, diuretic therapy in patients with cirrhosis and ascites [36], alcohol-induced impaired absorption, and changes in the protein and amino acid metabolism. Furthermore, endotoxins and cytokines (IL6) may play a role [37].

Since the liver is the key organ in the metabolism of zinc, liver disease can affect zinc levels and, vice versa, zinc deficiency can affect the liver. Reduced zinc levels can have a negative impact on several liver functions and impair the regeneration capacity of the liver. However, independent of the stage of cirrhosis, zinc stores in in liver, bone and muscle can be replenished over the course of six or more months [37]. In patients with cirrhosis, supplementation of zinc in combination with branched-chain amino acids (BCAA) for six months with [38] and without [39] hepatic encephalopathy has demonstrated a positive effect on blood ammonia levels. However, an increase in albumin could be demonstrated only in one of the two studies [38].

2.4.4. Selenium

The essential micronutrient selenium is incorporated in at least 25 selenoproteins. Deficiency of selenium can be found in some patients with advanced chronic liver disease. In addition to a nutritional deficit, reduced selenium levels may reflect an impaired metabolism of selenomethionine to selenide in the liver. In a study by Burk et al., selenoprotein P, a protein that is mainly formed in the liver and that transports selenium to extrahepatic tissues, was reduced in parallel with the severity of the liver disease [40].

2.5. Bone Disease

Osteopenia and osteoporosis are common findings in patients with cirrhosis, with a prevalence of up to 68% for osteopenia and a range from 11% to 55% for osteoporosis [41]. Consequently, fractures are common in patients with chronic liver disease, and occur in up to 40% of patients with cirrhosis [42].

The pathophysiology is complex and, in addition to an altered vitamin D and calcium metabolism, other factors may be important. Hypogonadism is associated with an increased osteoclast activity, leading to accelerated bone loss. An excess of unconjugated bilirubin negatively affects the differentiation of primary osteoblasts into their primary function. Chronic glucocorticoid therapy in patients with autoimmune hepatitis is associated with osteoporosis, and environmental factors, such as chronic alcohol consumption, smoking, low BMI, sedentary lifestyle and poor nutrition have an additional negative effect on bone turnover [43].

Screening for osteopenia and osteoporosis should be considered in all patients suffering from liver cirrhosis, and be part of the standard procedure in patients that are evaluated for liver transplantation. A timely diagnosis is important to prevent fractures as typical osteoporosis-related complications. Bone mineral density screening should be repeated on a yearly basis in patients with cholestatic liver disease and/or multiple risk factors and every two to three years in other patients with liver cirrhosis [41].

3. Therapeutic Approach to Treat Nutritional Deficits

3.1. Caloric, Protein and Lipid Supplementation

In patients with advanced cirrhosis, nutrition is of paramount importance. A nutritional assessment should be performed on a regular basis and corrective measures implemented as soon as a deficit is observed. If available, a clinical nutrition specialist should perform the nutritional assessment. The aim is to identify daily deficits and to define daily nutritional requirements. This assessment should include caloric and protein intake as well as vitamins and micronutrients.

In patients with cirrhosis, a daily intake of 30–35 kcal and of 1.2 to 1.5 g protein per kg body weight (BW) is recommended [44,45]. In obese patients with liver cirrhosis, a moderately hypocaloric diet (−500–800 kcal/d), respectively a reduced daily caloric intake of 20–25 kcal/kg BW, should be combined with an increase in protein intake (>1.5 g, up to 2.5 g/kg BW) [44–46], Table 1.

Regarding lipids, no specific recommendations are provided in the guidelines for patients with liver cirrhosis [44,45]. Compared to the glucose and protein metabolism, alterations in the lipid metabolism seem to be of minor importance in patients with liver cirrhosis. This is illustrated by the finding that the elimination of lipid emulsions containing long-chain or long-chain and medium-chain triglycerides, and the release of free fatty acids thereof were not altered in patients with chronic hepatic failure compared to healthy controls [47,48].

Table 1. Nutrition management in patients with advanced liver cirrhosis.

	Cirrhosis with Malnutrition	**Cirrhosis with Sarcopenic Obesity**
Caloric intake	30–35 kcal/kg BW	20–25 kcal/kg BW
Protein intake	1.2 to 1.5 g/kg BW	>1.5 g, up to 2.5 g/kg BW
Lipid intake	No specific recommendation	No specific recommendation
Vitamins		
Vitamin A *	Supplement if decreased	Supplement if decreased
Vitamin D	Supplement if decreased	Supplement if decreased
Micronutrients		
Zinc	Supplement if decreased	Supplement if decreased
Selenium	Supplement if decreased	Supplement if decreased

BW: body weight. * avoid oversubstitution.

Ideally, the nutritional goals can be achieved by regular meals, if required, by reducing the size and increasing the frequency of meals. A late evening snack is recommended to compensate for the reduced glycogen production and storage, and to prevent muscle proteolysis in patients with advanced cirrhosis [49]. The snack should comprise at least 50 g of complex carbohydrates [46]. If required, protein-enriched oral drinks can be added.

In patients that cannot achieve the nutritional goals with oral substitution, placement of an enteral tube should be considered. The presence of non-bleeding esophageal varices is not a contraindication for enteral tube feeding [44,45]. In contrast, a percutaneous enteral gastrostomy (PEG) is associated with an elevated risk of complications, especially bleeding, and is therefore not recommended in patients with chronic advanced liver disease [44,45].

Periods of prolonged fasting should be avoided whenever possible. Risk situations are prolonged waiting time for interventions or surgery, and situations in which a patient is temporarily not able to maintain oral nutrition, e.g., during a stay in the intensive care unit. If oral or enteral feeding is not possible, parenteral nutrition should be considered early [44,45], Figure 1.

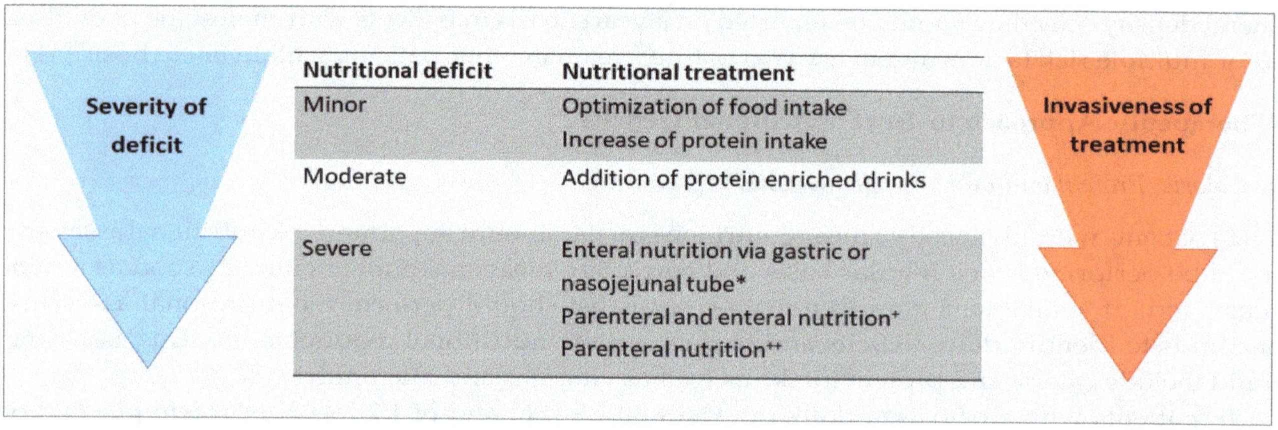

Figure 1. Nutrition management in malnourished patients with liver cirrhosis. * Non-bleeding esophageal varices are not a contraindication for enteral tube feeding, + if enteral nutrition is insufficient, ++ if enteral nutrition is not possible.

In patients with liver cirrhosis, restriction of protein intake is not indicated [44,45], since this promotes muscle proteolysis [50] and increased the risk of mortality on the waiting list for liver transplants [51]. Intolerance of mixed proteins with consecutive development of hepatic encephalopathy is very rare. In this specific situation, a diet with vegetable proteins may be beneficial [44], since vegetable proteins are rich in BCAA compared to animal proteins, and BCAA remove one mole of ammonia per mole of BCAA [52]. Alternatively, BCAA or leucine-enriched BCAA supplementation can be considered, the latter showing a stimulatory, and therefore beneficial, effect on mTORC1 in the skeletal muscle of patients with alcoholic liver cirrhosis [53]. After an episode of overt hepatic encephalopathy, BCAA supplementation improved muscle mass and minimal HE, but did not decrease recurrence of overt hepatic encephalopathy [45,54].

3.2. *Albumin*

From a nutritionist point of view, there is no indication for the substitution of albumin in patients with liver cirrhosis. However, albumin is used in patients with refractory ascites to prevent the circulatory dysfunction syndrome following paracentesis, in the setting of hepatorenal syndrome and in case of infection, especially spontaneous bacterial peritonitis (SBP) [55]. Whether long-term albumin infusions have a significant effect on morbidity and mortality in patients with advanced liver cirrhosis is currently being debated. In the ANSWER study, patients receiving albumin on a weekly basis had a lower mortality and complication rate than patients in the placebo group [56]. However, there were some concerns regarding the methodology of this trial (open label study, different management of the two treatment arms). No effect on the complication rate in patients with cirrhosis awaiting liver transplantation was found in the MACHT trial, that investigated the addition of midodrine and albumin to the standard of care treatment [57].

3.3. *Vitamins and Micronutrients*

Vitamin D has a broad impact not only on bone metabolism, but also on several hepatic cells and functions. Therefore, supplementation in case of reduced levels (<20 ng/mL) is indicated to prevent the risk of fractures that is increased in patients with cirrhosis [42], and to maintain Vitamin D related liver functions. A level of >30 ng/mL should be the therapeutic target [58,59].

For vitamin A, there is no generally accepted opinion regarding supplementation. Due to the negative effect on the liver in case of long-term high-dose substitution (>40,000 IU per day), some authors recommend against supplementation of vitamin A [34]. Taking into account the linear relationship between low serum retinol and vitamin A storage, and the association of HCC with very low vitamin A levels [33], low level substitution for a limited period of time in case of reduced vitamin A levels can be considered.

Zinc deficiency is frequent in patients with chronic liver disease and has been associated with insulin resistance, hepatic steatosis, iron overload and hepatic encephalopathy. Consequently, zinc levels should be measured in patients with cirrhosis and zinc supplemented in case of reduced levels [37,60].

Since cirrhosis causes functional selenium deficit in some patients, and, taking into account that the prevalence of selenium deficit rises with the severity of cirrhosis, supplementation in case of a confirmed deficit can be considered. However, to date, data regarding positive or negative effects of selenium substitution in patients with advanced liver cirrhosis are missing and, consequently, no general recommendation is possible. If selenium is supplemented, selenite and not selenomethionine should be prescribed, due to the altered metabolism in patients with cirrhosis [61].

3.4. *General Management*

Patients with malnutrition and sarcopenia should be followed on a regular basis by a clinical nutrition specialist, and nutritional status as well as measures to correct malnutrition and sarcopenia should be periodically reassessed. Furthermore, nutritional aspects should be integrated in the assessment and the clinical decision-making process by the multidisciplinary medical team treating patients with advanced chronic liver disease.

4. Conclusions

Patients with advanced liver cirrhosis are prone to malnutrition. Reasons for malnutrition are a reduced intake of food and especially proteins, a decreased synthetic function of the liver, impaired glycogen production and storage, proteolysis in the muscle, and loss of proteins via paracenteses, the kidneys or the GI tract.

A comprehensive management of patients with advanced chronic liver disease should aim at the identification of malnutrition in general and selective nutritional deficits in particular. Due to ascites and general fluid overload, body weight and body mass index may be misleading in cirrhotic patients, and a more in-depth analysis of body composition and function is indicated. SGA is an easy to perform nutritional assessment in patients with liver cirrhosis. However, in overweight and obese patients, its performance is limited, due to a weak concordance with sarcopenia [10].

Sarcopenia, a common complication in patients with advanced liver cirrhosis, is at least partially the consequence of malnutrition. Ideally, it can be diagnosed from cross-sectional abdominal images. Sarcopenic obese patients need special attention, since nutritional and muscularity deficits may be overlooked.

Treatment of patients with advanced liver cirrhosis should be comprehensive and address the individual patients' caloric and protein requirements, as well as the correction of vitamin and micronutrient deficits. Whether continuous administration of albumin is helpful in malnourished cirrhotic patients is currently not clear, since study results are discordant.

There is certainly a need for more randomized studies, to better assess the effect of a comprehensive nutritional management on mortality and morbidity, and, in particular, on the evolution of sarcopenia and other cirrhosis-associated complications.

Author Contributions: Conceptualization, J.S. and G.S.; methodology, J.S and G.S.; writing—original draft preparation, J.S. and G.S.; writing—review and editing, J.S. and G.S.

References

1. Ge, P.S.; Runyon, B.A. Treatment of Patients with Cirrhosis. *N. Engl. J. Med.* **2016**, *375*, 767–777. [CrossRef] [PubMed]
2. Cheung, K.; Lee, S.S.; Raman, M. Prevalence and mechanisms of malnutrition in patients with advanced liver disease, and nutrition management strategies. *Clin. Gastroenterol. Hepatol.* **2012**, *10*, 117–125. [CrossRef] [PubMed]
3. Ockenga, J.; Bischoff, S.C.; Tillmann, H.L.; Rifai, K.; Widjaja, A.; Boker, K.H.; Manns, M.P.; Brabant, G. Elevated bound leptin correlates with energy expenditure in cirrhotics. *Gastroenterology* **2000**, *119*, 1656–1662. [CrossRef] [PubMed]
4. Ockenga, J.; Widjaja, A.; Holtmannspotter, M.; Schmidt, R.E.; Brabant, G. Bound leptin is regulated by tumour necrosis factor-alpha in HIV-infected patients: A potential mediator of wasting? *AIDS* **1998**, *12*, 2233–2235.
5. Buechler, C.; Haberl, E.M.; Rein-Fischboeck, L.; Aslanidis, C. Adipokines in Liver Cirrhosis. *Int. J. Mol. Sci.* **2017**, *18*, 1392. [CrossRef]
6. Chander Roland, B.; Garcia-Tsao, G.; Ciarleglio, M.M.; Deng, Y.; Sheth, A. Decompensated cirrhotics have slower intestinal transit times as compared with compensated cirrhotics and healthy controls. *J. Clin. Gastroenterol.* **2013**, *47*, 888–893. [CrossRef]
7. Bergheim, I.; Parlesak, A.; Dierks, C.; Bode, J.C.; Bode, C. Nutritional deficiencies in German middle-class male alcohol consumers: Relation to dietary intake and severity of liver disease. *Eur. J. Clin. Nutr.* **2003**, *57*, 431–438. [CrossRef]
8. Merli, M.; Giusto, M.; Gentili, F.; Novelli, G.; Ferretti, G.; Riggio, O.; Corradini, S.G.; Siciliano, M.; Farcomeni, A.; Attili, A.F.; et al. Nutritional status: Its influence on the outcome of patients undergoing liver transplantation. *Liver Int.* **2010**, *30*, 208–214. [CrossRef]
9. Stephenson, G.R.; Moretti, E.W.; El-Moalem, H.; Clavien, P.A.; Tuttle-Newhall, J.E. Malnutrition in liver transplant patients: Preoperative subjective global assessment is predictive of outcome after liver transplantation. *Transplantation* **2001**, *72*, 666–670. [CrossRef]
10. Moctezuma-Velazquez, C.; Ebadi, M.; Bhanji, R.A.; Stirnimann, G.; Tandon, P.; Montano-Loza, A.J. Limited performance of subjective global assessment compared to computed tomography-determined sarcopenia in predicting adverse clinical outcomes in patients with cirrhosis. *Clin. Nutr.* **2018**. [CrossRef]
11. Child, C.G.; Turcotte, J.G. Surgery and portal hypertension. *Major Prob. Clin. Surg.* **1964**, *1*, 1–85.
12. Arroyo, V.; Garcia-Martinez, R.; Salvatella, X. Human serum albumin, systemic inflammation, and cirrhosis. *J. Hepatol.* **2014**, *61*, 396–407. [CrossRef]
13. Rondana, M.; Milani, L.; Merkel, C.; Caregaro, L.; Gatta, A. Value of prealbumin plasma levels as liver test. *Digestion* **1987**, *37*, 72–78. [CrossRef] [PubMed]
14. Liu, F.; Cai, L.Y.; Zhong, L.; Chen, C.; Xu, F.; Zhao, Z.X.; Chen, X.M. Model for end-stage liver disease combined with serum prealbumin to predict the prognosis of patients with decompensated liver cirrhosis. *J. Dig. Dis.* **2010**, *11*, 352–357. [CrossRef] [PubMed]
15. Huang, L.; Li, J.; Yan, J.J.; Liu, C.F.; Wu, M.C.; Yan, Y.Q. Prealbumin is predictive for postoperative liver insufficiency in patients undergoing liver resection. *World J. Gastroenterol.* **2012**, *18*, 7021–7025. [CrossRef]
16. Wen, X.; Yao, M.; Lu, Y.; Chen, J.; Zhou, J.; Chen, X.; Zhang, Y.; Lu, W.; Qian, X.; Zhao, J.; et al. Integration of Prealbumin into Child-Pugh Classification Improves Prognosis Predicting Accuracy in HCC Patients Considering Curative Surgery. *J. Clin. Trans. Hepatol.* **2018**, *6*, 377–384. [CrossRef] [PubMed]
17. Alberino, F.; Gatta, A.; Amodio, P.; Merkel, C.; Di Pascoli, L.; Boffo, G.; Caregaro, L. Nutrition and survival in patients with liver cirrhosis. *Nutrition* **2001**, *17*, 445–450. [CrossRef]

18. Englesbe, M.J.; Patel, S.P.; He, K.; Lynch, R.J.; Schaubel, D.E.; Harbaugh, C.; Holcombe, S.A.; Wang, S.C.; Segev, D.L.; Sonnenday, C.J. Sarcopenia and mortality after liver transplantation. *J. Am. Coll. Surg.* **2010**, *211*, 271–278. [CrossRef]
19. Golse, N.; Bucur, P.O.; Ciacio, O.; Pittau, G.; Sa Cunha, A.; Adam, R.; Castaing, D.; Antonini, T.; Coilly, A.; Samuel, D.; et al. A new definition of sarcopenia in patients with cirrhosis undergoing liver transplantation. *Liver Transpl.* **2017**, *23*, 143–154. [CrossRef]
20. Montano-Loza, A.J. Muscle wasting: A nutritional criterion to prioritize patients for liver transplantation. *Curr. Opin. Clin. Nutr. Metab. Care* **2014**, *17*, 219–225. [CrossRef]
21. Durand, F.; Buyse, S.; Francoz, C.; Laouenan, C.; Bruno, O.; Belghiti, J.; Moreau, R.; Vilgrain, V.; Valla, D. Prognostic value of muscle atrophy in cirrhosis using psoas muscle thickness on computed tomography. *J. Hepatol.* **2014**, *60*, 1151–1157. [CrossRef] [PubMed]
22. Ebadi, M.; Wang, C.W.; Lai, J.C.; Dasarathy, S.; Kappus, M.R.; Dunn, M.A.; Carey, E.J.; Montano-Loza, A.J.; From the Fitness, Life Enhancement, and Exercise in Liver Transplantation (FLEXIT) Consortium. Poor performance of psoas muscle index for identification of patients with higher waitlist mortality risk in cirrhosis. *J. Cachexia Sarcopenia Muscle* **2018**, *9*, 1053–1062. [CrossRef] [PubMed]
23. Montano-Loza, A.J.; Angulo, P.; Meza-Junco, J.; Prado, C.M.M.; Sawyer, M.B.; Beaumont, C.; Esfandiari, N.; Ma, M.; Baracos, V.E. Sarcopenic obesity and myosteatosis are associated with higher mortality in patients with cirrhosis. *J. Cachexia Sarcopenia Muscle* **2016**, *7*, 126–135. [CrossRef] [PubMed]
24. Romeiro, F.G.; Augusti, L. Nutritional assessment in cirrhotic patients with hepatic encephalopathy. *World J. Hepatol.* **2015**, *7*, 2940–2954. [CrossRef]
25. Sinclair, M.; Hoermann, R.; Peterson, A.; Testro, A.; Angus, P.W.; Hey, P.; Chapman, B.; Gow, P.J. Use of Dual X-ray Absorptiometry in men with advanced cirrhosis to predict sarcopenia-associated mortality risk. *Liver Int.* **2019**, *39*, 1089–1097. [CrossRef]
26. Giusto, M.; Lattanzi, B.; Albanese, C.; Galtieri, A.; Farcomeni, A.; Giannelli, V.; Lucidi, C.; Di Martino, M.; Catalano, C.; Merli, M. Sarcopenia in liver cirrhosis: The role of computed tomography scan for the assessment of muscle mass compared with dual-energy X-ray absorptiometry and anthropometry. *Eur. J. Gastroenterol. Hepatol.* **2015**, *27*, 328–334. [CrossRef]
27. Kamath, P.S.; Wiesner, R.H.; Malinchoc, M.; Kremers, W.; Therneau, T.M.; Kosberg, C.L.; D'Amico, G.; Dickson, E.R.; Kim, W.R. A model to predict survival in patients with end-stage liver disease. *Hepatology* **2001**, *33*, 464–470. [CrossRef]
28. Montano-Loza, A.J.; Duarte-Rojo, A.; Meza-Junco, J.; Baracos, V.E.; Sawyer, M.B.; Pang, J.X.Q.; Beaumont, C.; Esfandiari, N.; Myers, R.P. Inclusion of Sarcopenia Within MELD (MELD-Sarcopenia) and the Prediction of Mortality in Patients with Cirrhosis. *Clin. Trans. Gastroenterol.* **2015**, *6*, e102. [CrossRef]
29. Zuniga, S.; Firrincieli, D.; Housset, C.; Chignard, N. Vitamin D and the vitamin D receptor in liver pathophysiology. *Clin. Res. Hepatol. Gastroenterol.* **2011**, *35*, 295–302. [CrossRef]
30. Konstantakis, C.; Tselekouni, P.; Kalafateli, M.; Triantos, C. Vitamin D deficiency in patients with liver cirrhosis. *Ann. Gastroenterol.* **2016**, *29*, 297–306. [CrossRef]
31. Putz-Bankuti, C.; Pilz, S.; Stojakovic, T.; Scharnagl, H.; Pieber, T.R.; Trauner, M.; Obermayer-Pietsch, B.; Stauber, R.E. Association of 25-hydroxyvitamin D levels with liver dysfunction and mortality in chronic liver disease. *Liver Int.* **2012**, *32*, 845–851. [CrossRef] [PubMed]
32. Olson, J.A. Serum levels of vitamin A and carotenoids as reflectors of nutritional status. *J. Natl. Cancer Inst.* **1984**, *73*, 1439–1444. [PubMed]
33. Newsome, P.N.; Beldon, I.; Moussa, Y.; Delahooke, T.E.; Poulopoulos, G.; Hayes, P.C.; Plevris, J.N. Low serum retinol levels are associated with hepatocellular carcinoma in patients with chronic liver disease. *Aliment. Pharmacol. Ther.* **2000**, *14*, 1295–1301. [CrossRef] [PubMed]
34. Chaves, G.V.; Peres, W.A.; Goncalves, J.C.; Ramalho, A. Vitamin A and retinol-binding protein deficiency among chronic liver disease patients. *Nutrition* **2015**, *31*, 664–668. [CrossRef]
35. Geubel, A.P.; De Galocsy, C.; Alves, N.; Rahier, J.; Dive, C. Liver damage caused by therapeutic vitamin A administration: Estimate of dose-related toxicity in 41 cases. *Gastroenterology* **1991**, *100*, 1701–1709. [CrossRef]
36. Barry, M.; Keeling, P.W.; Feely, J. Tissue zinc status and drug elimination in patients with chronic liver disease. *Clin. Sci.* **1990**, *78*, 547–549. [CrossRef]
37. Grungreiff, K.; Reinhold, D.; Wedemeyer, H. The role of zinc in liver cirrhosis. *Ann. Hepatol.* **2016**, *15*, 7–16. [CrossRef]

38. Takuma, Y.; Nouso, K.; Makino, Y.; Hayashi, M.; Takahashi, H. Clinical trial: Oral zinc in hepatic encephalopathy. *Aliment. Pharmacol. Ther.* **2010**, *32*, 1080–1090. [CrossRef]
39. Hayashi, M.; Ikezawa, K.; Ono, A.; Okabayashi, S.; Hayashi, Y.; Shimizu, S.; Mizuno, T.; Maeda, K.; Akasaka, T.; Naito, M.; et al. Evaluation of the effects of combination therapy with branched-chain amino acid and zinc supplements on nitrogen metabolism in liver cirrhosis. *Hepatol. Res.* **2007**, *37*, 615–619. [CrossRef]
40. Burk, R.F.; Early, D.S.; Hill, K.E.; Palmer, I.S.; Boeglin, M.E. Plasma selenium in patients with cirrhosis. *Hepatology* **1998**, *27*, 794–798. [CrossRef]
41. Patel, N.; Munoz, S.J. Bone disease in cirrhosis. *Clin. Liver Dis.* **2015**, *6*, 96–99. [CrossRef] [PubMed]
42. Nakchbandi, I.A. Osteoporosis and fractures in liver disease: Relevance, pathogenesis and therapeutic implications. *World J. Gastroenterol.* **2014**, *20*, 9427–9438. [PubMed]
43. Handzlik-Orlik, G.; Holecki, M.; Wilczynski, K.; Dulawa, J. Osteoporosis in liver disease: Pathogenesis and management. *Ther. Adv. Endocrinol. Metab.* **2016**, *7*, 128–135. [CrossRef] [PubMed]
44. Plauth, M.; Bernal, W.; Dasarathy, S.; Merli, M.; Plank, L.D.; Schutz, T.; Bischoff, S.C. ESPEN guideline on clinical nutrition in liver disease. *Clin. Nutr.* **2019**, *38*, 485–521. [CrossRef]
45. EASL. Clinical Practice Guidelines on nutrition in chronic liver disease. *J. Hepatol.* **2019**, *70*, 172–193. [CrossRef]
46. Amodio, P.; Bemeur, C.; Butterworth, R.; Cordoba, J.; Kato, A.; Montagnese, S.; Uribe, M.; Vilstrup, H.; Morgan, M.Y. The nutritional management of hepatic encephalopathy in patients with cirrhosis: International Society for Hepatic Encephalopathy and Nitrogen Metabolism Consensus. *Hepatology* **2013**, *58*, 325–336. [CrossRef]
47. Druml, W.; Fischer, M.; Pidlich, J.; Lenz, K. Fat elimination in chronic hepatic failure: Long-chain vs medium-chain triglycerides. *Am J Clin Nutr.* **1995**, *61*, 812–817. [CrossRef] [PubMed]
48. Xu, Z.; Li, Y.; Wang, J.; Wu, B.; Li, J. Effect of omega-3 polyunsaturated fatty acids to reverse biopsy-proven parenteral nutrition-associated liver disease in adults. *Clin. Nutr.* **2012**, *31*, 217–223. [CrossRef] [PubMed]
49. Tsien, C.D.; McCullough, A.J.; Dasarathy, S. Late evening snack: Exploiting a period of anabolic opportunity in cirrhosis. *J. Gastroenterol. Hepatol.* **2012**, *27*, 430–441. [CrossRef]
50. Cordoba, J.; Lopez-Hellin, J.; Planas, M.; Sabin, P.; Sanpedro, F.; Castro, F.; Esteban, R.; Guardia, J. Normal protein diet for episodic hepatic encephalopathy: Results of a randomized study. *J. Hepatol.* **2004**, *41*, 38–43. [CrossRef]
51. Ney, M.; Abraldes, J.G.; Ma, M.; Belland, D.; Harvey, A.; Robbins, S.; Den Heyer, V.; Tandon, P. Insufficient Protein Intake Is Associated with Increased Mortality in 630 Patients with Cirrhosis Awaiting Liver Transplantation. *Nutr. Clin. Pract.* **2015**, *30*, 530–536. [CrossRef] [PubMed]
52. Dasarathy, S.; Merli, M. Sarcopenia from mechanism to diagnosis and treatment in liver disease. *J. Hepatol.* **2016**, *65*, 1232–1244. [CrossRef]
53. Tsien, C.; Davuluri, G.; Singh, D.; Allawy, A.; Ten Have, G.A.; Thapaliya, S.; Schulze, J.M.; Barnes, D.; McCullough, A.J.; Engelen, M.P.; et al. Metabolic and molecular responses to leucine-enriched branched chain amino acid supplementation in the skeletal muscle of alcoholic cirrhosis. *Hepatology* **2015**, *61*, 2018–2029. [CrossRef] [PubMed]
54. Les, I.; Doval, E.; Garcia-Martinez, R.; Planas, M.; Cardenas, G.; Gomez, P.; Flavià, M.; Jacas, C.; Mínguez, B.; Vergara, M.; et al. Effects of branched-chain amino acids supplementation in patients with cirrhosis and a previous episode of hepatic encephalopathy: A randomized study. *Am. J. Gastroenterol.* **2011**, *106*, 1081–1088. [CrossRef] [PubMed]
55. EASL. Clinical Practice Guidelines for the management of patients with decompensated cirrhosis. *J. Hepatol.* **2018**, *69*, 406–460. [CrossRef]
56. Caraceni, P.; Riggio, O.; Angeli, P.; Alessandria, C.; Neri, S.; Foschi, F.G.; Levantesi, F.; Airoldi, A.; Boccia, S.; Svegliati-Baroni, G.; et al. Long-term albumin administration in decompensated cirrhosis (ANSWER): An open-label randomised trial. *Lancet* **2018**, *391*, 2417–2429. [CrossRef]
57. Sola, E.; Sole, C.; Simon-Talero, M.; Martin-Llahi, M.; Castellote, J.; Garcia-Martinez, R.; Moreira, R.; Torrens, M.; Márquez, F.; Fabrellas, N.; et al. Midodrine and albumin for prevention of complications in patients with cirrhosis awaiting liver transplantation. A randomized placebo-controlled trial. *J. Hepatol.* **2018**, *69*, 1250–1259. [CrossRef]

58. Holick, M.F.; Binkley, N.C.; Bischoff-Ferrari, H.A.; Gordon, C.M.; Hanley, D.A.; Heaney, R.P.; Murad, M.H.; Weaver, C.M.; Endocrine Society. Evaluation, treatment, and prevention of vitamin D deficiency: An Endocrine Society clinical practice guideline. *J. Clin. Endocrinol. Metab.* **2011**, *96*, 1911–1930. [CrossRef]
59. Elangovan, H.; Chahal, S.; Gunton, J.E. Vitamin D in liver disease: Current evidence and potential directions. *Biochim. Biophys. Acta* **2017**, *1863*, 907–916. [CrossRef]
60. Grungreiff, K. Branched Amino Acids and Zinc in the Nutrition of Liver Cirrhosis. *J. Clin. Exp. Hepatol.* **2018**, *8*, 480–483. [CrossRef]
61. Burk, R.F.; Hill, K.E.; Motley, A.K.; Byrne, D.W.; Norsworthy, B.K. Selenium deficiency occurs in some patients with moderate-to-severe cirrhosis and can be corrected by administration of selenate but not selenomethionine: A randomized controlled trial. *Am. J. Clin. Nutr.* **2015**, *102*, 1126–1133. [CrossRef] [PubMed]

9

Economic Challenges in Nutritional Management

Emilie Reber [1,*,†], Kristina Norman [2,3,†], Olga Endrich [4], Philipp Schuetz [5], Andreas Frei [6] and Zeno Stanga [1]

1 Department for Diabetes, Endocrinology, Nutritional Medicine and Metabolism, Bern University Hospital, and University of Bern, 3010 Bern, Switzerland
2 Department of Nutrition and Gerontology, German Institute for Human Nutrition Potsdam-Rehbrücke, 14558 Nuthetal, Germany
3 Research Group on Geriatrics, Charité Universitätsmedizin Berlin, Corporate Member of Freie Universität Berlin, Humboldt-Universität zu Berlin, and Berlin Institute of Health, 13347 Berlin, Germany
4 Health Data Management and Health Economics, Medical Directorate, Bern University Hospital, and University of Bern, 3010 Bern, Switzerland
5 Medical University Department, Division of General Internal and Emergency Medicine, Kantonsspital Aarau, 5001 Aarau, Switzerland
6 Freelance Health Economist, 4133 Pratteln, Switzerland
* Correspondence: emilie.reber@insel.ch
† Equally contributing first authors.

Abstract: Disease-related malnutrition (DRM) is a highly prevalent independent risk and cost factor with significant influence on mortality, morbidity, length of hospital stay (LOS), functional impairment and quality of life. The aim of our research was to estimate the economic impact of the introduction of routinely performed nutritional screening (NS) in a tertiary hospital, with subsequent nutritional interventions (NI) in patients with potential or manifest DRM. Economic impact analysis of natural detection of inpatients at risk and estimation of the change in economic activity after the implementation of a systematic NS were performed. The reference population for natural detection of DRM is about 20,000 inpatients per year. Based on current data, DRM prevalence is estimated at 20%, so 4000 patients with potential and manifest DRM should be detected. The NI costs were estimated at CHF 0.693 million, with savings of CHF 1.582 million (LOS reduction) and CHF 0.806 million in additional revenue (SwissDRG system). Thus, the introduction of routine NS generates additional costs of CHF 1.181 million that are compensated by additional savings of CHF 2.043 million and an excess in additional revenue of CHF 2.071 million. NS with subsequent adequate nutritional intervention shows an economic potential for hospitals.

Keywords: economic challenges; nutritional management; malnutrition

---

1. Introduction

Disease-related malnutrition (DRM) is a debilitating, important and frequently occurring problem with an estimated prevalence of 20–50% on hospital admission [1–5]. The consequences of DRM are well known: Increases in morbidity, complication and mortality rates, resource use for inpatient treatment, prolonged hospital length of stay (LOS), decreased quality of life (QoL) and decreased body function. Many studies have shown the positive effects of nutritional interventions (NI), mainly in the reduction of complication rates, LOS, or rates of non-elective re-hospitalizations [3,6–10]. The recently published study by Schuetz et al.—a multicenter study with 2088 medical patients at nutritional risk, from eight Swiss hospitals—showed a significant reduction in serious complications and mortality as well as an improvement in physical function and quality of life after 30 days [11]. The study by Deutz et al. also showed a significant reduction in mortality after 90 days [12]. Available studies on cost-effectiveness clearly show that NI can save money and that the costs of NI are more than offset by the savings [7,9,13].

Since 2012, hospitals in Switzerland are remunerated using per-case rates for inpatients through the Swiss Diagnosis Related Groups (SwissDRG) system. In the SwissDRG it is possible to take DRM into account by coding it as a principal or secondary diagnosis. This requires optimal nutritional management from the hospitals, with an initial screening and adequate therapy in the course of treatment. Coding DRM may have the effect that a certain percentage of the patients will be assigned to a DRG with a higher cost-weight, generating additional revenue for the hospital (like a bonus system). Aeberhard et al. investigated the financial effects of coding DRM in the SwissDRG system, including all inpatients from the years 2013 to 2016 in our university hospital. During the observation period, 3.2% of the patients were coded with DRM. In 8.3% of these cases, the coding led to the attribution of a DRG with an increased cost-weight. This resulted in total additional revenue of circa CHF 3.5 million, which was offset by costs of CHF 2.8 million for assessment and treatment of DRM [1]. Thus, the costs of screening and treatment of DRM were already overcompensated for as a result of the DRM coding and changes in SwissDRG attribution. These results have been confirmed in similar studies [14,15].

As regularly performed nutritional risk screening is not established at the Bern University Hospital, these results reflect the natural detection (ND) of DRM. If nutritional screening (NS) is performed routinely on all patients, the detection rate of DRM will likely increase, leading to earlier detection and treatment. Performing routine screening will generate further costs. Besides that, the same costs for each patient at nutritional risk occurs when the NS is performed, as in the natural detection of DRM. However, due to an increased detection rate, the number of patients with treated and coded DRM will rise, with NI costs increasing as a consequence, but with additional revenues generated [16,17]. If DRM is detected and adequately treated, three types of consequences will occur:

- There will be costs for the detection of DRM and consequently for nutritional treatment,
- Treatment of DRM will lead to improvements in clinical outcomes that transfer to savings in the costs of basic treatment, and
- Patients may be attributed to DRGs with increased cost-weights, causing additional revenues for the hospital.

Previous economic analyses have always compared either the costs of NI with savings in the costs of basic nutritional treatments [3,7,13] or with the additional revenues due to DRG changes [14,16,17]. No study is known to have compared costs with a combination of both savings and additional revenue.

The objective of this study was to estimate the economic impact of the introduction of a systematically performed NS on all patients in our hospital, with subsequent NI in all patients at nutritional risk.

2. Materials and Methods

The data for this economic impact analysis were collected from the electronic patient record system of the Bern University Hospital in Bern, Switzerland, between 1 January and 31 December 2018. This is a cost-minimization analysis of the short-term economic consequences of inpatient hospitalization for the year 2018. Included were direct medical costs for NS and NI, cost savings due to NI, and additional revenues due to DRM coding and DRG changes. Using a population-based approach, the economic effects of a systematically performed NS were projected and compared with the existing situation reflecting the natural detection of DRM and routine nutritional management. To this end, a flow chart was created, and the patient flows and resource use were assessed. The costs of ND were subtracted from those of a systematic NS. Furthermore, the number of additional staff needed to perform routine NS was estimated. Data were obtained through analyses of the literature, the use of secondary statistics, and data collection at the Bern University Hospital. In cases of unclear or controversial data, assumptions were made. The flow chart is presented in Figure 1.

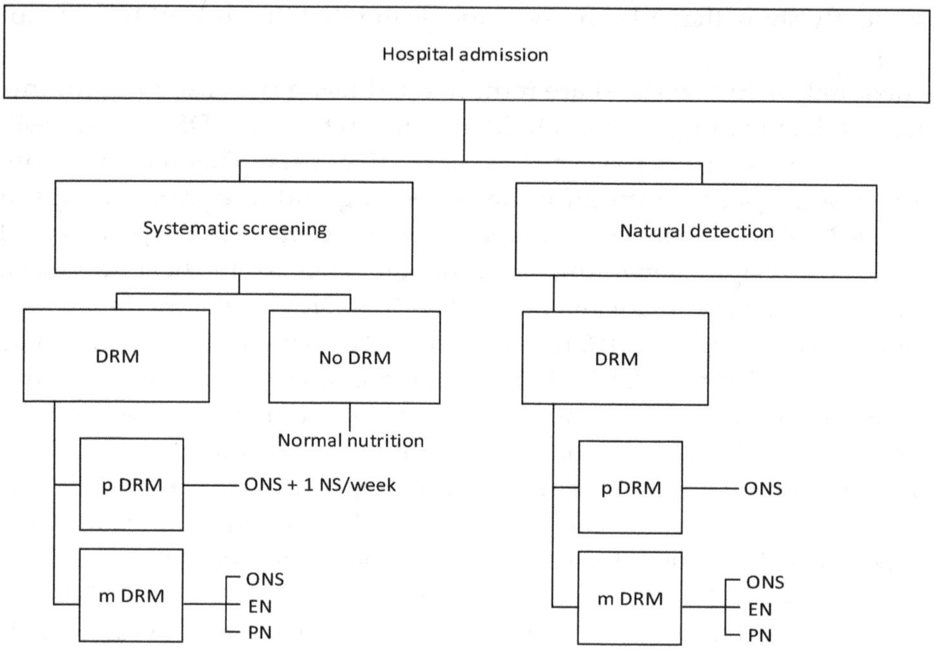

Figure 1. Nutritional screening (NS) and natural detection (ND). DRM: Disease-related malnutrition; p DRM: potential DRM; m DRM: manifest DRM; ONS: oral nutritional supplements; EN: enteral nutrition; PN: parenteral nutrition.

In a systematic NS, all patients are screened on admission to the hospital using a validated tool—in our case, the Nutritional Risk Screening 2002 (NRS 2002) [18]. Patients with an NRS score of 2 points or less are likely to be unaffected. Patients with an NRS score of 3 are considered at risk of DRM, and those with a score >3 points are considered to have manifest DRM. Patients with potential DRM undergo NS once per week. Patients with potential DRM will receive oral nutritional supplements (ONS) in addition to the customary nutrition and will also undergo NS once per week. Patients with manifest DRM will receive specific NI such as ONS, enteral nutrition (EN), or parenteral nutrition (PN) as needed and indicated in addition to the customary hospital nutrition. Their nutritional status will be regularly observed so that in these patients no additional NS will be needed [19].

3. Input Data

In Table 1 the input data are summarized.

Table 1. Overview of the input data.

Item	Both	Natural Detection	Nutritional Screening
Target population		Variable	20,000
Detection rate DRM		6.4%	20.0%
Proportions p DRM:m DRM		25% vs. 75%	45% vs. 55%
Number of nutritional screenings			No DRM, m DRM: 1; p DRM: 2
Nutritional interventions			
p DRM: ONS	100%	25%	45%
m DRM: ONS	45%	34%	25%
m DRM: EN	39%	29%	21%
m DRM: PN	16%	12%	9%
Reduction LOS in mDRM, days	1.2		
SwissDRG attribution change		8.3%	15.0%
Average increase cw		0.694	0.44

DRM: disease-related malnutrition; p DRM: potential DRM; m DRM: manifest DRM; ONS: oral nutritional supplements; EN: enteral nutrition; PN: parenteral nutrition; LOS: length of hospital stay; SwissDRG: Swiss diagnosis-related group, cw: cost-weight.

3.1. Target Population

For a systematic NS with subsequent NI, patients with an expected LOS of >3 days were considered eligible. In 2018, this amounted to 21,819 patients (information from Bern University Hospital). The average LOS of these patients was 10.01 days. This number also included healthy newborns. Therefore, it was assumed that the target population for a systematic NS at the Bern University Hospital would amount to approximately 20,000 patients yearly. Even though Aeberhard et al. [1] included all inpatients, it is unlikely that DRM was detected in patients with a LOS ≤3. Therefore, the reference population for ND patients with DRM was also assumed to be about 20,000 patients per year.

3.2. Detection Rate

Detection rates of 19% and 25.6% were obtained from two German studies [16,17]. The latter, however, also included patients with NRS ≥2, and the rate of patients with NRS >3 was computed at 20.7%. A Dutch study found that NS could increase the detection rate of DRM from 50% to 80% given a DRM prevalence of 32% [20]. Based on these data, the detection rate was estimated at 20%. For natural detection, we doubled the rate of 3.2% from Aeberhard et al. [1], using 6.4%.

3.3. Proportions with Potential and Manifest DRM

In patients with NS, the proportion of potential versus manifest DRM was estimated at 45%:55% based on [17]. In the naturally detected patients, these proportions were assumed to be 25%:75% as in [1].

3.4. Number of Screenings

Patients potentially having DRM are screened on admission and then once weekly. Patients with manifest DRM are only screened once on admission [19].

The number of screenings therefore depends on the proportions of patients with potential and manifest DRM and their expected LOS. Two studies showed that LOS in patients with DRM is longer than in well-nourished patients (11 vs. 7 days [16], 14 vs. 7.6 days [17]). Thus, it was assumed that LOS in patients without DRM was one week or less, and that LOS detected in DRM patients detected by NS was 12–14 days (1–2 weeks). Therefore, it was assumed that patients without DRM receive one NS, patients with potential DRM receive two NS, and patients with manifest DRM receive one.

3.5. Types and Proportions of NI

We distinguish between three types of NI: ONS, EN, and PN. In the study by Aeberhard et al., 59% of ND patients received ONS, 29% received EN, and 12% received PN [1]. All patients with potential DRM received ONS. Of the 59% of patients prescribed ONS, 25% were patients with potential DRM and 34% were patients with manifest DRM. The proportions of potential and manifest DRM differ in patients with NS. This implies that 45% with potential DRM will be prescribed ONS. In addition, of the 55% with manifest DRM, 25% will receive ONS, 21% will receive EN, and 9% will receive PN.

3.6. Reduction of LOS

Available data suggest that hospital LOS can be reduced by NI. However, it is difficult to quantify the amount. It seems that this effect is more likely to occur in patients with manifest DRM than with potential DRM and that it is more pronounced in connection with severe DRM [5,20–22]. Based on the findings of Elia et al. (−13.8% in relation to 22.5 hospital days) [3], Sriram et al. (−10% in relation to 6 days) [5] and Bally et al. (0%, calculated −3.2% of 13 days, not significant) [6], it was assumed here that NS will reduce LOS in patients with manifest DRM by 10%. This results in a reduction in LOS of 1.2 days. The same assumption is also made for ND patients.

3.7. DRG Changes

In ND, coding of a case of DRM led to a DRG change in 8.3% of all coded cases [1]. In patients with NS this proportion was substantially higher, amounting to 27% [16] and 15% [17]. Therefore, it was conservatively estimated to be 15%.

3.8. Increase in Cost-Weight

The average amount of additional revenue per case with a DRG change amounted to CHF 7564 [1]. Given a base rate of CHF 10,900, this corresponds to an average increase in the cost-weight of 0.694. However, in patients with NS, the average increase was clearly smaller (0.44) [16,17].

3.9. Ethics

This study was conducted in accordance with the ethical guidelines of the 1957 Declaration of Helsinki and approved by the Bernese Cantonal Ethics committee (BASEC ID 2017-00480), Bern, Switzerland.

4. Cost and Savings

4.1. Cost of NS

The costs of NS were calculated based on the time needed in minutes multiplied by the cost per minute of nursing staff. According to Wenger et al., the time needed to administer NS is about 5 min [19]. The costs per minute were calculated from an hourly rate (gross wage including employers' contributions to social insurance, information University Hospital Bern) and amounted to CHF 3.93.

4.2. Costs per Patient with NI

Therapy costs per patient for NI patients with DRM included daily personnel and materials costs multiplied by the duration of NI in days. In the case of EN and PN, one-time costs per therapy were added (Table 2). These values were based on Aeberhard et al. [1] and updated for 2019.

For ONS, the time expended by staff members was 10 min for a nutritional therapist, 10 min for nursing staff, and 2 min for a physician; for EN it was 10 min for a nutritional therapist, 40 min for nursing staff, and 2 min for a physician; and for PN it was 12 min for a nutritional therapist, 70 min for nursing staff, and 2.4 min for physicians. The costs were CHF 41.40 per hour for a nutritional therapist, CHF 47.11 per hour for nursing staff, and CHF 78.24 per hour for physicians (information provided by the Bern University Hospital). Data on materials costs, duration of NI and one-time costs were obtained from Aeberhard et al. [1]. Thus, the costs per patient for NI were calculated as CHF 187.57 for ONS, CHF 842.96 for EN, and CHF 1557.84 for PN.

Table 2. Costs of nutritional interventions (NI) per patient and intervention.

	ONS	EN	PN
Per day			
Personnel costs, CHF	17.36	40.91	66.37
Materials costs, CHF	4.97	40.09	75.02
Personnel and materials costs, CHF	22.33	81.00	141.39
Per therapy			
Duration of therapy, days	8.4	10.3	9.6
Personnel and material costs, CHF	187.57	834.35	1357.36
One-time costs, CHF		8.61	200.48
Total therapy costs, CHF	187.57	842.96	1557.84

ONS: oral nutritional supplements; EN: enteral nutrition; PN: parenteral nutrition.

4.3. *Savings per Prevented Inpatient Day*

It was assumed that the reduction of LOS occurred at the end of the hospitalization period. The costs then were mainly related to accommodation, food, medical care, follow-up visits, hospital buildings and the like. Such LOS-dependent costs are also used for the remuneration of hospital services in DRG outliers. In such cases, in addition to the per-case rate, the hospital is reimbursed a daily rate for each day exceeding the upper trim point delimiting inlier LOS. These daily rates are based on cost-weights per day. The cost-weight per day was calculated at 0.126 as a weighted average across the SwissDRGs based on Aeberhard et al. [1]. This was multiplied by the base rate of the Bern University Hospital (CHF 10,900). Thus, the cost per prevented hospital day was estimated at CHF 1373.

4.4. *Additional Revenue due to SwissDRG Change*

The number of patients with SwissDRG changes were multiplied by the average increases in the cost-weights and the CHF 10,900 base rate of the Bern University Hospital.

5. Results

5.1. *Effect of a Systematic NS*

The patient flow and performance of systematic NS are summarized in Table 3.

Table 3. Patient flow and resource use in connection with a systematic nutritional screening (NS).

Patients Flow and Performance	Proportion/Rate	Number
Target population	20,000	
Detection rate, of which:	20%	4000
- proportion p DRM	0.45	1800
- proportion m DRM	0.55	2200
Number of systematic nutritional screenings		
- On hospital admission	1	20,000
- Weekly in cases with p DRM	1	1800
Total screenings		21,800
Nutritional interventions		
p DRM		
- ONS	45.0%	1800
m DRM		
- ONS	24.9%	997
- EN	21.3%	851
- PN	8.8%	352
Total nutritional interventions	100.0%	4000
Saved hospital days	Per Patient	Total
expected LOS	12	
reduction %	10%	
Reduction LOS, days	1.2	2640
Swiss DRG changes	Detected Cases	
Changes in DRG attribution	0.15	600

DRM: disease-related malnutrition; p DRM: potential DRM; m DRM: manifest DRM; ONS: oral nutritional supplements; EN: enteral nutrition; PN: parenteral nutrition; LOS: length of hospital stay; DRG: diagnosis-related groups.

For a systematic NS, 20,000 patients per year would have to be screened on hospital admission. Assuming a detection rate of 20%, 4000 patients (including potential and manifest DRM) would be detected. Of these, 45% (1800) will have potential DRM and 55% (2200) will have manifest DRM. Patients with potential DRM and a projected LOS of 12 days will experience a second instance of NS in the second week of their hospital stay. So, in total, 21,800 NS will be performed. The 1800 patients with potential DRM and an absolute 24.9% of the 2200 patients with manifest DRM (=997 patients) will receive ONS. Furthermore, 21.3% (=851 patients) will receive EN, and 8.8% (=352 patients) will receive PN. These NI will effect a reduction of LOS of 1.2 days per case in patients with manifest DRM. This will result in global savings of 2640 hospital days in 2200 patients.

In all 4000 DRM patients, DRM will be coded as a complication or comorbidity in the DRG system. This coding will cause a DRG change in 15% of all DRM coded cases (i.e., 600 patients). The resulting costs are summarized in Table 4.

A total of 21,800 NS will be performed per year at a cost of CHF 3.93 per unit of NS. Thus, the costs of NS will amount to CHF 85,583. The costs of NI are calculated in a similar way using the number of patients multiplied by the NI costs per patient. The costs for all 2797 patients with ONS (1800 with potential, 997 with manifest DRM) were calculated as CHF 524,694, the costs of the 851 patients with EN as CHF 717,076, and those of the 352 patients with PN as CHF 548,358. Overall, the costs of NI amount to CHF 1,790,128. Combined with the costs of NS, global costs amount to 1,875,711. These costs are balanced by savings of CHF 3,625,930 due to the reduction of LOS. Furthermore, additional revenue of CHF 2,877,600 results from DRG changes. So, after deduction of the costs, there is a net monetary gain of CHF 4,627,818 for the hospital.

Table 4. Costs resulting from a systematic NS.

	Number	Value	Costs
Costs			
Systematic nutritional screening	21,800	3.93	85,583
Nutritional interventions			
ONS	2797	187.57	524,694
EN	851	842.96	717,076
PN	352	1557.84	548,358
Total nutritional interventions	4000		1,790,128
Total costs			1,875,711
Savings (LOS reduction) (−)	2640	1373.46	−3,625,930
Additional revenue (SwissDRG) (−)	600	4796.00	−2,877,600
Net effect			−4,627,818

Costs are indicated with positive (+), savings and additional revenue with negative (−) prefix. DRM: disease-related malnutrition; p DRM: potential DRM; m DRM: manifest DRM; ONS: oral nutritional supplements; EN: enteral nutrition; PN: parenteral nutrition.

5.2. *Effects of ND, Treatment and Coding of DRM*

Table A1 (Appendix A) shows the patient flow in the case of natural detection of DRM. In relation to the target population of 20,000 patients, the detection rate is 6.4%, which results in 1280 patients per year with DRM detected, treated and coded. Of these, 25% (320 patients) will be patients with potential DRM and 75% (960 patients) will be with manifest DRM. ONS will be provided to 755 patients (59%), EN to 371 patients (29%), and PN to 154 patients (12%).

It can be assumed that the average LOS in patients with naturally detected DRM would have been longer if they had not been treated for DRM and if NI had not reduced this LOS in the 960 patients with manifest DRM by 1.2 days. This amounts to a savings of 1152 hospital days. In 8.33% of the patients, i.e., in 107 cases, there is a DRG change.

Table A2 (Appendix A) shows the costs related to natural detection of DRM. The costs of NI amounts to CHF 141,652 for the treatment of 755 patients with ONS, CHF 312,906 for the 371 patients with EN, and CHF 239,284 for the 154 patients with PN. Total costs amount to CHF 693,842 per year. The savings due to a reduction of LOS amounted to CHF 1,582,224. The additional revenue resulting from SwissDRG changes amounts to CHF 806,579. The costs are overcompensated for by the savings and the additional revenue, resulting in an overall net savings of CHF 1,694,961.

5.3. Costs, Savings, and Additional Revenue Attributable to NS

As compared with the actual state of a natural detection, a systematic NS would generate additional costs of CHF 85,583 for screening and CHF 1,096,286 for NI, totaling CHF 1,181,869. These would be compensated for by savings of CHF 2,043,706 due to a reduction in LOS and by additional revenue of CHF 2,071,021 arising from coding and DRG changes (Table 5).

Table 5. Net monetary effects of the introduction of a systematic NS.

	Nutritional Screening	Natural Detection	Extra Costs/ Savings NS
Costs			
Systematic screening	85,583		85,583
Nutritional interventions	1,790,128	693,842	1,096,286
Total costs	1,875,711	693,842	1,181,869
Savings (reduction LOS) (−)	−3,625,930	−1,582,224	−2,043,706
Additional revenue (SwissDRG) (−)	−2,877,600	−806,579	−2,071,021
Net effect	−4,627,818	−1,694,961	−2,932,858

5.4. Staff Needed

Table A3 shows (Appendix A) the calculation of the staff needed, broken down by professional group. The total number of working hours and days was based on the time needed per day and the duration of the therapy in days (see Table 1) and on the number of patients undergoing therapy. Details are given in Table A4 (Appendix A). The number of positions was calculated using an average working day of 8.4 h, 220 working days per year and a fulltime position, and a productivity of 80%.

For a systematic NS, 4.09 positions for nutritional therapists, 9.27 positions for nursing staff, and 0.82 positions for physicians is needed. The treatment of naturally detected patients with DRM presently requires 1.35 positions for nutritional therapists, 3.6 positions for nursing staff, and 0.27 positions for physicians. Thus, the additional staff needed amounts to 2.75 positions for nutritional therapists, 5.66 positions for nursing staff and 0.55 positions for physicians.

5.5. Scenario Analyses

The results show that the savings and the additional revenue are each separately greater than the costs. Scenario analyses were performed based on few important assumptions to determine the minimum savings or additional revenues needed in order to cover only the costs. To find a best estimate for the reduction of LOS, the value of a saved hospital day, the proportion of DRG changes, and the average increases in the cost-weights, the following scenario analyses were performed:

Analysis 1, cost consequences in case the savings = 0, shows that even if no savings could be realized, NS could still achieve a net benefit through the additional revenue of CHF 1,001,889.

Analysis 2, cost consequences if additional revenue = 0, reveals that, even if no additional revenue were realized, NS would still lead to net savings of CHF 1,750,218.

Analysis 3, minimal additional revenue needed if savings = 0, shows that, in order to compensate for the costs, additional revenue of CHF 1,875,711 is needed. This could be achieved (1) by reducing the proportion of cases with changes in DRG attribution to 9.8% while keeping the increase in the cost-weight constant, or (2) by leaving the percentage of cases with changes in DRG attribution unchanged while increasing the average cost-weight by only 0.29.

Analysis 4 shows that a 5% reduction in LOS with a constant value per day would be sufficient to achieve the minimum required savings of CHF 1,875,711. On the other hand, if the reduction of LOS were left unchanged, a valuation of CHF 710 per saved hospital day would be sufficient.

6. Discussion

The introduction of a systematic NS would be accompanied by yearly costs of CHF 1.875 million. These costs would be compensated for by savings of CHF 3.635 million from a reduction in LOS and by additional revenue of CHF 2.877 million due to changes in documentation and coding of DRM. These numbers include the costs, savings and additional revenue produced by natural detection of DRM. These were estimated at CHF 0.693 million for the costs, CHF 1.582 million for the savings, and CHF 0.806 million for the additional revenue. Thus, the introduction of a systematic NS would generate additional costs of CHF 1.181 million that would be compensated for by additional savings of CHF 2.043 million and additional revenue of CHF 2.071 million.

These figures are based on projections using data from literature analyses, use of secondary statistics and data collected from the Bern University Hospital. It is notable that the savings per se are almost twice the costs, and the additional revenue alone is about 1.5 times the costs. These results are based on a few central assumptions about the data collected. The most important of these are discussed here.

The detection rate of NS was estimated to be 20%. Compared with data from the literature showing prevalence rates of 20–50% and even greater, this is a cautious assumption. The assumption regarding the size of the target population seems well justified, as only patients with an expected LOS of >3 days were considered. In estimating the expected LOS of patients with DRM, neither the average LOS (barely 6 days) of all patients from the Bern University Hospital nor the LOS (20 days) of the naturally detected patients in the study by Aeberhard et al. [1] can be considered representative. The expected LOS in patients with DRM (12 days) is plausible given that the average LOS of the target population is 10 days.

The costs of NS are very low compared with those of NI. The costs as well as the savings and the additional revenue are determined by the detection rate and the number of patients with DRM. Varying the assumptions relating to the detection rate will therefore result in a corresponding almost proportional variation in the difference between the costs and the savings and the additional revenue. This difference depends strongly on the assumptions regarding the savings and the additional revenue.

The projected savings are based on assumptions about the reduction of LOS due to NI. These are based on the results of meta-analyses, reviews and single studies. The literature is not consistent, but it shows evidence of or tendencies toward reduction of LOS, complication rates or rates of non-elective rehospitalizations [5,6,10–13]. However, for an economic assessment, available data on types and frequencies of avoided complications are not specific enough. Reductions in rehospitalizations are also difficult to evaluate because of varying follow-up periods. Therefore, it seems justified to use the reduction in LOS as a proxy for the many and various effects, with evidence of an improvement in clinical and economic outcomes due to NI.

For each one-day reduction in LOS, CHF 1371 was saved. This reflects the high costs associated with medical care in Switzerland and at university hospitals. A Danish study found the costs of outliers to be $224 per day in 2006. A Dutch study from the year 2005 estimated these costs at 476 €, and a US study reported costs of $1770 in 2018. The global average costs per hospital day at the Bern University Hospital amounted to CHF 2848 (information provided by the Federal Office of Public Health). So, valuing the LOS-dependent cost with per diem additional rates for DRG outliers seems justified.

The amount of additional revenues received is determined by the proportion of cases with DRG changes and the resulting increase in the average cost-weight in these cases. In the study by Aeberhard et al. [1], the proportion with changes in DRG attribution amounted to 8.3%. Compared with other studies in patients without NS, this is quite low. The average increase in the cost-weight was 0.694, a figure confirmed by other studies as well. In patients with NS, these numbers are not valid. The proportion of cases with changes in DRG attributions was assumed to be 15%. This is a conservative estimate and corresponds with the lower of two values from studies with NS (15% and 27%). The average increase in the cost-weight in these patients was lower, amounting to circa 0.44 in both studies, a figure, which was therefore applied in the current study.

7. Cost Effectiveness of Nutritional Therapy in the Post-Hospital or Community Setting: A Brief Statement

Prevalence of malnutrition has been studied less often in the community setting due to the lack of systematic or standardized screening programs, for example at healthcare institutions or in the offices of general practitioners. It is well established, however, that between 20% and 40% of patients admitted from the community setting to a hospital are already malnourished. Also, nutritional status frequently worsens during a hospital stay, which means that a large proportion of patients, particularly those older than 60 years, are discharged to a community setting or to other institutions with malnutrition. It is estimated that only around 10% of malnourished patients are in fact hospital patients, with the rest dwelling in a community or nursing home setting [23].

Few studies have addressed the costs of malnutrition and the economic impact of nutritional support in these settings [24]. Due to feasibility, the majority of studies investigating cost effectiveness of nutritional therapy are in-hospital analyses, but these only reflect a short period in terms of the patients' needs for nutritional therapy. Malnourished patients, particularly those who are old, frequently need continued nutritional support. This is a challenge for the analysis of cost effectiveness, as the costs of management in one setting may be offset by greater cost savings in another setting, such as when patients are moving from one care setting to another and a more comprehensive perspective is needed. Not surprisingly, nutritional therapy is frequently discontinued after a hospital stay. Most studies that have assessed cost effectiveness of NI in the community-dwelling population are initiated at hospital discharge [25–28]. These frequently use oral nutritional supplements and are carried out for 3–6 months after a hospital stay. Studies of community-dwelling or nursing home residents more frequently address further types of nutritional support, such as dietary counseling, snacks between meals, or multi-component nutritional support.

Table A5 (Appendix A) gives an overview of the type and design of studies investigating the cost effectiveness of nutritional support following hospital discharge in the community-dwelling elderly or in nursing home residents. Despite the different methodologies used, nutritional therapy was generally found to be cost effective, with the higher costs incurred by nutritional support being ultimately associated with decreased use of health care resources and improved quality of life.

8. Conclusions

This is the first study to compare the costs of a systematic NS and subsequent adequate NI, with the combined effects of savings due to reduced LOS and additional revenue resulting from SwissDRG changes. The costs of the intervention could be separately compensated for by savings in the costs of basic treatment and by the additional revenue generated. NS with subsequent adequate NI is thus associated with high economic potential for the hospital. Moreover, the EFFORT trial was able to demonstrate an impressive effect of NI, with a significant reduction in mortality and severe complications as well as improvement of physical function and quality of life in medical inpatients [11]. These clinical benefits, in terms of savings in supplemental hospital costs, were not included in the current economic impact analysis. If they had been, this would have greatly increased the financial efficacy.

Author Contributions: Conceptualization, E.R. and Z.S.; data analysis and curation, O.E. and A.F.; writing—original draft preparation, E.R. and K.N.; writing—review and editing, A.F. and O.E. and P.S. and Z.S.; supervision, Z.S.

Appendix A

Table A1. Patient flow and resource use in connection with ND.

Patients Flow and Performance	Proportion/Rate	Number
Target population	20,000	
	Proportion/Rate	*n*
Detection rate, of which:	6.4%	1280
proportion p DRM	0.25	320
proportion m DRM	0.75	960
Nutritional interventions		
	Proportion	*n*
ONS	59%	755
EN	29%	371
PN	12%	154
Saved hospital days	Per Patient	total
Reduction in LOS, days	1.2	1152
SwissDRG changes	Detected Cases	
	Proportion	*n*
Changes in DRG attribution	0.0833	107

DRM: disease-related malnutrition; p DRM: potential DRM; m DRM: manifest DRM; ONS: oral nutritional supplements; EN: enteral nutrition; PN: parenteral nutrition; LOS: length of hospital stay; DRG: diagnosis-related groups.

Table A2. Consequences of the costs of ND.

	Number	Value	Costs
Costs nutritional Interventions			
ONS	755	187.57	141,652
EN	371	842.96	312,906
PN	154	1557.84	239,284
Total costs	1280		693,842
Savings (reduction LOS) (−)	1152	1373.46	−1582,224
Additional revenue (SwissDRG) (−)	107	7564.70	−806,579
Net effect			−1,694,961

Costs are indicated with positive (+), savings and additional revenue with negative (−) prefix. DRM: disease-related malnutrition; p DRM: potential DRM; m DRM: manifest DRM; ONS: oral nutritional supplements; EN: enteral nutrition; PN: parenteral nutrition.

Table A3. Hours, workdays and positions needed for NI in the case of systematic NS, ND and additional needs for systematic NS.

	Nutritional Therapy	Nursing	Physician
	Systematic nutritional screening		
Hours total	6052	13,700	1210
Days total	721	1631	144
Positions needed	4.09	9.27	0.82
Natural Detection			
Hours total	1989	5327	398
Days total	237	634	47
Positions needed	1.35	3.60	0.27
	Additional needs for systematic nutritional screening		
Hours total	4063	8373	813
Days total	484	997	97
Positions needed	2.75	5.66	0.55

Table A4. Staff time per nutritional intervention and professional group.

		Dietician	Nursing Staff	Physician
ONS				
Duration of therapy, days	8.4			
Minutes/patient/day		10	10	2
Minutes/patient		84	84	16.8
N patients NS	2797			
Minutes for NS		234,976	234,976	46,995
N patients ND	755			
Minutes for ND		63,437	63,437	12,687
EN				
Duration of therapy, days	10.3			
Minutes/patient/day		10	40	2
Minutes/patient		103	412	20.6
N patients NS	851			
Minutes for NS		87,619	350,475	17,524
N patients ND	371			
Minutes for ND		38,234	152,934	7647
PN				
Duration of therapy, days	9.6			
Minutes/patient/day		12	70	2.4
Minutes/patient		115.2	672	23.04
N patients NS	352			
Minutes for NS		40,550	236,544	8110
N patients ND	154			
Minutes for ND		17,695	103,219	3539

DRM: disease-related malnutrition; p DRM: potential DRM; m DRM: manifest DRM; ONS: oral nutritional supplements; EN: enteral nutrition; PN: parenteral nutrition.

Table A5. Studies addressing the economic impact of nutritional support after hospital discharge in the community or nursing home setting.

Author	Population	Type of Study	Cost Analysis	Results
Nutritional Support After Hospital Discharge				
Author	**Population**	**Type of Study**	**Cost Analysis**	**Results**
Edington et al., 2004 [29] United Kingdom	mixed malnourished ≥ 65 y, (n = 100)	RCT intervention ONS for 8 weeks, 24 weeks follow-up	Cost-effectiveness analysis, direct and indirect costs	No difference regarding quality of life, post-hospital health care resource use or cost
Norman et al., 2011 [25] Germany	gastrointestinal disease, malnourished (n = 114)	RCT intervention Dietary counseling at discharge and high-protein ONS for months vs. dietary counseling at discharge	Cost-effectiveness analysis, direct costs of nutritional support	Intervention patients: increase in quality of life after 3 months ICER: EUR9497–12099/QALY
Neelemaat et al., 2012 [26] The Nederlands	mixed, malnourished ≥ 60 y (n = 210)	RCT: ONS, dietary counseling, vitamin D for 3 months after hospital discharge vs. usual care	Cost-effectiveness analysis, direct and indirect costs	No significant difference in QALYs at 3 months follow-up, intervention group: improvement in functional limitations, EUR618/functional limitation improvement (0.95 probability the intervention is cost effective)
Zhong et al., 2016 [27] United States of America	Mixed, malnourished ≥ 65 y (n = 622)	RCT: high-protein ONS, enriched b-hydroxy-b-methylbutyrate for 3 months after hospital discharge compared to placebo	Cost-effectiveness analysis, direct and indirect costs	Intervention group: increase in quality of life ICER: USD 33,818/QALY lifetime ICER: USD 524/LY
Nutritional support in the community or nursing home setting				
Author	Population	Type of study	Cost analysis	Results
Arnaud-Battandier et al., 2004 [30] France	Malnourished ≥ 70 y community or nursing home residents (n = 287)	prospective, cohort study of patients from 2 groups of physicians (high vs. low ONS prescription rate), 12-month follow-up	Comparison of direct costs	Higher costs of ONS in intervention group (EUR M, but lower costs of medical care: hospital admissions (EUR1631 vs. EUR 2203) and medical visits (EUR 299 vs. EUR 462)
Lorefält et al., 2011 [31] Sweden	nursing home residents, ≥ 65 y (n = 109)	Prospective cohort study of nutrition education and care (individualized meals) for 3 months	Comparison of direct costs	Higher costs in intervention group (EUR 830 vs. EUR 760 for nutritional support, EUR 652 vs. EUR 402 for education program)
Freijer et al., 2013 [32] The Nederlands	malnourished ≥ 65 y; community or nursing home residents (n = 720,223)	Health economic evaluation of published studies	Budget impact analysis	Annual cost savings of EUR 11.62 million due to intervention with ONS
Schilp et al., 2014 [28] The Nederlands	malnourished ≥ 65 y; community-dwelling old (n = 146)	RCT, dietary counseling vs. usual care	Cost-effectiveness analysis	No differences regarding gain in weight, QALY or costs
Simmons et al., 2015 [33] United States of America	Malnourished/at risk ≥ 65 y, nursing home residents (n = 154)	3-arm RCT: ONS vs. in-between snacks vs. usual care for 6 months	Cost-effectiveness analysis	No change in body weight, intervention costs per person per day; ONS group 2.54 and snack group 3.85; ICER: 103 kcal/USD in ONS group vs. 79 kcal/USD in snack group
van der Pols-Vijlbrief et al., 2017 [34] The Nederlands	community-dwelling older adults receiving home care with or at risk of malnutrition ≥65 y (n = 155)	RCT, multifactorial personalized intervention for 6 months	Cost-effectiveness analysis	No differences regarding gain in weight, functional status, QALY or costs
Elia et al., 2018 [35] United Kingdom	Malnourished, nursing home residents ≥65 y (n = 104)	RCT, comparing ONS versus dietary advice for 3 months	Cost effectiveness analysis with direct and indirect costs	Intervention group improved quality of life: ICER: GBP 10,961/QALY

ONS: oral nutritional supplements; QALY: quality of life adjusted life year; ICER: incremental cost-effectiveness ratio.

References

1. Aeberhard, C.; Abt, M.; Endrich, O.; Aubry, E.; Leuenberger, M.S.; Schütz, P.; Sterchi, A.B.; Stanga, Z. Auswirkung, der Kodierung der Mangelernährung im SwissDRGSystem. *Aktuell. Ernährungsmed.* **2018**, *43*, 92–100.
2. Aeberhard, C.; Birrenbach, T.; Joray, M.; Muhlebach, S.; Perrig, M.; Stanga, Z. Simple training tool is insufficient for appropriate diagnosis and treatment of malnutrition: A pre-post intervention study in a tertiary center. *Nutrition* **2016**, *32*, 355–361. [CrossRef] [PubMed]
3. Elia, M. The Cost of Malnutrition in England and Potential Cost Savings from Nutritional Interventions (short version). BAPEN. 2015. Available online: www.bapen.org.uk/pdfs/economic-report-short.pdf (accessed on 8 July 2019).
4. Imoberdorf, R.; Meier, R.; Krebs, P.; Hangartner, P.J.; Hess, B.; Staubli, M.; Wegmann, D.; Rühlin, M.; Ballmer, P.E. Prevalence of undernutrition on admission to Swiss hospitals. *Clin. Nutr.* **2010**, *29*, 38–41. [CrossRef] [PubMed]
5. Sriram, K.; Sulo, S.; VanDerBosch, G.; Partridge, J.; Feldstein, J.; Hegazi, R.A.; Summerfelt, W.T. A Comprehensive Nutrition-Focused Quality Improvement Program Reduces 30-Day Readmissions and Length of Stay in Hospitalized Patients. *JPEN J. Parenter. Enteral Nutr.* **2017**, *41*, 384–391. [CrossRef] [PubMed]
6. Bally, M.R.; Blaser Yildirim, P.Z.; Bounoure, L.; Gloy, V.L.; Mueller, B.; Briel, M.; Schuetz, P. Nutritional Support and Outcomes in Malnourished Medical Inpatients: A Systematic Review and Meta-analysis. *JAMA Int. Med.* **2016**, *176*, 43–53. [CrossRef] [PubMed]
7. Elia, M.; Normand, C.; Laviano, A.; Norman, K. A systematic review of the cost and cost effectiveness of using standard oral nutritional supplements in community and care home settings. *Clin. Nutr.* **2016**, *35*, 125–137. [CrossRef] [PubMed]
8. National Institute for Health and Care Excellence (NICE). Nutritional support for adults: oral nutrition support, enteral tube feeding and parenteral nutrition. Clinical Guideline 32, published February 2006m last modified August 2017. Available online: https://www.nice.org.uk/Guidance/CG32 (accessed on 8 July 2019).
9. Stratton, R.J.; Green, C.J.; Elia, M. *Disease-Related Malnutrition: An Evidence-Based Approach to Treatment*; CABI: Wallingford, UK, 2003; pp. 1128–1129.
10. Stratton, R.J.; Hebuterne, X.; Elia, M. A systematic review and meta-analysis of the impact of oral nutritional supplements on hospital readmissions. *Ageing Res. Rev.* **2013**, *12*, 884–897. [CrossRef]
11. Schuetz, P.; Fehr, R.; Baechli, V.; Geiser, M.; Deiss, M.; Gomes, F.; Bilz, S.; Sigrist, S.; Brändle, M.; Benz, C.; et al. Individualised nutritional support in medical inpatients at nutritional risk: A randomised clinical trial. *Lancet* **2019**, *393*, 8–14. [CrossRef]
12. Deutz, N.E.; Matheson, E.M.; Matarese, L.E.; Luo, M.; Baggs, G.E.; Nelson, J.L.; Hegazi, R.A.; Tappenden, K.A.; Ziegler, T.R. NOURISH Study Group. Readmission and mortality in malnourished, older, hospitalized adults treated with a specialized oral nutritional supplement: A randomized clinical trial. *Clin. Nutr.* **2016**, *35*, 18–26. [CrossRef]
13. Muscaritoli, M.; Krznaric, Z.; Singer, P.; Barazzoni, R.; Cederholm, T.; Golay, A.; Van Gossum, A.; Kennedy, N.; Kreymann, G.; Laviano, A.; et al. Effectiveness and efficacy of nutritional therapy: A systematic review following Cochrane methodology. *Clin. Nutr.* **2017**, *36*, 939–957. [CrossRef]
14. Voltz, C.; Seegler, S.; Keil, J.-P.; Fleßa, S. Malnutrition in Hospital Care – Potential Revenues of Nutrition. *Aktuelle Ernährungsmedizin.* **2016**, *41*, 187–189.
15. Vonzun, N.; Sterchi, A.-B.; Imoberdorf, R.; Rühlin, M. Malnutrition and DRG—The Swiss Solution. *Aktuell. Ernährungsmed.* **2014**, *39*, 392–396.
16. Ockenga, J.; Freudenreich, M.; Zakonsky, R.; Norman, K.; Pirlich, M.; Lochs, H. Nutritional assessment and management in hospitalised patients: Implication for DRG-based reimbursement and health care quality. *Clin. Nutr.* **2005**, *24*, 913–919. [CrossRef]
17. Reinbold, T.; Broß, I.; Lenfers, B. Malnutrition in the G-DRG-System—Effects of a Structured Nutritional Management on Codification and Revenues. *Aktuell. Ernährungsmed.* **2013**, *38*, 24–29.
18. Kondrup, J.; Rasmussen, H.H.; Hamberg, O.; Stanga, Z. Nutritional risk screening (NRS 2002): A new method based on an analysis of controlled clinical trials. *Clin. Nutr.* **2003**, *22*, 321–336. [CrossRef]

19. Wenger, C.; Hischier, T.; Rhyner, A.; Iff, S.; Sterchi, A.-B.; Stanga, Z. Introduction of Malnutrition Management on two Specialized University Clinics. *Aktuell. Ernährungsmed.* **2008**, *33*, 296–301. [CrossRef]
20. Kruizenga, H.M.; Van Tulder, M.W.; Seidell, J.C.; Thijs, A.; Ader, H.J.; Van Bokhorst-de van der Schueren, M.A. Effectiveness and cost-effectiveness of early screening and treatment of malnourished patients. *Am. J. Clin. Nutr.* **2005**, *82*, 1082–1089. [CrossRef]
21. Holyday, M.; Daniells, S.; Bare, M.; Caplan, G.A.; Petocz, P.; Bolin, T. Malnutrition screening and early nutrition intervention in hospitalised patients in acute aged care: A randomised controlled trial. *J. Nutr. Health Aging* **2012**, *16*, 562–568. [CrossRef] [PubMed]
22. Somanchi, M.; Tao, X.; Mullin, G.E. The facilitated early enteral and dietary management effectiveness trial in hospitalized patients with malnutrition. *JPEN J. Parenter. Enteral Nutr.* **2011**, *35*, 209–216. [CrossRef] [PubMed]
23. Elia, M.; Russell, C. *Combating Malnutrition: Recommendations for Action*; Nutrition Advisory Group on Malnutrition Led by BAPEN 2009; BAPEN: Redditch, UK, 2009.
24. Abizanda, P.; Sinclair, A.; Barcons, N.; Lizan, L.; Rodriguez-Manas, L. Costs of Malnutrition in Institutionalized and Community-Dwelling Older Adults: A Systematic Review. *J. Am. Med. Dir. Assoc.* **2016**, *17*, 17–23. [CrossRef] [PubMed]
25. Norman, K.; Pirlich, M.; Smoliner, C.; Kilbert, A.; Schulzke, J.D.; Ockenga, J.; Lochs, H.; Reinhold, T. Cost-effectiveness of a 3-month intervention with oral nutritional supplements in disease-related malnutrition: A randomised controlled pilot study. *Eur. J. Clin. Nutr.* **2011**, *65*, 735–742. [CrossRef] [PubMed]
26. Neelemaat, F.; Bosmans, J.E.; Thijs, A.; Seidell, J.C.; van Bokhorst-de van der Schueren, M.A. Oral nutritional support in malnourished elderly decreases functional limitations with no extra costs. *Clin. Nutr.* **2012**, *31*, 183–190. [CrossRef] [PubMed]
27. Zhong, Y.; Cohen, J.T.; Goates, S.; Luo, M.; Nelson, J.; Neumann, P.J. The Cost-Effectiveness of Oral Nutrition Supplementation for Malnourished Older Hospital Patients. *Appl. Health Econ. Health Policy.* **2017**, *15*, 75–83. [CrossRef] [PubMed]
28. Schilp, J.; Bosmans, J.E.; Kruizenga, H.M.; Wijnhoven, H.A.H.; Visser, M. Is dietetic treatment for undernutrition in older individuals in primary care cost-effective? *J. Am. Med. Dir. Assoc.* **2014**, *15*, 226.e7–226.e13. [CrossRef] [PubMed]
29. Edington, J.; Barnes, R.; Bryan, F.; Dupree, E.; Frost, G.; Hickson, M.; Lancaster, J.; Mongia, S.; Smith, J.; Torrance, A.; et al. A prospective randomised controlled trial of nutritional supplementation in malnourished elderly in the community: Clinical and health economic outcomes. *Clin. Nutr.* **2004**, *23*, 195–204. [CrossRef]
30. Arnaud-Battandier, F.; Malvy, D.; Jeandel, C.; Schmitt, C.; Aussage, P.; Beaufrere, B.; Cynober, L. Use of oral supplements in malnourished elderly patients living in the community: A pharmaco-economic study. *Clin. Nutr.* **2004**, *23*, 1096–1103. [CrossRef] [PubMed]
31. Lorefalt, B.; Andersson, A.; Wirehn, A.B.; Wilhelmsson, S. Nutritional status and health care costs for the elderly living in municipal residential homes–an intervention study. *J. Nutr. Health Aging* **2011**, *15*, 92–97. [CrossRef] [PubMed]
32. Freijer, K.; Nuijten, M.J.; Schols, J.M. The budget impact of oral nutritional supplements for disease related malnutrition in elderly in the community setting. *Front. Pharmacol.* **2012**, *3*, F78. [CrossRef] [PubMed]
33. Simmons, S.F.; Keeler, E.; An, R.; Liu, X.; Shotwell, M.S.; Kuertz, B.; Silver, H.J.; Schnelle, J.F. Cost-Effectiveness of Nutrition Intervention in Long-Term Care. *J. Am. Geriatr. Soc.* **2015**, *63*, 2308–2316. [CrossRef] [PubMed]
34. van der Pols-Vijlbrief, R.; Wijnhoven, H.A.H.; Bosmans, J.E.; Twisk, J.W.R.; Visser, M. Targeting the underlying causes of undernutrition. Cost-effectiveness of a multifactorial personalized intervention in community-dwelling older adults: A randomized controlled trial. *Clin. Nutr.* **2017**, *36*, 1498–1508. [CrossRef] [PubMed]
35. Elia, M.; Parsons, E.L.; Cawood, A.L.; Smith, T.R.; Stratton, R.J. Cost-effectiveness of oral nutritional supplements in older malnourished care home residents. *Clin. Nutr.* **2018**, *37*, 651–658. [CrossRef] [PubMed]

10

Early Supplemental Parenteral Nutrition in Critically Ill Children

An Jacobs, Ines Verlinden, Ilse Vanhorebeek and Greet Van den Berghe *

Clinical Division and Laboratory of Intensive Care Medicine, Department of Cellular and Molecular Medicine, KU Leuven University Hospital, 3000 Leuven, Belgium; an.jacobs@kuleuven.be (A.J.); ines.verlinden@kuleuven.be (I.V.); ilse.vanhorebeek@kuleuven.be (I.V.)

* Correspondence: greet.vandenberghe@kuleuven.be

Abstract: In critically ill children admitted to pediatric intensive care units (PICUs), enteral nutrition (EN) is often delayed due to gastrointestinal dysfunction or interrupted. Since a macronutrient deficit in these patients has been associated with adverse outcomes in observational studies, supplemental parenteral nutrition (PN) in PICUs has long been widely advised to meeting nutritional requirements. However, uncertainty of timing of initiation, optimal dose and composition of PN has led to a wide variation in previous guidelines and current clinical practices. The PEPaNIC (Early versus Late Parenteral Nutrition in the Pediatric ICU) randomized controlled trial recently showed that withholding PN in the first week in PICUs reduced incidence of new infections and accelerated recovery as compared with providing supplemental PN early (within 24 h after PICU admission), irrespective of diagnosis, severity of illness, risk of malnutrition or age. The early withholding of amino acids in particular, which are powerful suppressors of intracellular quality control by autophagy, statistically explained this outcome benefit. Importantly, two years after PICU admission, not providing supplemental PN early in PICUs did not negatively affect mortality, growth or health status, and significantly improved neurocognitive development. These findings have an important impact on the recently issued guidelines for PN administration to critically ill children. In this review, we summarize the most recent literature that provides evidence on the implications for clinical practice with regard to the use of early supplemental PN in critically ill children.

Keywords: Pediatric Intensive Care Unit; enteral nutrition; early parenteral nutrition; critical illness

---

1. Introduction

Optimal nutritional support is considered of paramount importance for critically ill children admitted to the pediatric intensive care unit (PICU), since malnutrition and inadequate nutrient delivery have been associated with worse clinical outcome [1,2]. Moreover, critically ill children have limited macronutrient stores and relatively higher energy requirements than adults admitted to the intensive care unit (ICU), which can lead to substantial caloric and macronutrient deficits [2–4]. The feeding is thought to attenuate the metabolic stress response, prevent oxidative cellular injury and modulate immune responses, and has led to a shift from nutritional support as adjunctive care to actual therapy of the critically ill child [5]. The enteral route is preferred for providing nutrition [5]. However, critically ill children are often too ill to be fed normally by mouth, and nasogastric or nasoduodenal tube feeding is often not tolerated because of gastric dysmotility or ileus. Interruption of enteral feeding also occurs frequently for various reasons, like medical or surgical contraindications, or radiology, bedside or surgical procedures [6]. Therefore, parenteral nutrition (PN) is often initiated to supplement the insufficient enteral intake. Nonetheless, official guidelines on timing and thresholds of initiation, composition and doses of supplemental PN vary widely [5,7–9]. Moreover, concerns about overfeeding have led to even more uncertainty [9]. A recent survey showed significant differences in nutritional practices in PICUs worldwide, in terms of macronutrient goals, estimation of energy requirements, timing of nutrient delivery and thresholds for starting supplemental PN [10]. In this review, we summarize the most recent literature findings affecting evidence and clinical practices with regard to the use of early PN in critically ill children. We searched PubMed up to April 2019, without language restrictions, using different combinations of the search terms "parenteral nutrition", "PICU", "early" and "pediatric critical illness". We focused on publications of the last eight years, discussed in the context of earlier work.

2. Timing of PN Initiation

Several observational studies have shown that malnutrition is associated with worse clinical outcome [1,2,11]. A macronutrient deficit has been associated with infections, weakness, prolonged mechanical ventilation and delayed recovery. For that reason, guidelines used to recommend that when provision of enteral nutrition (EN) is insufficient, impossible or contraindicated, supplemental PN should be initiated [7,12,13]. However, observational studies cannot assign causality to an association. Hence, the association between inadequate nutrition and worse clinical outcome might merely exist because of a non-optimal nutritional support for the sickest children, which are at the highest risk of adverse outcome. Although it seems intuitive that providing early nutrition will be beneficial, it does not necessarily mean that nutritional support in the early phase of critical illness will improve clinical outcome [9]. In critically ill adults, the large multicenter EPaNIC (Early versus Late Parenteral Nutrition in ICU, $n = 4640$) randomized controlled trial (RCT) showed that withholding supplemental PN until day eight of an ICU stay (late PN), and thus accepting a substantial macronutrient deficit, was associated with fewer ICU infections, a shorter duration of mechanical ventilation and renal-replacement therapy and a shorter ICU and total hospital stay as compared with initiating supplemental PN early (within 48 h after ICU admission) [14]. Data generated by the broad international yearly survey of clinical nutrition practices "nutritionDay" revealed an important change in the pattern of PN prescription after publication of the EPaNIC results (Personal communication kindly shared by Prof. Dr. M. Hiesmayr, nutritionDay Project Leader). As compared with adults, critically ill children have limited stores of energy, fat and protein, as well as relatively higher energy requirements [2,3]. Since this makes them more vulnerable to a substantial caloric and macronutrient deficit, the effect of withholding supplemental PN in critically ill children could be different than in adults. Therefore, a multicenter PEPaNIC RCT (Early versus Late Parenteral Nutrition in the Pediatric ICU) was conducted [15] that investigated the same intervention in 1440 critically ill children aged 0–17 years in three PICUs in Belgium, the Netherlands and Canada. Withholding supplemental PN during the first week in critically ill children resulted in fewer new infections, a shorter dependency on mechanical ventilation and general intensive care and a shorter hospital stay as compared with providing PN early (within 24 h after PICU admission; see Figure 1). The clinical superiority of late PN was more pronounced in children than it was in adults, and was shown irrespective of diagnosis, severity of illness, risk of malnutrition or age of the child [15]. This last finding was surprising, since neonates are more susceptible to macronutrient deficits than older children [7], raising concerns by experts [16–18]. To address these concerns, a secondary analysis of the PEPaNIC trial was performed to investigate the effects of withholding PN for one week in 209 critically ill neonates who did not (or could hardly) tolerate EN [19]. Analyses were performed for term neonates aged up to four weeks, up to one week and younger than one day. Late PN resulted in fewer nosocomial infections in neonates aged up to one week and younger than one day, and in shorter dependency on intensive care and mechanical ventilation for all studied age groups of neonates. Hence, term neonates also benefited from withholding PN during the first week in the PICU, which is in agreement with findings for older children and adults [14,15]. Moreover, there was a more pronounced benefit of late PN in the youngest children, as shown in Figure 1. Since a macronutrient deficiency is presumed to be more detrimental during acute illness in undernourished children [5], a second subanalysis of the PEPaNIC RCT was performed, investigating the effects of withholding supplemental PN during the first PICU week in a subgroup of critically ill children who were undernourished upon admission to the PICU [20]. Undernourishment was defined as a weight-for-age z score lower than −2 in children younger than one year, and a body mass index-for-age z score lower than −2 in children one year or older. This identified 289 of 1440 PEPaNIC patients (20%) with undernourishment upon PICU admission. Among the undernourished patients, late PN reduced the absolute risk of new infections and shortened the duration of PICU stay. These effect sizes of late PN were even larger than in the main trial cohort of the PEPaNIC RCT. Late PN did not affect the safety outcomes of mortality, incidence of hypoglycemia or weight deterioration during PICU stay in the undernourished patients. A larger longitudinal study of all PEPaNIC patients with weight z scores available on admission and on the last day in the PICU showed that weight deterioration during PICU stay was associated with worse clinical outcomes, but that withholding supplemental PN during the first week did not alter weight z score deterioration during the PICU stay [21].

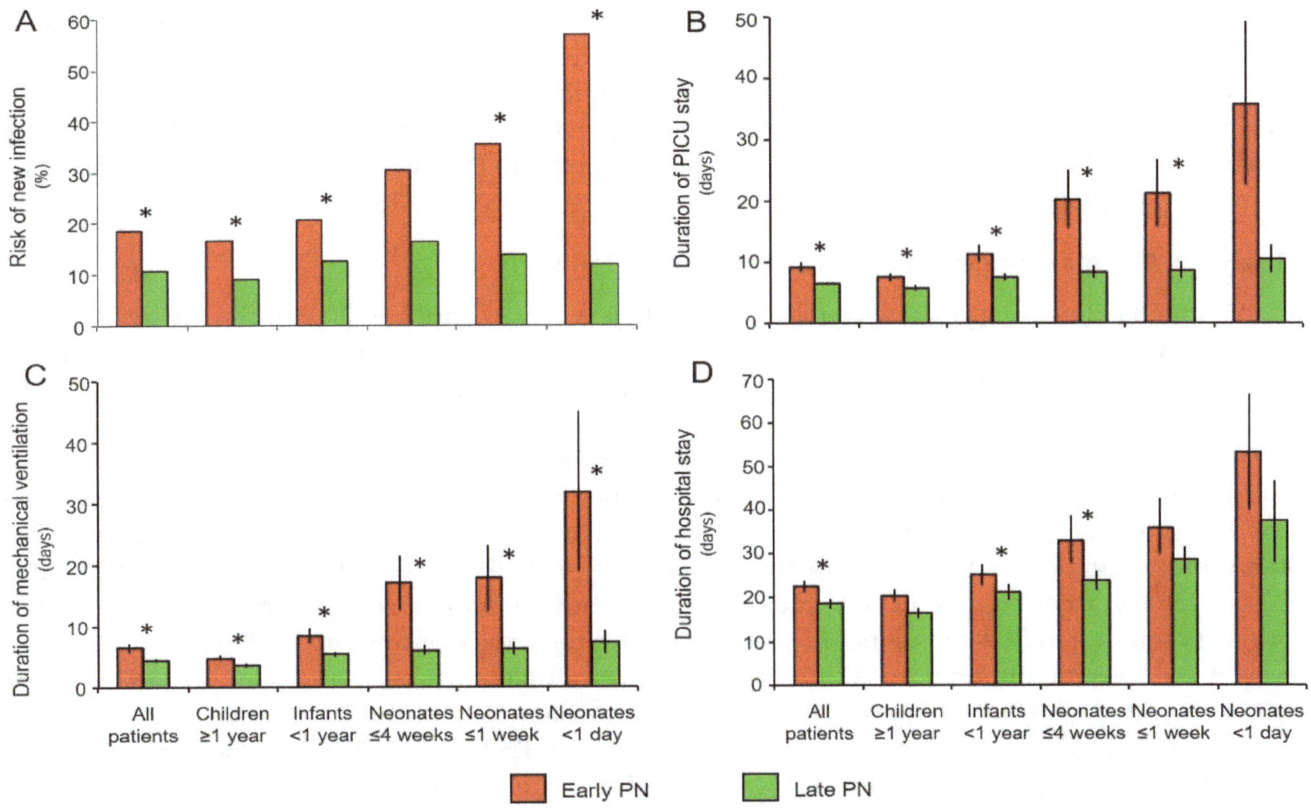

Figure 1. Bars represent incidence of (**A**) the risk of acquiring a new infection in PICUs (percentage), (**B**) duration (days) of PICU stay, (**C**) duration (days) of mechanical ventilation, and (**D**) duration (days) of total hospital stay. Whiskers indicate standard errors of the mean. Asterisks represent p values < 0.05 obtained with multivariable analysis adjusting for baseline risk factors (treatment center, age, risk of malnutrition (STRONGkids score), diagnosis upon admission and severity of illness (Pediatric Logistic Organ Dysfunction (PeLOD) score, and Pediatric Risk of Mortality 2 (PIM2) score) for all patients; treatment center, risk of malnutrition, diagnosis upon admission and severity of illness for children and infants; and treatment center, type of illness upon admission (medical, surgical cardiac, surgical other), severity of illness and weight for age z score for neonates).

The benefits of withholding supplemental PN during the first week in the PICU appeared not only present from a clinical point of view, but also from a health–economic perspective. A cost-effectiveness study indeed showed that the total direct medical costs were considerably lower with late PN as compared with early supplemental PN initiation [22]. This cost saving was beyond the expected lower costs for the use of PN itself, since avoidance of new infections by late PN yielded the largest cost reduction.

A possible limitation of the PEPaNIC RCT is the use of standard equations for the estimation of energy requirements instead of indirect calorimetry [23]. However, the use of indirect calorimetry for estimating energy expenditure does not seem to be accurate [24], or feasible [25], and is not frequently used in daily practice [10,26].

Apart from the PEPaNIC RCT, no other randomized controlled trial investigating the use or timing of supplemental PN in critically ill children has been published in the last eight years. A limited number of observational studies on the use of supplemental PN and over- and underfeeding in PICUs showed different results [2,24,27]. A retrospective single center study showed that late initiation of supplemental PN was associated with a higher nosocomial infection rate as compared with early initiation of supplemental PN [27]. In contrast, an observational study in 31 PICUs showed that the use of PN in general was associated with higher mortality [2]. Another retrospective study determining the incidence of over- and underfeeding in 139 children admitted to a tertiary PICU showed that underfeeding was associated with shorter durations of PICU and hospital stays, as well as with fewer ventilation days, as compared with appropriately fed and overfed patients [24]. However, the observational design of these studies holds a risk of bias by confounding variables, especially in nutritional research [28]. Therefore, comparison with the results of the PEPaNIC RCT is challenging. Further randomized controlled trials are warranted to determine the ideal time point for initiation of supplemental PN in PICUs.

3. Early PN Composition and the Role of Macronutrients

Although extensive guidelines on the composition of PN in critically ill children are available [5], a recent survey on nutritional practices in PICUs worldwide showed a wide variation in parenterally administered doses of protein, lipids and glucose [10]. Protein targets in particular seem to be a point of discussion. Several studies have assessed the association between protein delivery to and clinical outcome of critically ill children [2,29,30]. In an observational international cohort study that included 500 critically ill children, mortality at 60 days was higher in patients who received PN independently of the amount of energy or protein intake [2]. However, an important severity of illness bias has to be taken into account, since patients who are less sick are more likely to better tolerate EN. The study adjusted for severity of illness using admission scores, but data for calculating this severity of illness score were missing in 31% of the included patients, and the choice of severity of illness score differed between the participating centers [2]. Another large multicenter observational study of the same group showed an association between higher enteral protein intake and lower odds of mortality in more than 1200 mechanically ventilated critically ill children [29]. The effect was dose-dependent, and independent of energy intake. Again, the incomplete datasets and the lack of uniform usage for severity of illness scores, and the substantial number of patients who received EN, could potentially bias these observations. The authors reasoned that an increased demand in amino acids in catabolic disease, such as critical illness, could contribute to increased higher protein degradation from muscle to ensure bodily functions [29], which is associated with poor outcome [31]. By providing proteins, the synthesis of muscle proteins might be boosted, and thereby muscle loss could be prevented, possibly limiting the severity of intensive care unit-acquired weakness [32]. Nevertheless, a preplanned secondary analysis of the adult EPaNIC study did not support this concept, as increased macronutrient intake with early PN, including more amino acids, did not counteract muscle atrophy and actually increased the risk of developing clinically relevant muscle weakness in the ICU [33]. Interestingly, in a preplanned secondary analysis of the PEPaNIC RCT, the dose of amino acids was actually associated with more infections and a longer dependency on mechanical ventilation and other intensive medical care in children admitted to the PICU [30]. This risk of harm associated with early amino acid administration was elevated even at low doses of administered amino acids. A possible explanation for the difference between these results and the ones from the previously cited observational studies is the randomized design of the PEPaNIC trial, in which the doses of macronutrients differed from patient to patient and ranged widely [30]. In critically ill adults, three RCTs could not show benefits from early amino acid supplementation [34–37], but clinical trials on the effects of amino acid administration on clinical outcome in critically ill children in a randomized manner are lacking [38]. In contrast with the harm of amino acid administration, the secondary analysis of the PEPaNIC RCT suggested a benefit of glucose and lipid administration. Indeed, administering more glucose during the first three days of PICU stay was independently associated with fewer infections, and administering more lipids was independently associated with earlier PICU discharge [30]. Clearly, large-scale prospective RCTs in critically ill children are needed to identify the optimal composition of supplemental PN [9,38].

4. Impact of Early PN on Long-Term Outcome

Because of new insights in diagnostic and therapeutic measures in the field of pediatric critical care medicine [39], centralization of care [40] and specialized staff training and education [41,42], there has been an important decline in the mortality rate in PICUs over the last decades [43,44]. However, this improved survival has led towards a shift to considerable long-term morbidity, years after discharge [45,46]. This has been most thoroughly documented in regards to impairment of neurocognitive development, but it also includes growth retardation and may comprise poor physical functioning and reduced quality of life [47–50]. The fact that children are treated in the PICU during crucial developmental phases likely plays a role. Interestingly, it appears that, to a certain extent, neurocognitive outcome is modifiable, as shown by the attenuation of neurocognitive impairment with the prevention of hyperglycemia during intensive care [51]. Treatments in PICUs that have been shown to cause neurodevelopmental harm, such as anesthetic and analgesic agents [52,53] and toxicants such as phthalates that leach from indwelling medical devices [54], may also be targets for research into safer alternatives. Concerning nutrition in PICUs, in relation to long-term outcome, experts were concerned about the safety of withholding early supplemental PN in neonates in view of the more frequent episodes of hypoglycemia observed in the late PN arm of the PEPaNIC RCT [15,17]. However, in a previous large randomized controlled trial investigating the effect of tight glycemic control on morbidity and mortality in PICUs and on long-term neurocognitive development, a high incidence of brief hypoglycemia with tight glycemic control was not associated with harm to neurocognitive development, as documented four years later [51]. The proportion of neonates included in the PEPaNIC RCT was similar to that in the tight glycemic control trial [15,55]. In a preplanned two-year follow-up study, in which all patients included in the PEPaNIC RCT were approached for possible assessment of physical and neurocognitive development, exposure to hypoglycemia also did not associate with the investigated long-term outcomes [53]. Moreover, the main results of this follow-up study showed no adverse effects of withholding supplemental PN during the first week in PICUs on survival, anthropometrics, health status and neurocognitive development. In fact, omitting early supplemental PN in PICUs improved parent-reported executive functioning (inhibition, working memory, metacognition and overall executive functioning), externalizing behavioral problems and visual-motor integration two years later, as compared with early supplemental PN. In particular, a better inhibitory control was observed (Figure 2). Since poor inhibitory control in children contributes to impulsive and destructive behaviors that upset or harm others [56], delaying supplemental PN can have important consequences on daily life and social environments later in life. The long-term effects of late versus early supplemental PN were more pronounced in patients who were younger than one year of age at the time of PICU admission as compared with older children. This age-dependent vulnerability supports the hypothesis that the harm induced by early supplemental PN might be caused by a direct metabolic insult to the developing brain, since it was not statistically explained by the acute effects of the intervention itself, such as the increased incidence of new infections or delayed recovery. However, further research is warranted to unravel the underlying mechanisms that would provide support for this hypothesis. Although long-term outcomes and quality-of-life years after PICU discharge have gained great importance in research [45,46], investigating these outcomes is logistically challenging, expensive and time-consuming. To investigate whether these long-term effects persist or change over time, a four-year follow-up study of the PEPaNIC RCT is currently ongoing, of which the results are expected by 2020.

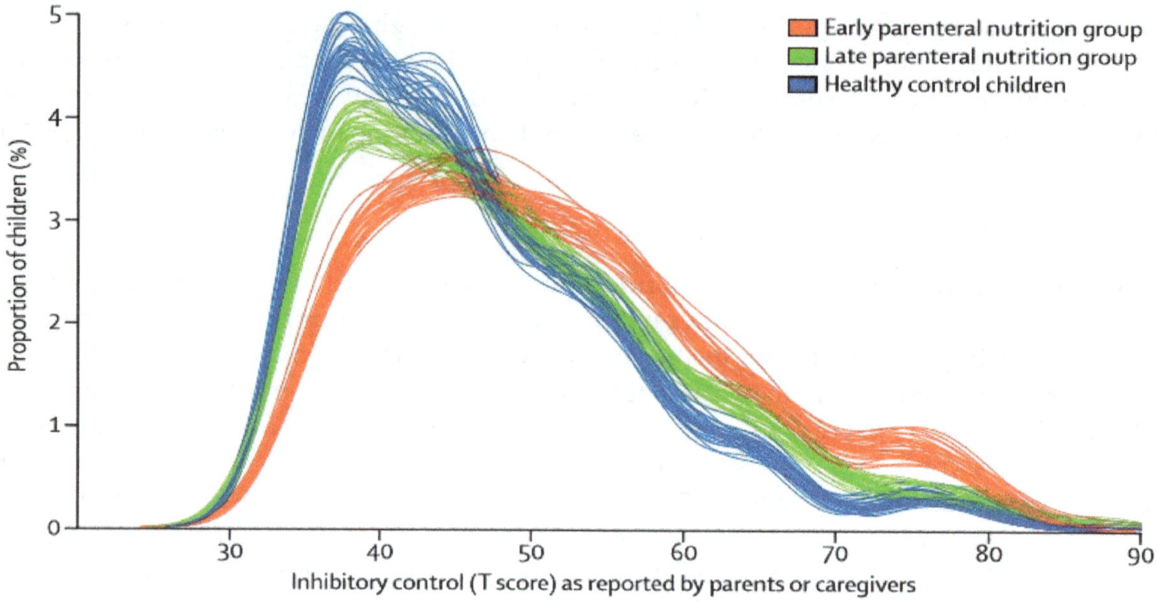

Figure 2. Density estimates for inhibitory function as reported by parents or caregivers. Densities, which correspond to the proportions of children with a certain score (equivalent to a smoothed histogram), are shown separately for healthy control children and for PEPaNIC participants who were randomly assigned to receive late PN or early PN. Higher scores indicate worse functioning. Each line corresponds to one of 31 imputed datasets. Figure reprinted from [53] with permission from Elsevier.

5. Potential Mechanisms Underlying Harm by Early PN

Several mechanisms may contribute to an adverse clinical impact of administering PN in the early phase of critical illness in children. As early PN has affected both short-term and long-term outcomes of patients, carryover effects persisting in the long term must play a role.

5.1. Potential Mechanisms Underlying the Adverse Impact of Early PN on Short-Term Outcome

As discussed, it was the administration of more amino acids that was associated with adverse short-term outcomes evoked by early PN in the PEPaNIC study [30]. The mechanisms underlying the potential harm of amino acids in this context remain to be unraveled, but it is possible to speculate. First, amino acids are powerful suppressors of autophagy [57], a pathway shown to be crucial in critically ill humans and animals for innate immunity and the removal of cellular damage [58,59]. Autophagy activation appeared suppressed in muscle from randomized adult patients exposed to early PN as compared with late PN in the EPaNIC trial, and amino acids in particular suppressed autophagy activation in a rabbit model of prolonged critical illness [33,58,59]. Second, macronutrients and amino acids in particular have long been assumed to counteract the hypercatabolic response to critical illness, which mobilizes amino acids by (mainly muscle) protein breakdown to guarantee substrate delivery to vital tissues [60]. More specifically, administration of exogenous amino acids was thought to circumvent the need for endogenous amino acid release and to stimulate muscle protein synthesis. However, once amino acid doses exceed anabolic capacity, they no longer stimulate muscle protein synthesis but are shuttled towards the liver for production of urea [61]. Such increased plasma urea concentrations were observed in early PN patients in the PEPaNIC RCT as compared with late PN patients [15]. In critically ill adults who received early PN, the administered amino acids did not counteract muscle wasting [33], but increased plasma urea and urinary nitrogen excretion (with a net waste of 63% of the extra nitrogen intake from early PN in the first two weeks) [62], which can cause harm to both liver and kidney. These results are in line with the EAT-ICU trial (Early goal-directed nutrition in ICU patients) results, in which increased urea production—but no beneficial effect on outcome—was seen with early goal-directed nutrition versus standard nutritional care in critically ill adults [63]. Altogether, these findings suggest that muscle wasting during the acute phase of critical illness may be considered an adaptive response designed to provide substrates for gluconeogenesis in order to meet the energy requirements of vital organs [32].

5.2. Potential Mechanisms Underlying the Adverse Impact of Early PN on Long-Term Outcome

Underlying mechanisms of the long-term harm caused by early PN in the context of critical illness remain largely unraveled. The clinical benefits of late PN observed far beyond the intervention window suggests that early PN induces carry-over "memory" effects with a negative impact on long-term outcome. Poor long-term outcomes in other conditions have been related to accelerated telomere shortening and the induction of aberrant so-called "epigenetic" changes. Importantly, inadequate nutrition may cause both adverse effects. Hence, these processes may also play a role in the developmental impairment of critically ill children and the adverse impact of early PN on neurocognitive development.

Telomeres are nucleoprotein complexes at the end of human chromosomes that shorten with each cell cycle. Telomere shortening can be accelerated by environmental and lifestyle factors [64,65], including excessive food consumption and/or unhealthy nutrition [66,67]. It has been demonstrated that critically ill children enter the PICU with significantly shorter leukocyte telomeres than matched healthy children [68]. More importantly, early PN had a telomere-shortening effect as compared with late PN in critically ill children between PICU admission and discharge, independent of baseline risk factors and post-randomization factors. Whether this accelerated telomere shortening contributes to long-term developmental impairment, and particularly the neurocognitive impairment caused by early PN, remains to be investigated.

The involvement of aberrant epigenetic changes in long-term consequences after acute events in life appears plausible. Epigenetics refers to the study of heritable changes in gene expression that do not involve changes in the underlying DNA sequence. Epigenetic changes play an important role in physical and neurocognitive development [69–72]. The most stable epigenetic change is the methylation or de-methylation of DNA. This is the attachment to or removal of a methyl group from a nucleotide, which occurs almost exclusively at the 5′ carbon in the cytosine residue of a CpG dinucleotide [69,70]. Alterations in DNA methylation have been implicated in the adverse effects of various environmental stressors, such as inadequate nutrition (both undernutrition and overfeeding), that have been shown to impact long-term health and disease [73]. Particularly during early life, DNA methylation changes may bring about long-term effects [71,72,74]. Data are needed on whether nutritional management in the early phase of critical illness induces aberrant changes in DNA methylation, which could explain the adverse impact of early PN on neurocognitive development.

6. Conclusions and Newest Guidelines

Nutritional support is considered to be an important aspect of patient care in PICUs [26], with large differences in PICUs worldwide regarding practices of supplemental PN for patients in whom EN as the preferred route is insufficient or impossible [5,10]. A large multicenter RCT showed that withholding supplemental PN throughout the first week in the PICU was clinically superior for short-term outcome as compared with initiating supplemental PN within 24 h after admission [19]. This was the case independent of age [19] or nutritional status [20]. The administered amino acids in particular appeared to explain the adverse impact of early provision of PN, possibly via suppression of required autophagy activation and the shuttling of amino acids to urea production with harmful effects to the liver and kidney. In the long-term, omitting PN during the first week of pediatric critical illness did not show harm, and actually improved executive functioning, behavioral problems and visual-motor integration, as compared with administering PN early. These findings had an important impact on recent ESPGHAN (European Society for Pediatric Gastroenterology Hepatology and Nutrition) pediatric PN guidelines [60], in which it is advised to consider withholding PN, including amino acids, for one week in critically ill infants, children and adolescents. However, the lack of other RCTs in this specific field makes it challenging to compare these findings with other available recent studies. Further research, in the form of multicenter RCTs, is warranted to determine the optimal composition and ideal timing of initiation of supplemental PN in critically ill children.

Author Contributions: A.J., I.V. (Ilse Vanhorebeek) and G.V.d.B. were responsible for the design of the review article. A.J. performed comprehensive literature search. A.J., I.V. (Ines Verlinden) and I.V. (Ilse Vanhorebeek) wrote the article. G.V.d.B. revised it carefully and gave a significant scientific contribution to its content.

References

1. Pollack, M.M.; Ruttimann, U.E.; Wiley, J.S. Nutritional depletions in critically ill children: Associations with physiologic instability and increased quantity of care. *JPEN J. Parenter. Enter. Nutr.* **1985**, *9*, 309–313. [CrossRef] [PubMed]
2. Mehta, N.M.; Bechard, L.J.; Cahill, N.; Wang, M.; Day, A.; Duggan, C.P.; Heyland, D.K. Nutritional practices and their relationship to clinical outcomes in critically ill children–An international multicenter cohort study. *Crit. Care Med.* **2012**, *40*, 2204–2211. [CrossRef] [PubMed]
3. Oosterveld, M.J.; Van Der Kuip, M.; De Meer, K.; De Greef, H.J.; Gemke, R.J. Energy expenditure and balance following pediatric intensive care unit admission: A longitudinal study of critically ill children. *Pediatr. Crit. Care Med.* **2006**, *7*, 147–153. [CrossRef] [PubMed]
4. Joosten, K.F.; Kerklaan, D.; Verbruggen, S.C. Nutritional support and the role of the stress response in critically ill children. *Curr. Opin. Clin. Nutr. Metab. Care* **2016**, *19*, 226–233. [CrossRef] [PubMed]
5. Mehta, N.M.; Skillman, H.E.; Irving, S.Y.; Coss-Bu, J.A.; Vermilyea, S.; Farrington, E.A.; McKeever, L.; Hall, A.M.; Goday, P.S.; Braunschweig, C. Guidelines for the provision and assessment of nutrition support therapy in the pediatric critically Ill patient: Society of critical care medicine and american society for parenteral and enteral nutrition. *Pediatr. Crit. Care Med.* **2017**, *18*, 675–715. [CrossRef] [PubMed]
6. Mehta, N.M.; McAleer, D.; Hamilton, S.; Naples, E.; Leavitt, K.; Mitchell, P.; Duggan, C. Challenges to optimal enteral nutrition in a multidisciplinary pediatric intensive care unit. *JPEN J. Parenter. Enter. Nutr.* **2010**, *34*, 38–45. [CrossRef] [PubMed]
7. Koletzko, B.; Goulet, O.; Hunt, J.; Krohn, K.; Shamir, R.; Parenteral Nutrition Guidelines Working Group; European Society for Clinical Nutrition and Metabolism; European Society of Paediatric Gastroenterology, Hepatology and Nutrition. 1. guidelines on paediatric parenteral nutrition of the European Society of Paediatric Gastroenterology, Hepatology and Nutrition (ESPGHAN) and the European Society for Clinical Nutrition and Metabolism (ESPEN), supported by the European Society of Paediatric Research (ESPR). *J. Pediatr. Gastroenterol. Nutr.* **2005**, *41* (Suppl. 2), S1–S4. [PubMed]
8. Fivez, T.; Kerklaan, D.; Mesotten, D.; Verbruggen, S.; Joosten, K.; Van den Berghe, G. Evidence for the use of parenteral nutrition in the pediatric intensive care unit. *Clin. Nutr.* **2017**, *36*, 218–223. [CrossRef] [PubMed]
9. Joffe, A.; Anton, N.; Lequier, L.; Vandermeer, B.; Tjosvold, L.; Larsen, B.; Hartling, L. Nutritional support for critically Ill children. *Cochrane Database Syst. Rev.* **2016**. [CrossRef]
10. Kerklaan, D.; Fivez, T.; Mehta, N.M.; Mesotten, D.; van Rosmalen, J.; Hulst, J.M.; Van den Berghe, G.; Joosten, K.F.; Verbruggen, S.C. Worldwide survey of nutritional practices in PICUs. *Pediatr. Crit. Care Med.* **2016**, *17*, 10–18. [CrossRef]
11. Martinez, E.E.; Mehta, N.M. The science and art of pediatric critical care nutrition. *Curr. Opin. Crit. Care* **2016**, *22*, 316–324. [CrossRef]
12. Joffe, A.; Anton, N.; Lequier, L.; Vandermeer, B.; Tjosvold, L.; Larsen, B.; Hartling, L. Nutritional support for critically Ill children. *Cochrane Database Syst. Rev.* **2009**. [CrossRef]

13. Mehta, N.M.; Compher, C.; ASPEN Board of Directors. ASPEN clinical guidelines: Nutrition support of the critically ill child. *JPEN J. Parenter. Enter. Nutr.* **2009**, *33*, 260–276. [CrossRef]
14. Casaer, M.P.; Mesotten, D.; Hermans, G.; Wouters, P.J.; Schetz, M.; Meyfroidt, G.; Van Cromphaut, S.; Ingels, C.; Meersseman, P.; Muller, J.; et al. Early versus late parenteral nutrition in critically ill adults. *N. Engl. J. Med.* **2011**, *365*, 506–517. [CrossRef]
15. Fivez, T.; Kerklaan, D.; Mesotten, D.; Verbruggen, S.; Wouters, P.J.; Vanhorebeek, I.; Debaveye, Y.; Vlasselaers, D.; Desmet, L.; Casaer, M.P.; et al. Early versus late parenteral nutrition in critically Ill children. *N. Engl. J. Med.* **2016**, *374*, 1111–1122. [CrossRef]
16. Goulet, O.; Jochum, F.; Koletzko, B. Early or late parenteral nutrition in critically Ill children: Practical implications of the PEPaNIC trial. *Ann. Nutr. Metab.* **2017**, *70*, 34–38. [CrossRef]
17. Groenendaal, F. Early versus late parenteral nutrition in critically Ill children. *N. Engl. J. Med.* **2016**, *375*, 384. [CrossRef]
18. Vichayavilas, P.; Gist, K.; Kaufman, J. More and sooner, but not necessarily better. *J. Thorac. Dis.* **2016**, *8*, 1877–1879. [CrossRef]
19. Van Puffelen, E.; Vanhorebeek, I.; Joosten, K.F.M.; Wouters, P.J.; Van den Berghe, G.; Verbruggen, S. Early versus late parenteral nutrition in critically ill, term neonates: A preplanned secondary subgroup analysis of the PEPaNIC multicentre, randomised controlled trial. *Lancet Child Adolesc. Health* **2018**, *2*, 505–515. [CrossRef]
20. Van Puffelen, E.; Hulst, J.M.; Vanhorebeek, I.; Dulfer, K.; Van den Berghe, G.; Verbruggen, S.C.A.T.; Joosten, K.F.M. Outcomes of delaying parenteral nutrition for 1 week vs initiation within 24 h among undernourished children in pediatric intensive care: A subanalysis of the PEPaNIC randomized clinical trial. *JAMA Netw. Open* **2018**, *1*, e182668. [CrossRef]
21. Van Puffelen, E.; Hulst, J.M.; Vanhorebeek, I.; Dulfer, K.; Van den Berghe, G.; Joosten, K.F.M.; Verbruggen, S. Effect of late versus early initiation of parenteral nutrition on weight deterioration during PICU stay: Secondary analysis of the PEPaNIC randomised controlled trial. *Clin. Nutr.* **2019**. [CrossRef] [PubMed]
22. Van Puffelen, E.; Polinder, S.; Vanhorebeek, I.; Wouters, P.J.; Bossche, N.; Peers, G.; Verstraete, S.; Joosten, K.F.M.; Van den Berghe, G.; Verbruggen, S.; et al. Cost-effectiveness study of early versus late parenteral nutrition in critically ill children (PEPaNIC): Preplanned secondary analysis of a multicentre randomised controlled trial. *Crit. Care* **2018**, *22*, 4. [CrossRef] [PubMed]
23. Li, Y.; Huang, Y. Early versus late parenteral nutrition in critically Ill children. *N. Engl. J. Med.* **2016**, *375*, 384–385. [CrossRef] [PubMed]
24. Larsen, B.M.K.; Beggs, M.R.; Leong, A.Y.; Kang, S.H.; Persad, R.; Garcia Guerra, G. Can energy intake alter clinical and hospital outcomes in PICU? *Clin. Nutr. ESPEN* **2018**, *24*, 41–46. [CrossRef] [PubMed]
25. Beggs, M.R.; Garcia Guerra, G.; Larsen, B.M.K. Do PICU patients meet technical criteria for performing indirect calorimetry? *Clin. Nutr. ESPEN* **2016**, *15*, 80–84. [CrossRef] [PubMed]
26. Van der Kuip, M.; Oosterveld, M.J.; van Bokhorst-de van der Schueren, M.A.; de Meer, K.; Lafeber, H.N.; Gemke, R.J. Nutritional support in 111 pediatric intensive care units: A European survey. *Intensive Care Med.* **2004**, *30*, 1807–1813. [CrossRef]
27. Wang, D.; Lai, X.; Liu, C.; Xiong, Y.; Zhang, X. Influence of supplemental parenteral nutrition approach on nosocomial infection in pediatric intensive care unit of Emergency Department: A retrospective study. *Nutr. J.* **2015**, *14*, 103. [CrossRef]
28. Ioannidis, J.P.A. The challenge of reforming nutritional epidemiologic research. *J. Am. Med. Assoc.* **2018**, *320*, 969–970. [CrossRef]
29. Mehta, N.M.; Bechard, L.J.; Zurakowski, D.; Duggan, C.P.; Heyland, D.K. Adequate enteral protein intake is inversely associated with 60-d mortality in critically ill children: A multicenter, prospective, cohort study. *Am. J. Clin. Nutr.* **2015**, *102*, 199–206. [CrossRef]
30. Vanhorebeek, I.; Verbruggen, S.; Casaer, M.P.; Gunst, J.; Wouters, P.J.; Hanot, J.; Guerra, G.G.; Vlasselaers, D.; Joosten, K.; Van den Berghe, G. Effect of early supplemental parenteral nutrition in the paediatric ICU: A preplanned observational study of post-randomisation treatments in the PEPaNIC trial. *Lancet Respir Med.* **2017**, *5*, 475–483. [CrossRef]
31. Fan, E.; Dowdy, D.W.; Colantuoni, E.; Mendez-Tellez, P.A.; Sevransky, J.E.; Shanholtz, C.; Himmelfarb, C.R.; Desai, S.V.; Ciesla, N.; Herridge, M.S.; et al. Physical complications in acute lung injury survivors: A two-year longitudinal prospective study. *Crit. Care Med.* **2014**, *42*, 849–859. [CrossRef]

32. Preiser, J.C. High protein intake during the early phase of critical illness: Yes or no? *Crit. Care* **2018**, *22*, 261. [CrossRef]
33. Hermans, G.; Casaer, M.P.; Clerckx, B.; Guiza, F.; Vanhullebusch, T.; Derde, S.; Meersseman, P.; Derese, I.; Mesotten, D.; Wouters, P.J.; et al. Effect of tolerating macronutrient deficit on the development of intensive-care unit acquired weakness: A subanalysis of the EPaNIC trial. *Lancet Respir Med.* **2013**, *1*, 621–629. [CrossRef]
34. Doig, G.S.; Simpson, F.; Bellomo, R.; Heighes, P.T.; Sweetman, E.A.; Chesher, D.; Pollock, C.; Davies, A.; Botha, J.; Harrigan, P.; et al. Intravenous amino acid therapy for kidney function in critically ill patients: A randomized controlled trial. *Intensive Care Med.* **2015**, *41*, 1197–1208. [CrossRef]
35. Ferrie, S.; Allman-Farinelli, M.; Daley, M.; Smith, K. Protein requirements in the critically Ill: A randomized controlled trial using parenteral nutrition. *JPEN J. Parenter. Enter. Nutr.* **2016**, *40*, 795–805. [CrossRef]
36. Rugeles, S.J.; Rueda, J.D.; Diaz, C.E.; Rosselli, D. Hyperproteic hypocaloric enteral nutrition in the critically ill patient: A randomized controlled clinical trial. *Indian J. Crit. Care Med.* **2013**, *17*, 343–349. [CrossRef]
37. Gunst, J.; Vanhorebeek, I.; Thiessen, S.E.; Van den Berghe, G. Amino acid supplements in critically ill patients. *Pharmacol. Res.* **2018**, *130*, 127–131. [CrossRef]
38. Coss-Bu, J.A.; Hamilton-Reeves, J.; Patel, J.J.; Morris, C.R.; Hurt, R.T. Protein requirements of the critically Ill pediatric patient. *Nutr. Clin. Pract.* **2017**, *32*, 128S–141S. [CrossRef]
39. Carcillo, J.A. What's new in pediatric intensive care. *Crit. Care Med.* **2006**, *34*, S183–S190. [CrossRef]
40. Pearson, G.; Shann, F.; Barry, P.; Vyas, J.; Thomas, D.; Powell, C.; Field, D. Should paediatric intensive care be centralised? Trent versus Victoria. *Lancet* **1997**, *349*, 1213–1217. [CrossRef]
41. Gupta, P.; Tang, X.; Rettiganti, M.; Lauer, C.; Kacmarek, R.M.; Rice, T.B.; Markovitz, B.P.; Wetzel, R.C. Association of house staff training with mortality in children with critical illness. *Acta Paediatr.* **2016**, *105*, e60–e66. [CrossRef] [PubMed]
42. Pollack, M.M.; Patel, K.M.; Ruttimann, E. Pediatric critical care training programs have a positive effect on pediatric intensive care mortality. *Crit. Care Med.* **1997**, *25*, 1637–1642. [CrossRef] [PubMed]
43. Burns, J.P.; Sellers, D.E.; Meyer, E.C.; Lewis-Newby, M.; Truog, R.D. Epidemiology of death in the PICU at five U.S. teaching hospitals. *Crit. Care Med.* **2014**, *42*, 2101–2108. [CrossRef] [PubMed]
44. Namachivayam, P.; Shann, F.; Shekerdemian, L.; Taylor, A.; van Sloten, I.; Delzoppo, C.; Daffey, C.; Butt, W. Three decades of pediatric intensive care: Who was admitted, what happened in intensive care, and what happened afterward. *Pediatr. Crit. Care Med.* **2010**, *11*, 549–555. [CrossRef] [PubMed]
45. Rennick, J.E.; Childerhose, J.E. Redefining success in the PICU: New patient populations shift targets of care. *Pediatrics* **2015**, *135*, e289–e291. [CrossRef] [PubMed]
46. Verstraete, S.; Van den Berghe, G.; Vanhorebeek, I. What's new in the long-term neurodevelopmental outcome of critically ill children. *Intensive Care Med.* **2018**, *44*, 649–651. [CrossRef]
47. Aspesberro, F.; Mangione-Smith, R.; Zimmerman, J.J. Health-related quality of life following pediatric critical illness. *Intensive Care Med.* **2015**, *41*, 1235–1246. [CrossRef]
48. Madderom, M.J.; Reuser, J.J.; Utens, E.M.; van Rosmalen, J.; Raets, M.; Govaert, P.; Steiner, K.; Gischler, S.J.; Tibboel, D.; van Heijst, A.F.; et al. Neurodevelopmental, educational and behavioral outcome at 8 years after neonatal ECMO: A nationwide multicenter study. *Intensive Care Med.* **2013**, *39*, 1584–1593. [CrossRef]
49. Sterken, C.; Lemiere, J.; Vanhorebeek, I.; Van den Berghe, G.; Mesotten, D. Neurocognition after paediatric heart surgery: A systematic review and meta-analysis. *Open Heart* **2015**, *2*, e000255. [CrossRef]
50. Buysse, C.M.; Vermunt, L.C.; Raat, H.; Hazelzet, J.A.; Hop, W.C.; Utens, E.M.; Joosten, K.F. Surviving meningococcal septic shock in childhood: Long-term overall outcome and the effect on health-related quality of life. *Crit. Care* **2010**, *14*, R124. [CrossRef]
51. Mesotten, D.; Gielen, M.; Sterken, C.; Claessens, K.; Hermans, G.; Vlasselaers, D.; Lemiere, J.; Lagae, L.; Gewillig, M.; Eyskens, B.; et al. Neurocognitive development of children 4 years after critical illness and treatment with tight glucose control: A randomized controlled trial. *J. Am. Med. Assoc.* **2012**, *308*, 1641–1650. [CrossRef] [PubMed]
52. Van Zellem, L.; Utens, E.M.; de Wildt, S.N.; Vet, N.J.; Tibboel, D.; Buysse, C. Analgesia-sedation in PICU and neurological outcome: A secondary analysis of long-term neuropsychological follow-up in meningococcal septic shock survivors. *Pediatr. Crit. Care Med.* **2014**, *15*, 189–196. [CrossRef] [PubMed]
53. Verstraete, S.; Verbruggen, S.C.; Hordijk, J.A.; Vanhorebeek, I.; Dulfer, K.; Guiza, F.; van Puffelen, E.; Jacobs, A.; Leys, S.; Durt, A.; et al. Long-term developmental effects of withholding parenteral nutrition for 1 week in

the paediatric intensive care unit: A 2-year follow-up of the PEPaNIC international, randomised, controlled trial. *Lancet Respir Med.* **2018**. [CrossRef]

54. Verstraete, S.; Vanhorebeek, I.; Covaci, A.; Guiza, F.; Malarvannan, G.; Jorens, P.G.; Van den Berghe, G. Circulating phthalates during critical illness in children are associated with long-term attention deficit: A study of a development and a validation cohort. *Intensive Care Med.* **2016**, *42*, 379–392. [CrossRef] [PubMed]
55. Vlasselaers, D.; Milants, I.; Desmet, L.; Wouters, P.J.; Vanhorebeek, I.; van den Heuvel, I.; Mesotten, D.; Casaer, M.P.; Meyfroidt, G.; Ingels, C.; et al. Intensive insulin therapy for patients in paediatric intensive care: A prospective, randomised controlled study. *Lancet* **2009**, *373*, 547–556. [CrossRef]
56. Utendale, W.T.; Hubert, M.; Saint-Pierre, A.B.; Hastings, P.D. Neurocognitive development and externalizing problems: The role of inhibitory control deficits from 4 to 6 years. *Aggress. Behav.* **2011**, *37*, 476–488. [CrossRef] [PubMed]
57. Meijer, A.J. Amino acid regulation of autophagosome formation. *Methods Mol. Biol.* **2008**, *445*, 89–109. [CrossRef]
58. Deretic, V.; Saitoh, T.; Akira, S. Autophagy in infection, inflammation and immunity. *Nat. Rev. Immunol.* **2013**, *13*, 722–737. [CrossRef]
59. Derde, S.; Vanhorebeek, I.; Guiza, F.; Derese, I.; Gunst, J.; Fahrenkrog, B.; Martinet, W.; Vervenne, H.; Ververs, E.J.; Larsson, L.; et al. Early parenteral nutrition evokes a phenotype of autophagy deficiency in liver and skeletal muscle of critically ill rabbits. *Endocrinology* **2012**, *153*, 2267–2276. [CrossRef]
60. Van Goudoever, J.B.; Carnielli, V.; Darmaun, D.; Sainz de Pipaon, M.; The ESPGHAN/ESPEN/ESPR/CSPEN Working Group on Pediatric Parenteral Nutrition. ESPGHAN/ESPEN/ESPR/CSPEN guidelines on pediatric parenteral nutrition: Amino acids. *Clin. Nutr.* **2018**, *37*, 2315–2323. [CrossRef]
61. Rennie, M.J.; Bohe, J.; Wolfe, R.R. Latency, duration and dose response relationships of amino acid effects on human muscle protein synthesis. *J. Nutr.* **2002**, *132*, 3225S–3227S. [CrossRef] [PubMed]
62. Gunst, J.; Vanhorebeek, I.; Casaer, M.P.; Hermans, G.; Wouters, P.J.; Dubois, J.; Claes, K.; Schetz, M.; Van den Berghe, G. Impact of early parenteral nutrition on metabolism and kidney injury. *J. Am. Soc. Nephrol.* **2013**, *24*, 995–1005. [CrossRef] [PubMed]
63. Allingstrup, M.J.; Kondrup, J.; Wiis, J.; Claudius, C.; Pedersen, U.G.; Hein-Rasmussen, R.; Bjerregaard, M.R.; Steensen, M.; Jensen, T.H.; Lange, T.; et al. Early goal-directed nutrition versus standard of care in adult intensive care patients: The single-centre, randomised, outcome assessor-blinded EAT-ICU trial. *Intensive Care Med.* **2017**, *43*, 1637–1647. [CrossRef] [PubMed]
64. Blackburn, E.H.; Epel, E.S.; Lin, J. Human telomere biology: A contributory and interactive factor in aging, disease risks, and protection. *Science* **2015**, *350*, 1193–1198. [CrossRef] [PubMed]
65. Epel, E.S.; Blackburn, E.H.; Lin, J.; Dhabhar, F.S.; Adler, N.E.; Morrow, J.D.; Cawthon, R.M. Accelerated telomere shortening in response to life stress. *Proc. Natl. Acad. Sci. USA* **2004**, *101*, 17312–17315. [CrossRef]
66. Pendergrass, W.R.; Penn, P.E.; Li, J.; Wolf, N.S. Age-related telomere shortening occurs in lens epithelium from old rats and is slowed by caloric restriction. *Exp. Eye Res.* **2001**, *73*, 221–228. [CrossRef]
67. Crous-Bou, M.; Fung, T.T.; Prescott, J.; Julin, B.; Du, M.; Sun, Q.; Rexrode, K.M.; Hu, F.B.; De Vivo, I. Mediterranean diet and telomere length in Nurses' Health Study: Population based cohort study. *Br. Med. J.* **2014**, *349*, g6674. [CrossRef]
68. Verstraete, S.; Vanhorebeek, I.; van Puffelen, E.; Derese, I.; Ingels, C.; Verbruggen, S.C.; Wouters, P.J.; Joosten, K.F.; Hanot, J.; Guerra, G.G.; et al. Leukocyte telomere length in paediatric critical illness: Effect of early parenteral nutrition. *Crit. Care* **2018**, *22*, 38. [CrossRef]
69. Qureshi, I.A.; Mehler, M.F. Understanding neurological disease mechanisms in the era of epigenetics. *JAMA Neurol.* **2013**, *70*, 703–710. [CrossRef]
70. Radford, E.J. Exploring the extent and scope of epigenetic inheritance. *Nat. Rev. Endocrinol.* **2018**, *14*, 345–355. [CrossRef]
71. Groom, A.; Elliott, H.R.; Embleton, N.D.; Relton, C.L. Epigenetics and child health: Basic principles. *Arch. Dis. Child.* **2011**, *96*, 863–869. [CrossRef] [PubMed]
72. Relton, C.L.; Groom, A.; St Pourcain, B.; Sayers, A.E.; Swan, D.C.; Embleton, N.D.; Pearce, M.S.; Ring, S.M.; Northstone, K.; Tobias, J.H.; et al. DNA methylation patterns in cord blood DNA and body size in childhood. *PLoS ONE* **2012**, *7*, e31821. [CrossRef] [PubMed]

11

Pharmaceutical Aspects of Artificial Nutrition

Emilie Reber [1,*], Markus Messerli [2], Zeno Stanga [1] and Stefan Mühlebach [3]

[1] Department for Diabetes, Endocrinology, Nutritional Medicine and Metabolism, Bern University Hospital and University of Bern, 3010 Bern, Switzerland; zeno.stanga@insel.ch

[2] Department of Pharmaceutical Sciences, Pharmaceutical Care Research Group, University of Basel, 4050 Basel, Switzerland; markus.messerli@unibas.ch

[3] Department of Pharmaceutical Sciences, Division of Clinical Pharmacy & Epidemiology/Hospital Pharmacy, University of Basel, 4050 Basel, Switzerland; stefan.muehlebach@viforpharma.com

* Correspondence: emilie.reber@insel.ch

Abstract: Artificial nutrition, including enteral (EN) and parenteral (PN) nutrition, is indicated whenever adequate oral nutrition fails to sufficiently supply the necessary nutrients to the body. It is a convenient, efficacious, safe, and well-tolerated form of clinical nutrition in the hospital and home setting. EN is administered via nasogastric tube or ostomies while PN usually requires a central venous access for administration, straight into the blood stream. The infused nutrients can then be taken up directly by the different organs. PN is targeted as a single daily portion formulated as an oil-in-water emulsion providing the necessary substrates for the catabolic and anabolic metabolism including macro- and micronutrients and fluids. PN has a complex pharmaceutical composition—all-in-one admixture—and its compounding or ready-to-use preparation. The use of PN is more challenging and more expensive compare to the use of EN, commercially available as ready-to-use formulations. EN and concomitant medication is highly challenging. Upon incorrect handling and administration, PN is associated with potentially severe or even fatal complications, mostly relating to the central venous access (e.g., catheter-related sepsis) or to a metabolic intolerance (e.g., hyperglycemia, refeeding syndrome) because of inappropriate administration. A correct order of admixing, correct dosing, and administration of the artificial is crucial for safety and efficacy; clinical and biochemical monitoring of the patient and treatment regimen adaption are necessary. The high number of reactive solutes allow only limited stability of a ready-to-use PN admixture. The potential for numerous incompatibilities and interactions renders PN admixtures generally unsuitable as drug vehicle. Laboratory compatibility and stability testing and pharmaceutical expertise are a prerequisite to define the PN composition including nutrients or even drugs admixed to define the appropriate and individualized nutrition and medication regimen. The aim of this narrative review is to present the actual state-of-the-art to deliver best quality artificial nutrition with special regard on pharmaceutical aspects such as instabilities, incompatibilities, and concomitant co-medication.

Keywords: parenteral nutrition; enteral nutrition; artificial nutrition; all-in-one parenteral admixture; compatibility; stability; pharmaceutical expertise; drug admixing; drug administration

---

1. Introduction

Enteral nutrition (EN) is used whenever the gastrointestinal tract is functioning and when oral access is impaired (e.g., chewing and/or swallowing issues). In patients with partial or total intestinal failure, nutrients may not or not be sufficiently absorbed from the intestine. Hence, parenteral nutrition (PN) has to be administered as a formulation, containing the necessary substrates, ready to be used in the intermediate metabolism. Intestinal failure may result from an extensive surgical bowel resection or a disease leading to reduced function of the intestine and/or impairment of motility, digestive or absorptive capacity (e.g., mesenteric infarction, laparoschisis, Morbus Hirschsprung). Table 1 shows recently published data from Pironi et al. regarding epidemiology of intestinal failure in 3239 patients across the world [1]. PN allows quantity- and quality-wise a full or partial nutritional support and can guarantee survival and good quality of life. EN and PN are the two forms of artificial nutrition, developed and introduced in the 1960s. EN and PN, or their combination, require an adapted and individualized nutrition regimen respecting the specific condition and requirements of the patient. Nowadays and in contrast to the early beginnings, EN and PN are mostly based on physico–chemically fully defined, balanced and stable products, manufactured in industry. While EN products can be delivered as stable ready-to-use formulations, total or partial PN has to be compounded or prepared ready-to-use for administration compliant with pharmaceutical good manufacturing practice (GMP) requirements. The available industrial PN premixes contain stable nutritional components mechanically separated from each other in chambers with breakable sealing. Upon ready-to-use preparation as all-in-one (AiO) admixture in a convenient, single container and for single line daily PN treatment, the sealing is mechanically broken and the content manually shaken. For safety and tolerance of administration of the usually hypertonic PN admixtures showing an osmolality exceeding 2000 mosm/kg, an inserted/implanted central intravenous access is required [2]. Consequently, PN and its prerequisites are more challenging, more expensive, and more prone for complications compared to EN. Nevertheless, a well-indicated PN according to existing guidelines shows good efficacy and safety in patients, also in long lasting home PN and if assisted by a nutrition support team (NST) [3–8].

Table 1. Epidemiologic data from 3239 patients with chronic intestinal failure in countries around the world, from Pironi et al. [1].

Type of Chronic Intestinal Failure	Underlying Disease
Benign chronic intestinal failure (n = 2919, 90.1%)	Crohn's disease (22.4%) Mesenteric ischemia (17.7%) Surgical complications (15.8%) Primary chronic intestinal pseudo-obstruction (9.7%) Post-radiation enteritis (7.3%) Others (21.3%, with <3% each-one) Not reported (5.9%)
Malignant chronic intestinal failure (n = 320, 9.9%)	Type of active cancer not specified (62%) Gastrointestinal cancer (28%) Extra-abdominal cancer (10%) Concurrent enteritis due to radio- or chemotherapy (5%) Peritoneal carcinomatosis (12%)

Databases such as PubMed and Cochrane were searched for guidelines, recommendations and registries, using filters for human studies in English only, and excluding children, as well as homepages from national and international nursing and nutritional societies. The aim of this narrative review is to present the actual state-of-the-art for artificial nutrition delivery with special regard on pharmaceutical aspects. This review aims to provide nutritionists dealing with artificial nutrition knowledge to deliver best quality PN, understanding of the concept and benefits of the AiO, and the pharmaceutical challenges of artificial nutrition (instabilities and incompatibilities, drug admixture).

2. Accesses for Artificial Nutrition

PN should be initiated at the latest after five to seven days of insufficient oral and/or enteral feeding. This may be initiated even earlier in case of severe malnutrition [5]. Preoperative PN and also EN have been for example been shown to improve surgical outcome in patients affected by Crohn's disease undergoing abdominal surgery [9,10]. The beneficial value of supplemental PN in critically ill patients has also been demonstrated in recent prospective studies [11]. EN may be administered via nasogastric tubes, nasojejunal tubes or percutaneous gastrostomy/jejunostomy (endoscopic or radiologic), Witzel fistulas or fine needle catheter jejunostomy, depending on the anticipated duration of the EN therapy and of the indication. The need for a central venous access for PN is obvious when for example calculating the individual daily requirements for electrolytes, which have to be contained in an AiO PN admixture. These alone increase the tonicity by more than 600–800 mosmol/kg, which is the maximal value for a peripherally administered intravenous infusion [5]. In long-term PN, tunneled subclavian or jugular catheters (e.g., Hickman catheters), implanted port systems or peripherally inserted central venous catheter (PICC) are used [6]. For short period of supplemental PN, the administration of peripheral PN admixtures through peripheral venous catheter is possible. Peripheral PN may be indicated for short-term use or as a supplement typically to maintain a previously well-nourished, patient or to serve as a bridge to centrally administered infusions or until adequate enteral feedings can be established [12,13]. The risk of microbial contamination and following growth is greater with peripheral PN than with PN, mainly due to the lower osmolarity in peripheral PN [14]. Moreover, the risk of phlebitis and extravasation is high and causes catheter removal [15].

3. Handling of Feeding Tubes and Catheters

The handling of feeding tubes is much less demanding than the catheter handling, as it does not require asepsis. It however largely depends on the type of tube. Regular dressing changes and slights moves of the tubes are however mandatory.

To minimize PN-associated complications, the appropriate central intravenous device has to be selected, placed, and inserted by a trained surgical team with experience. Together with good and regularly trained catheter handling, these are the two most important factors to keep the main intravenous access related complications in PN low. A rigorous aseptic technique is required for the manipulation and care of the catheters and the connections [2]. Blood drawing including aspiration through the central venous catheter has to be avoided. Suited trainings for patients and caregivers to learn the defined rules and best practices are essential and must be documented and evaluated [16]. Such education includes aseptic handling of the PN bag, of catheters, and its connections including also a rigorous handwashing procedure. Alcoholic chlorhexidine (0.5–2%) is recommended for skin disinfection; there are possible disinfectant alternatives in case of contraindications [2]. When a port system is used for PN, the giving set must be changed daily and in addition, the gripper needle has to be changed every three to seven days according to accepted standards. Evidence-based policies also apply for dressings of the exit sites [2]. The rinsing and plugging of the catheter with defined solutions are of critical importance and saline (0.9%) is the standard solution to be used. Heparin, initially recommended for port system rinsing, is still often used despite lacking appropriate compatibility documentation. Bozetti et al. showed a significant increase of catheter-related complication using heparin rinse compared to saline in HPN patients [17]. A recent Cochrane update analysis comparing saline against heparin for intermittent catheter locking in adults showed no evidence for a heparin benefit, as known from previous studies in children [18]. Heparin is prone to incompatibility reactions with many PN components, e.g., lipids, potentially leading to occlusion and/or infection of catheters. The use of heparin to rinse catheters lacks evidence regarding its effectiveness in reducing blood clotting. Moreover, it is prone to incompatibilities with lipids and emulsifiers from the PN admixtures. Even short and at low dose, heparin exposure in an intravenous line has shown emulsion cracking [19]. As a consequence of the cracking, lipid deposits form in catheters increasing risk for infectious complication and obstruction, possibly leading to catheter removal [6]. The potential risk to induce heparin hypersensitivity has also to be considered. In the actual PN guidelines, heparin is not more recommended for catheter rinsing and plugging [2,6,18]. A lock solution with taurolidine, a synthetic antimicrobial agent, might be considered in PN patients with repeated catheter-associated infections but should not be routinely used [20]. Other antibiotic lock solutions (vancomycin, gentamycin) are also used although the evidence for a preventing effect is low. Ethanol locks may be considered for secondary prevention in some cases. The use of in-line filters is not supported by the necessary evidence, similarly to heparin use or antibiotic prophylaxis [2]. Therefore, these methods are not considered as universal and compulsory preventive measures for all PN patients [5–7]. In-line filters may be used to (1) filter out precipitates or particles (reduce risk of embolism), (2) prevent pathogenic microorganisms to enter the bloodstream (reduce risk of infection), (3) hinder air to be infused into blood circulation (air embolization). In-line filters may however also create new problems [21]. They may themselves release particles or cause adsorption of nutrients or drugs reducing their systemic availability. In-line filters may thus also potentially be blocked and impair the PN administration. A fatality has even been associated with the use of in-line filters, as calcium phosphate precipitation occurred in the filtered admixture after warming up in the line [22]. There are no general recommendations for the use of in-line filters. German guidelines on PN settle beneficial effects of in-line filters in specific risk patient populations (e.g., children and immune-compromised patients) [23]. The ASPEN however recommends the use of 0.22 micron filter for lipid-free PN admixtures, and 1.2 micron filter for AiO admixtures [24]. The filter should be placed as close to the patient as possible and should be exchanged with each new PN container, as well as the administration set.

4. Complications of Enteral Nutrition

EN is generally efficient, safe and well tolerated. Small bore tubes made of more flexible materials, careful nursing and therapy monitoring contribute to decrease the complication rates. Risk factors for complications are among others neurological impairment, anatomical abnormalities, and advanced age [25]. Systematic antibiotic therapy before tube placement to prevent infectious complications (wounds and systemic infect) is controversially discussed. There is however good evidence for at-risk patients (e.g., immunocompromised patients) and placement of gastroscopic accesses [25]. Administration of a single dose of broad spectrum antibiotic half an hour before EN device placement has been shown to reduce peristomal infects by 22%. Complications rates vary according to the type of access, e.g., 0.3–15% for nasoenteric tubes, 1–4% for major and 13–40% for minor complications for endoscopic accesses. Complications rates are very low for surgical needle catheter jejeunostomies.

4.1. Gastrointestinal Complications

Gastrointestinal complications are frequent with enteral feeding [26]. Diarrhea may be the most common one, probably caused by adaption of the intestine after fasting period, by antibiotic therapy, or administration of too cold solutions. Delivery sites and rates influence may also influence the occurrence of diarrhea. Misplacement (too low) may be a further cause of diarrhea. Obstipation may also occur with enteral feeding solutions containing low or no dietary fibers, due to dehydration, immobility, or as a side effect of opiate therapy.

Nausea and vomiting may be due to tube dislocation, too fast administration or administration of too high volume. It may also be caused by the underlying disease or the related treatments, or due to medication containing sugar substitutes. Delayed gastric emptying and subsequent feeling of fullness are risk factor for aspiration and may also cause vomiting [25].

Reflux esophagitis and early dumping are further complications of EN.

4.2. Mechanical Complications

Feeding tubes may be misplaced, dislocate, or cause perforation (trachea or gastrointestinal tract), and nasal/gastrointestinal bleeding. Further, feeding tubes may be obstructed. Obstruction may be prevented by sufficient and consequent rinsing procedures, and by avoiding drug administration (as far as possible). There are various possibilities to re-open a tube, from warm water rinsing to rinsing with pancreatic enzymes and bicarbonate solutions. Feeding tubes may also cause irritation, and consecutive changes in the oral mucosa. Leaks or buried bumper syndrome may occur with PEG devices [25].

Aspiration is a rare complication (1–4%), causing fever and possibly pneumonia [25]. It may be silent or manifest with symptoms such as tachypnoea, tachycardia, and wheezing. Aspiration is however a great issue in critically ill patients [26]. It may be prevented elevating the head by 30–45° when lying [25].

4.3. Infectious Complications

Different infectious complications may occur during the EN therapy, such as pneumonia (arising from aspiration pneumonia), sinusitis, or bacterial contamination of the nutritional solution [26]. Some complications are related to the device, e.g., wound infection at the entry site with PEG devices and peritonitis with gastroenterostomies. Infections mostly require tube change/removal [25].

4.4. Metabolic Complication

The metabolic complications of the enteral nutrition are similar to the one of parenteral nutrition (e.g., the refeeding syndrome described in Section 5.3.1) but with much lower incidence and severity [25].

5. Complications of Parenteral Nutrition

5.1. Mechanical Complications

Catheters may sometimes dislocate or occlude, mainly due to incorrect manipulations. Reasons for catheter occlusions are manifold: PN admixture instabilities, incompatibilities with rinsing solutions and/or with other intravenous solutes administered through the catheter, etc. Taking blood samples through the central venous access must be prohibited since it is almost impossible to completely clear the line and the device afterwards. Moreover, blood samples from catheters often provide erroneous results because of residues of the PN in the catheters with high electrolyte or lipid concentrations. Blood clots may form and eventually mechanically occlude the catheter, being a possible origin of microbial colonization. Occluded catheters may be rinsed with saline solutions (10–20 mL) in a first step, applying slight pressure. If this is not successful, acidic or alkaline solutions may be applied according to defined procedures [2]. Reopening of occluded catheters is however discussed very controversially by the experts. It can be dangerous since clots may be microbially colonized. Blood stream infection may consecutively occur. Lipid deposits may be eliminated with ethanol or diluted sodium hydroxide. Thrombolytics are administered to eliminate an assumed blood clot [5,6]. Administration of PN with infusion pumps also helps to prevent catheter occlusions since the flow rate is kept constant [7].

5.2. Infectious Complications

In the beginning of PN history, infections and sepsis were frequent (affecting up to 40% of the patients) and thus a limitation to PN use [8]. By reducing the number of manipulations (e.g., AiO admixture administration), the incidence of catheter sepsis radically dropped (Table 1). Catheter-related sepsis occur at rates of 0.5–1 per catheter year in hospitals inpatients and 0.1–0.5 per catheter year in patients on home PN [5]. Gram-positive microbes (from the skin) are the mostly encountered microorganisms identified [2,27]. Catheter exit site-related or bloodstream infections are predominant complications and are associated with increased morbidity and mortality rates. Moreover, infectious complications contribute substantially to PN costs, causing additional hospitalizations and catheter removals.

5.3. Metabolic Complications

5.3.1. Refeeding Syndrome

The refeeding syndrome is a potentially life-threatening metabolic condition occurring in seriously malnourished patients or in patients recovering from severe catabolic diseases (e.g., sepsis, diabetic ketoacidosis) after start of a nutritional therapy. From a pathophysiological point of view, refeeding syndrome is an exaggerated response of the malnourished catabolic body to a nutritional therapy, indeed to anabolism [28,29]. Refeeding syndrome is characterized by severe electrolyte shifts (mainly hypophosphatemia, hypomagnesemia, and hypokalemia), vitamin deficiency (mainly thiamine), fluid overload and salt retention leading to organ dysfunction including cardiac arrhythmias up to death. Symptoms such as heart failure, peripheral edema and neurologic disorders can occur. The refeeding syndrome is most likely to appear within the first 72 h after initiation of the nutritional therapy. A risk stratification of patients before prior to start a nutritional intervention is recommended and can then by adapted according to the risk category [28,29]. Full energy requirements are targeted within five to ten days after initiation of the nutritional therapy depending on the risk category, starting at a low energy rate (5–15 kcal/kg/day) and increasing stepwise. Fluid management and sodium restriction may be necessary in patients belonging to higher risk categories. Thiamine (vitamin B1) has to be administrated as a 200–300 mg dose daily for three days, 30 min before the initiation of nutritional support. Finally, provision of trace elements and vitamins in the single and double recommended daily amounts of micronutrients, respectively, are recommended. Intensive clinical monitoring is mandatory to detect early signs of refeeding syndrome, such as organ failure and fluid overload. It should include vital signs, hydration status, and determinations of serum electrolyte levels.

5.3.2. Hyperglycemia

Hyperglycemia is another early and frequent complication affecting up to 50% of the patients upon PN initiation. Appropriate and initially frequent glycaemia testing is mandatory, since hyperglycemia has been linked with increased morbidity and mortality, especially in critically ill patients [30]. The targeted blood glucose level lies between 7.8 and 10.0 mM, (normoglycemia: 4.4–8.1 mM; 80–145 mg/100 mL) [31]. Insulin administration, optimally pump-assisted and in parallel to PN, may be necessary to control glycaemia (there is a dedicated specific article on this topic in this special issue [30]).

5.3.3. Liver-Associated Complications

Liver-associated PN complications are seen in up to 40% of the patients, especially in those with short bowl with less than 150 cm of remaining small intestine and in absence of colon (Table 2) [2]. In case of occurring liver-associated PN complications (e.g., hypertriglyceridemia, cholelithiasis, and cholestasis), it is recommended to administer PN formulations with reduced triglyceride (TG) content and a better fatty acids (FA) mix (e.g., by a higher monounsaturated FA (MUFA) content or an increased Ω-3 to Ω-6 ratio of the polyunsaturated FA (PUFA)) [2].

Table 2. Catheter- and parenteral nutrition (PN)-related complications [2].

Type	Rates Measures Per Catheter Year (95% Confidence Interval)
Catheter sepsis	0.34 (0.32–0.37)
Catheter occlusion	0.07 (0.06–0.08)
Central vein thrombosis	0.03 (0.02–0.03)
Liver/biliary issues	
Mild	0.42 (0.27–0.63)
Severe	0.02 (0.01–0.06)
Metabolic bone disease	0.05 (0.01–0.15)

5.3.4. Thrombosis

Central venous thrombosis is a common issue in PN patients with central venous access (up to 50% of PN patients) associated with high morbidity and mortality rates (Table 2). The localization is mostly proximal to the catheter. The frequency of thrombosis is linked to the experience and skills of the catheter insertion team as well as to the diameter of the catheter; small bore central venous catheters are therefore recommended. Low dose oral anticoagulants may be used in high-risk patients [6].

6. The Role of the Pharmacist and Specificities of Pharmaceutical Management

NSTs have multi-professional composition consisting of at least a physician, a specialized nurse, a dietician and a pharmacist, skilled to manage PN, and to deliver best nutritional support [16]. Pharmacists within the NST have an important role to play in selecting, preparing and instructing on the safe handling of nutritional products, especially PN. They have however also a clear role in optimizing medication for patients with EN (BN Group). Pharmacists provide medicinal products, care, and when necessary education and training related to artificial nutrition to the other NST members, to patients and their caregivers. Pharmacists are in charge for the logistic of the products and of their quality assurance. They check the drug and nutrients prescriptions from a pharmaceutical point of view, advising on the most effective and safe administration of drugs in order to prevent interactions and incompatibilities, in EN (administration via feeding tube) as well as in PN (admixture) [32]. Pharmacists are also in charge of the documentation and clarification of drug related adverse events, to increase treatment safety. Most patients on artificial nutrition also require drug treatment for their underlying diseases. This further complicates the overall treatment regimen aiming in given cases to combine the parenteral administration of nutrients and drugs, e.g., as the indication for (home) PN is extended to malignant chronic diseases or severe functional deficiency, often requiring additional complex medication in parallel to the artificial nutrition. This is a complicated endeavor, which needs a careful check of compatibility primarily respecting correct and suited dosing over time of both nutrition and medication to ensure safe and efficacious treatment requesting pharmaceutical skills [6,8,33]. Drug admixing issues are one of the main tasks of the pharmacist within the NST, who has to face and assess PN- and drug-related problems from the pharmaceutical perspective [32]. The pharmacist also contributes to define an appropriate nutritional and medical care plan, to avoid medication errors, and finally keeps responsibility that the right patient gets the right products administered in the right way [5,6,34].

7. Components of Artificial Nutrition

Standard commercial nutritional solutions for enteral use contain between 1 (isocaloric) and 2 kcal/mL (hypercaloric), with 15–20% proteins, 25–30% fats, and 50–60% carbohydrate, which represents a suitable macronutrients distribution for most patients. They may contain dietary fibers or not. Macromolecular and low-molecular weight solutions are available depending on the functionality of the gastrointestinal tract. Additionally, metabolically adapted solutions (e.g., high protein, low electrolyte content for kidney failure patients) or immunomodulating solutions (containing e.g., arginine or glutamine) are available. Organic amino acids (AA; protein), glucose (carbohydrate), different TG of FA (fat), and inorganic/organic electrolytes/nutrients together with water are the small molecular components of a PN [2]. Micronutrients, vitamins and trace elements have mostly to be added for a total PN as they are not necessarily included in industrial multi-chamber bags. Energy requirement in adults is 25–30 kcal/kg/day given as a mix of the most important universal fuel glucose and high caloric lipids. In contrast to EN, the AA content of PN is not calculated as energy as AA are primarily intended building components for protein synthesis which has to be considered when assessing the balance of EN and PN. The basic protein need in adults is 0.8–1 g/kg/day increasing to 1.2–1.5 g/kg/day in malnourished patients and even higher in special situations (e.g., 2.5 g/kg/day in burned patients or children). The energy need mainly depends the resting energy expenditure and on disease activity and severity (possibly increasing the requirements by 50%).

7.1. Amino Acids

In a severe catabolic state, glucose may be produced from AA over the formation of acetyl-CoA and through the Krebs cycle or over the pyruvate gluconeogenesis pathway (for glucose-dependent organs, e.g., brain), yielding in 1 g AA = 4 kcal. The protein (AA) breakdown may be estimated through the urine output, since nitrogen from the AA is eliminated as urea. One gram of urea contained in the urine matches 7.34 g of AA (0.47 g nitrogen). This calculation can be used for an intake-output estimate e.g., in well-monitored critically ill patients.

From the 21 AA, there are seven essential (isoleucine, leucine, lysine, methionine, phenylalanine, threonine, tryptophan, and valine) and four conditionally essential AA (histidine, tyrosine, cytosine, glutamine, and taurine). When AA show additional pharmacological effects, the term pharmaconutrition is used. This applies to glutamine, although the evidence for effectiveness is still debated. Commercial AA solutions for PN are traditionally crystalline solutions of L-AA (10%), despite differences between the manufacturers in the conditionally essential AA content (mainly glycine) [2]. AA in solutions are filled in airtight containers and protected by the antioxidant nitrogen gas, since oxygen oxidation (ambient air) is very likely to occur. AA and glucose put together in vitro can react and undergo Maillard reaction, which may influence their availability. Thus, a yellow to brownish colored product is then visible upon exposition to ambient conditions as e.g., beyond 24–48 h hanging time of ready-to-use AiO admixtures. The AA content in a daily dose of AiO PN admixture reaches 1.2–1.5 g/kg (100–150 g AA). In order to reverse catabolism (AA breakdown), AA should be administered together with fat/carbohydrates (mainly glucose). The suggested caloric intake is 20–27 kcal/g AA [5,7]. Optional admixtures of pharmaconutrients (e.g., 0.2 g glutamine/kg/day in trauma or burned patients) are dosed additionally to the necessary AA amount of the PN regimen and have to be taken into account in the nutrient balance.

7.2. Glucose

Around 66% of the body's energy fuel is normally provided by carbohydrates (1 g = 4 kcal), mainly by glucose, the primary and physiological energy substrate in the intermediate metabolism. It is prone to oxidative degradation when in solution. Some organs (e.g., blood and brain) fully depend on glucose for meet their energy requirements. Hence, mechanism such as gluconeogenesis ensures a minimal necessary glucose production (37 g/day) when external supply is insufficient or lacking and the restricted glycogen stores (150–300 g) empty [2]. Highly concentrated, hypertonic glucose solution is used to restrict the volume of an AiO PN admixtures and primarily contributing to their hyperosmolarity. Maximal infusion rate in adults is 3–6 g glucose/kg over 24 h. This rate is limiting the maximal infusion rate since the rate of glucose oxidation to pyruvate/acetyl-CoA/Krebs cycle in adults is limited to 5–7 mg/kg/min [2]. The level of blood glucose during PN has to be kept <10 mM and has to be regularly monitored, especially in the beginning of PN [31,35].

7.3. Lipids

Commercial intravenous lipid oil-in-water emulsions contain 100–200 g lipid/L [2]. The TG used are composed of different (PU)FA. The oil-in-water emulsion is stabilized with soya or egg yolk lecithin (12 g/L), a phosphatidylcholine with a negative surface charge resulting from the phosphate groups [36]. The surface charge is negative from the anionic phosphate moiety of the emulsifier at the surface of the oil droplets. This negative zeta potential keeps the emulsified oil droplets separated. The anionic charge of the phosphate lecithin moiety at the surface is critical for destabilizing incompatibilities, e.g., with (mainly polyvalent) cations. Intravenous lipid emulsions are nearly isotonic and contribute to decrease the osmolarity of an AiO PN admixture, e.g., in PN administered peripherally. Important to know, about 15 mmol phosphate are delivered from the emulsifier per liter of a commercial parenteral lipid emulsion [2]. TG are important energy fuels providing 9 kcal/g through the beta-oxidation of FA and the subsequent acetyl-CoA metabolism. Different FA types are contained in intravenous lipid emulsions, depending on the lipid sources. Nowadays, "structured lipids" are mostly being used, like SMOF lipids containing 30% soybean FA, 30% MCT, 25% olive oil FA, and 15% fish oil FA. Lipid emulsions dose in PN reaches 0.5–1.0 g/kg/day to cover about 33% of the patients' energy requirements. Lipids may be used to a higher extend in critically ill patients (up to 50%) to avoid insulin resistance issues [2]. Since they are partially essential FA, PUFAs must be included in AiO PN admixtures in the required doses. Ω-3 PUFAs like EPA (eicosatetraenoic acid) or DHA (docosahexaenoic acid) show anti-inflammatory effects through the synthesis of prostaglandins and leukotrienes and may be considered as pharmaconutrients. On the contrary, Ω-6 PUFAs shows pro-inflammatory effects forming arachidonic acid over the prostaglandins and leukotrienes pathways. Ω-9 MUFA have no action on these pathways and thus are neutral. Middle chain triglycerides (MCT) only contain non-essential saturated FA. They can be oxidized to produce energy directly in the mitochondria in absence of carnitine unlike long chain PUFAs. PUFAs are highly prone to peroxidation; resulting in toxic reaction products (e.g., radicals and aldehydes) contributing to the systemic inflammation and the oxidative stress of patients. Light and oxygen protection for storage and transport are therefore important to prevent peroxidation [37,38]. The oil droplet characteristics and distribution in the oil-in-water emulsion is a critical parameter. It should mimic the physiologic chylomicrons or lipoproteins with a critical upper diameter size of 5 μm correlating to a small blood vessel diameter. Larger droplets may eventually cause lipid embolism, while degradation products of lipid peroxidation may as radicals free cause DNA damages and contribute to inflammation [2,16].

7.4. Fluids and Electrolytes

Sufficient water and electrolytes doses have also to be provided by a nutrition regimen. Additional oral fluid or infusions to PN may be needed to reach the basic fluid requirements in adults of 30–40 mL/kg/day, but also to cover abnormal losses such as fever, vomiting, diarrhea, or stoma losses, burns and severe wounds [39]. The combination compatible amounts of (di- and trivalent) cations and anions in AiO admixture preventing instabilities e.g., by harmful precipitations of salts or deteriorated oil-in-water characteristics by interactions with the emulsifier is a pharmaceutical challenge.

7.5. Micronutrients

Daily administration of EN > 1500 mL covers the daily recommended micronutrients intake. Since most micronutrients are hydrophilic and body stores are limited, total PN must also cover vitamins and trace elements requirements from its initiation. Trace elements (polyvalent cations) show relevant and concentration-dependent physicochemical interactions e.g., with the oil-in-water emulsifier; they may also be catalyzers of chemical degradation processes (e.g., oxidation) [2]. This may become an issue since vitamins and trace elements are both infused into AiO PN bags. As an example, iron or copper catalyze the oxidation of the ascorbic acid (vitamin C), which then degrades within minutes. From an evidence-based standpoint, trace elements and vitamins should be administrated separately, e.g., trace elements admixed to the AA portion, and vitamins only given at the end of a PN administration limiting the exposure time of combined physical presence in the admixture [4–6].

7.6. The All-In-One Concept as the Pharmaceutical Formulation of Choice

PN is a complex, meta-stable, high quality pharmaceutical formulation defined by the pharmacopoeia. In presence of lipid, it represents an oil-in-water emulsion and contains various, partially ionized, reactive solutes, prone for physicochemical interactions. PN is highly concentrated (hypertonic) and its components are often close to their solubility limits as the volume is restricted [32]. A PN regimen has to be practicable and convenient, efficacious and safe, also upon long term use (home PN). Central venous access is needed for the administration and aseptic techniques are needed during ready-to-use preparation of industrial premixes or tailor-made compounding since PN has to be sterile and pyrogen-free [6]. Correct conditions for transport and storage and finally for the administration and hanging time are required to provide the right and ready to be metabolized amount of nutrients to fulfil the nutritional needs and to prevent and/or correct metabolic/physicochemical disturbances.

The PN composition and if needed its individualization has always been and is a challenge to ensure safety and optimal efficiency. The increased knowledge of disease and stress metabolism has contributed to diminish complications and to increase tolerance of PN [2]. Historically, PN started from the difficult to handle multi bottle to a convenient single container AiO system delivered as a ready-to-use complete daily portion enabling individualized, more physiologic and well-tolerated 24 h or cyclic co-administration of the nutrients (mostly overnight) [4,40].

Total PN admixtures and regimens contain over 50 individual solutes, mostly representing reactive species (Figure 1). This explains the stability issues and the important potential for physicochemical interactions such as degradation of components, generation of toxic products like reactive aldehydes from fatty acid degradation or harming precipitates formed from interacting electrolytes [2]. Additionally, a critically reduced homogeneity of the oil-in-water fat emulsion with eventual oiling out may cause serious adverse effects. The control and avoidance of microbial contamination are key issues to reduce infectious complications. Nowadays, pharmaceutical GMP rules are established and require for example to work in a laminar airflow bench for aseptic compounding/ready-to-use preparation. There are guidelines for correct labelling, storage, hanging time (24 h after ready to use preparation), transport and storage (2–8 °C) of AiO PN admixtures [4]. The combined admixing of potentially interacting or even incompatible microelements like trace elements with vitamins are still debated. Trace elements can catalyze oxidation and radical formation of e.g., vitamins [4,6] or of PUFA [37]. An acceptable, appropriately documented compromise has to be defined for the appropriate quality of the AiO admixture administered and the provision of the necessary amount of nutrients. Individualized compounding or ready-to-use preparation of a complete PN results in an AiO admixture, which cannot to be sterilized anymore by an established heating procedure [2].

Hence,in many countries, ready-to-use AiO PN has to be prepared according to the GMP rules and regulatory authorization is needed. There are however countries where extemporaneous parenteral nutrition preparations do not need any specific regulatory authorizations. The industrial approach with serial manufacturing targeted stable and storable PN products to overcome the stability issues of individually compounded AiO PN admixtures. This resulted in the development of different forms of special multi-chamber bags, separating the lipid emulsion, the AA and the glucose solutions from each other by mechanically separated chambers or compartments [2]. The bags materials are innovative multi-layered foils allowing vapor sterilization of the filled and sealed chambers representing AiO PN premixes which are with the additional air-tight wrapping including oxygen absorbing materials stable up to years as the main chemical destabilization by oxidative degradation of the nutrients is almost eliminated [40]. Ready-to-use preparation of these commercial AiO PN premixes includes mechanical breaking of the chamber sealing and manual shaking of the combined content still in a closed container envelop thus in aseptic conditions. Admixing of other needed components (electrolytes, micronutrients, or other intravenous supplements according to need and compatibility) into individual chambers require suited stability data, and defined and validated admixing procedures. The major part of PN adult patients can be treated with commercialized products. Therefore, PN treatment is sensibly facilitated. Nevertheless, individual PN compounding remains needed in selected patients, especially in children or neonates with their body growth requirements but also adults with home PN and/or after mesenteric infarction. However, such a service is available only in particular and experienced hospital pharmacies or compounding centers often also challenged for an appropriate logistic [2]. The evidence is still lacking whether an individualized tailor-made PN regime provides better outcome in neonates, acute critically ill patients or for patients in the home setting compared to a standardized commercial AiO PN. The debate concerning the individual energy, macro- and micronutrient requirements is still ongoing [41,42].

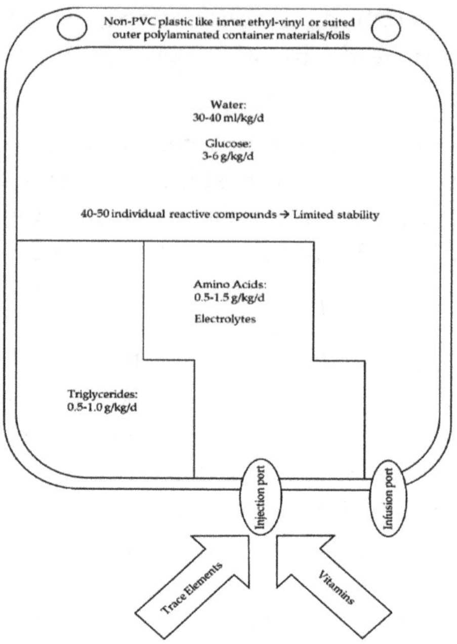

Figure 1. The all-in-one PN concept with adult nutrient requirement, adapted from [2].

8. Stability and Compatibility

Stability defines that the admixture components do not degrade in excess (e.g., <10%). Compatibility defines that these components do not physico–chemically interact with each other over a defined time. Stability and compatibility must last from compounding to delivery, up to the declared expiry date, and the administration under defined conditions. Both aspects are critical for the quality, efficacy and safety of the product [43] There are many physicochemical interactions occurring: instabilities (emulsion), solubility (precipitations), photo-induced (catalytic reactions), thermic reactions, material interactions (sorption, permeation), and chemical reactions (oxidation, reduction, hydrolysis, polymerization, decarboxylation, complexation, lipid peroxidation, Maillard reaction, etc.). A decrease in pH below 5.0 seriously compromises lipid emulsion stability. The first visible sign of decreased homogeneity of the oil-in-water emulsion is creaming (appearance of a white upper layer) [21]. Creaming is reversible by gentle mechanical shaking and occurs without a significant change in the mean particle size nor the particle size distribution. Such AiO PN admixture can be safely administered to the patient. The coalescence is the next deterioration step, which is not anymore reversible. Larger lipid droplets increasingly form over time and may be visible at the surface [21]. Coalescence may be measured by a light extinction method or validated microscopic analysis [44,45] Such emulsions should no more be administered to patients as they may induce adverse effects (e.g., inflammation from phagocytized fat globules, or embolism) [46]. The ultimate step of the on-going droplet enlargement is the emulsion breaking or cracking, where large fat globules separate from the dispersed oil-in-water phase [21]. Administration of such formulations is prohibited. These interactions occur between the components present in AiO PN admixture. They can become critical upon admixing and administration of higher amounts of electrolytes leading to precipitates when disrespecting the solubility product, which is influenced by specific conditions in the PN admixture (volume, pH, temperature, chelating components like AA for cations) [2]. Administration of parenterals containing precipitates may cause small vessels occlusion and consecutive organ damages, and may even become fatal when such precipitates are delivered e.g., into the lung [2]. Precipitates may as well occlude central venous catheter [2,16]. Critical concentrations of divalent cations (mainly Mg^{2+} and Ca^{2+}) in presence of inorganic phosphate lead to precipitation of insoluble phosphate salts. High requirements of such electrolytes exist in neonates but also in adults are incompatible in the amount needed since compatible concentrations for AiO PN admixture are overreached [2]. Such incompatibilities constitute medication errors and are preventable by careful expert proof and choice of appropriate formulations and dose of an individual AiO admixture by the pharmacist [34]. Replacing inorganic salts by organic ones may sometimes also prevent such insolubilities like organic (not hydrolyzed) glycerophosphates [6]. As a rule of thumb, monovalent (mainly Na^+ and K^+) and divalent (mainly Mg^{2+} and Ca^{2+}) cations concentrations in AiO admixtures should not exceed 130 mmol/L and 8 mmol/L, respectively (relative ratio of about 15 between mono- and divalent cations) [21,47].

Compatibility and stability of calcium and phosphate in PN admixtures depend on many factors, such as concentrations, pH, nature of the salts (inorganic or organic), presence/concentration of electrolytes, composition and concentration of the AA solution, lipid emulsion, mixing order, temperature, storage, and hanging time since admixing [21]. High concentrations of calcium and inorganic sodium or potassium phosphate (mono- or dibasic) salts show a greater risk of precipitation at room temperature due to the variation in solubility products at different pH (factor 60). The more acidic pH of peripheral PN admixtures (due to lower AA and/or glucose concentrations and increased lipid concentration) compared to central AiO PN admixtures (high osmolarity) also reduces calcium phosphate solubility [21]. Low infusion rates and room temperature, e.g., in PN admixtures for neonates, contribute to increase the risk of precipitation, eventually occurring during administration and consecutively causing severe organ damages, especially in the lungs. Calcium phosphate precipitation may also occur when iron dextran or bicarbonate are added to PN or infused through the same line without sufficient previous line rinsing [21]. Concentrations of organic calcium (e.g., gluconate) should not exceed 2.5 mmol/L in adult formulations with low osmolarity. Phosphate concentration (mono- and dibasic sodium phosphate salts) should not exceed 15 mmol/L [48]. Organic phosphate salts (e.g., glucoso-1-phosphate or glycerol phosphate) should be used in case of increased needs for calcium and phosphate (e.g., children or neonates). However, organic salts are prone to hydrolysis, possibly releasing highly incompatible inorganic phosphate [49].

Another critical reaction partner is the lipid emulsifier lecithin, a negatively charged natural, large molecular AiO PN component, important to control and stabilize the lipid droplet size, and their size distribution in intravenous formulations. Eventually, the stability of the emulsion is most decisive for the overall stability and safety of an individual AiO PN admixture. Polyvalent cations may react and neutralize the negatively charged phosphate moieties of lecithin at the lipid droplet surface (zeta potential) which is intended to hinder (reversible) aggregation of oil droplets (oil droplet agglomerates). Over time, agglomerates can further develop to irreversible oil droplet coalescence. The enlarged oil droplets (>5 μm diameter) are able to obstruct small blood vesicles (lipid embolism) [2]. Breaking apart of the emulsion and oiling out can occur, which has to be avoided strictly, whereas the initial oil droplet formation is potentially visible at the surface of an AiO PN admixture [2]. Their detection is challenging, and microscopic analysis might be a better approach [50]. Even though this microscopic technique is promising, it is not a recommended method to date. The United States pharmacopoeia recommends measuring the volume-weighted percent of fat droplets greater than 5 μm or PFAT5, must not exceed 0.05% of the total fat (PFAT5) [51] This measurement is usually performed by the manufacturer in an accredited laboratory and not in the daily analytical routine of hospital pharmacies [21]. Even small amounts of trace elements (μM concentration) or locally higher concentration upon admixing of components in a wrong order may influence the emulsion stability and safety. Solubilizers for lipophilic drugs used as vehicles in parenteral drug formulations when admixed or in contact with AiO PN may rise the emulsion stability. This negatively affects the lipid clearance in the body of administered TG from the AiO PN admixture since oil-in-water emulsion becomes meta-stable and thus resist to greater extent to enzymatic plasma lipid clearance [4].

8.1. Vitamin Stability

Some vitamins (e.g., vitamins A, B1, B2, B6, C and K) are chemically unstable and are easily oxidized with air and light. Vitamin A as a lipophilic compound may also interact with the PN container or the infusion set (absorption and/or adsorption). Vitamin B1 and B6 are unstable in presence of oxygen and in direct interaction with trace elements. Vitamin C is also easily degraded to oxalic acid reacting with calcium to form calcium oxalate precipitate [52]. Clinical deficiencies may occur due to such instabilities. Undesired degradation products (e.g., oxalate) may also be infused. Interactions between labile vitamins and PN components are manifold and therefore difficult to extrapolate in theory. Vitamins may only be added to PN AiO admixtures if specific and sufficient stability data are available. In best practice, vitamins should be added to AiO just before or at the very end of the PN administration [21]. This in order to reduce interaction time and eventual time-dependent degradation. Fat-soluble vitamins (A, D, E, K) can be added to lipid-containing AiO admixtures or into lipid infusions. They may be administered weekly or monthly (vitamin K) according to their storage in the body. Vitamins may be protected from light exposure and degradation by lipid emulsions, however, they are themselves prone to peroxidation. Light protection of AiO admixture containers containing vitamins is thus generally recommended during storage and administration [21]. Adding combined admixture of trace elements and vitamins hides high incompatibility potential (e.g., iron and vitamin C) and is therefore not recommended without specific stability data. Commercial multivitamin preparations can be safely administered as separate infusion or even as a slow bolus injection between daily administration of PN portions [53].

8.2. Trace Elements Compatibility

Copper cysteinate, iron phosphate, and formation of insoluble elemental selenium from selenite reduction with vitamin C are the best-known compatibility issues with trace elements [54]. Commercial trace elements solutions show very acidic pH (pH 2), which is critical for lipid stability. Emulsion stability and peroxidation are also negatively influenced by polyvalent cations (e.g., iron, copper, selenium, chrome and zinc) [38,49,55,56]. TG hydrolysis or admixing of trace elements may cause critical pH drop (below pH 5) hampering the emulsion stability. Trace elements should therefore never be added directly to lipid emulsion neither upon compounding nor in a multi-chamber bag. The pH of parenteral products may vary between manufacturers, making it difficult to extrapolate data from one brand to another. AA due to their pH buffering capacity may positively contribute to lipid emulsion stability. AA also have the ability to complex polyvalent cations like electrolytes or trace elements (chelation) avoiding bridging between negatively charged lipid droplets. During compounding or admixing, electrolytes and/or trace elements should therefore be added into the AA solution.

9. Artificial Nutrition and Drug Admixture

9.1. Drug Administration via Feeding Tube

Whenever drug administration occurs via a feeding tube, basic pharmaceutical questions arise to implement safe and efficient therapy: Can the tablet be crushed, or the capsule opened? How should a therapy plan ultimately be put into practice? Drug delivery via a feeding tube is an interprofessional challenge and requires special expertise from all involved stakeholders. Medical, nursing and pharmaceutical aspects have to be considered. The versatility of orally available drug formulations is large and includes specific forms with modified drug release or protective tablet coatings. Interactions between drugs, nutrients, and the human organism can lead to physicochemical reactions and pharmacological changes affecting treatment's efficacy and safety [57]. The prevention and handling of such interactions requires pharmaceutical advice and expertise. Incorrect administration of EN and/or medication due to improper handling must be considered as avoidable medication errors. While various international guidelines have been developed for the nutrition of patients, recommendations for the administration of drugs via feeding tubes are primarily based on empirical values [58]. Information on the accessibility of drugs to medications are not provided as standard information and therefore available only by means of extensive literature research. In 2012, Prohaska et al. found that information on the administration of antiretroviral drugs via feeding tube was only reported in 63% of the cases [59]. Significant problems may occur if drugs galenic is changed, e.g., when a tablet is crushed instead of swallowed. Fatalities have for example been reported after a retarded nifedipine preparation was repeatedly unduly crushed, and administered via feeding tube [60]. Enteral tubes are challenging for the caregivers, both during the hospital stay and after discharge. Resulting ambiguity in the care responsibility can endanger patient safety. Nowadays, tubes made of polyurethane or silicone should be used for EN. These materials guarantee a minimal foreign body sensation and good compatibility over a longer lying time. Polyvinyl chloride (PVC) should be used only for short periods because of the risk of pressure necrosis due to the washing out of the plasticizers [61,62]. Interactions between the tube material and the active ingredients of EN are common. PVC may for example retain relevant levels of carbamazepine, clonazepam, diazepam, phenytoin or tacrolimus, leading to treatment failure [63,64]. The position of the tube tip has a decisive influence on the release and absorption of active ingredients (pH stomach = 1–2, pH duodenum/jejunum = 7–8). Acid-sensitive drugs are destroyed in the acidic stomach environment. If a drug with an enteric coating is crushed and administered via a gastric tube, this leads to a loss of effect, since the drug is early degraded by the gastric acid. It is recommended to avoid administering medication through a jejunal or duodenal tube. In the case of jejunal feeding tube placement, the total amount of fluid used in drug administration should thus not exceed 50 mL. A time gap of 30 min should be kept between the individual bolus doses or the next application; otherwise, it can lead to diarrhea. It should further be taken into account that the tube tip does not have to be the site of the active ingredient intake, and that the passage time in the gastrointestinal tract differs significantly from the oral intake. Consequently, administration of drugs via feeding tube may result in a lower effectiveness or higher risk of side effects compared to the oral route. Blood/urine levels of drugs with narrow therapeutic range administered via a feeding tube should be regularly checked.

9.1.1. Administration of Drugs via Feeding Tube

From a methodical point of view, drug administration via feeding tube is challenging and offers the possibility of interprofessional medication review [65]. This is ideally be done before the final medication prescription, ensuring a safe and efficient administration. In the course of a visit on the ward or in the nursing home, the pharmacist clarify with the physician whether the patient really needs all prescribed drugs in his current situation. Any deprescribing relieves the patient and nursing staff, and reduces complications. Decision for the administration of drug via feeding tube is supported in a structured way as shown in Figure 2. The oral route should be preferred for the drug administration. The patient's ability to swallow has to be evaluated, and regularly promoted, as it may also depend on the form of the day. Depending on the patient's existing ability to swallow, solid dosage forms are replaced by sublingual, liquid, mouth-melting, or transdermal forms. If the patient can swallow liquids, medications should be offered in liquid form or as dispersible tablets (physiological route and less complication potential than via tube). Medicines in liquid dosage form are moreover uncomplicated to give over the tube than solid forms. Numerous interactions and reactions involving drug products, nutrients, and tube devices exist despite the use of solid drug formulation (lower reactivity compared to a dissolved drug delivery system).

Rectal, transdermal, nasal, sublingual or parenteral drug administration should be considered as alternatives to drug application via feeding tube [66]. If no alternative medication is available, an individualized formulation from the pharmacy may be considered. The tube system itself is equally crucial to further assessment. A PEG is more suitable for drug administration than a transnasal or a fine needle catheterized jejunostomy tube because of its brevity and width. The diameter and the location of the tip of the tube are just as important. The osmolality of enteral nutrition is on average 300 mosmol/kg and must not exceed 500–600 mosmol/kg. The stomach tolerates osmolality of up to 1000 mosmol/kg. Liquids with higher osmolality lead to diarrhea (due to a high volume of fluid and electrolyte that cannot be absorbed in the small intestine), nausea, flatulence (due to delayed gastric emptying), or vomiting. To prevent osmotic diarrhea or vomiting, drug formulations have to be diluted with water to isotonic or slightly hypertonic (<400–500 mosmol/kg) solutions to be given through the feeding tube. Even stricter isotonicity is required in case of small intestine tubes, due to the lack of dilution processes in the mouth, esophagus and stomach. Since the intestine, in contrast to the stomach has no storage function, no liquid amounts of more than 50 mL should be given as a bolus directly into the intestine. This significantly restricts the administration of several drugs with according tube position.

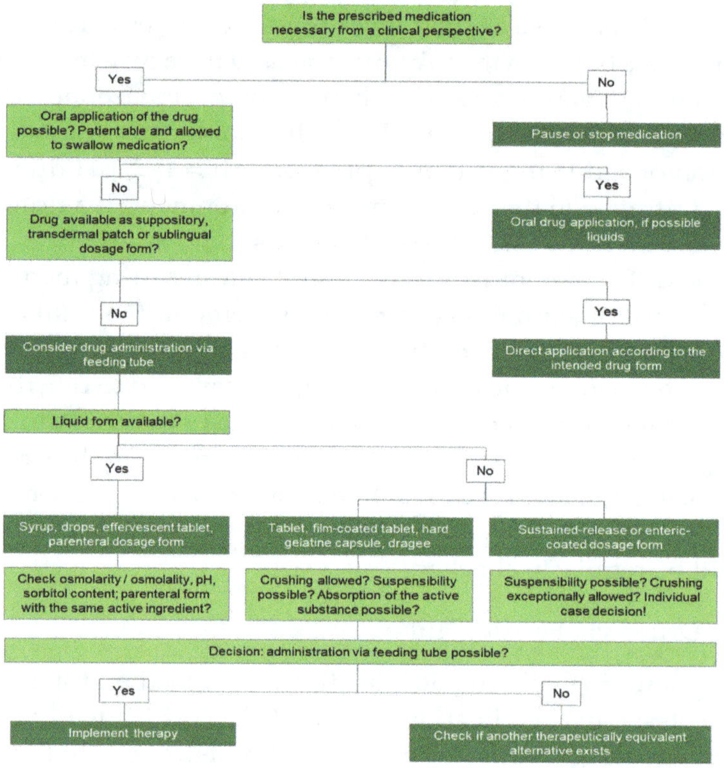

Figure 2. Algorithm for the evaluation of drug administration via feeding tube.

9.1.2. Safety Issues in the Administration of Drugs via Tube

The preparation and administration of carcinogenic, mutagenic drugs or drugs toxic to reproduction, so-called CMR drugs require special attention. Thus, the respective hazard risk handling with cytostatics, anti-infectives/virustatics, hormones, and immunosuppressants must be individually assessed. Work must then be carried out by trained staff, with the necessary protective measures (e.g., gloves, dust mask, protective googles). Patients' relatives and caregivers must be made aware of the relative risk potential. Pregnant or breastfeeding women have to be relieved of such activities. In addition, patients, relatives and caregivers must be informed about safer alternatives dosage forms as liquid dosage forms for example carry less risk than tablets that have to be divided or crushed. Open handling of CMR substances should always be avoided. Pharmacies having dedicated facilities may provide CMR drugs as capsules or pre-filled syringes to minimize drug exposure. The increasing number of oral cancer therapies on the drug market will lead to increased handling questions in the outpatient care.

9.2. Drug Admixture to PN

Extrapolation of AiO PN admixtures stability data from the literature is rarely possible because of the high number and concentration variabilities of components in an individual PN nutrition regimen (Table 3). This is even more complicated in case of drug admixing. The multitude and the concentration dependence of interactions create a multifactorial system not to be assessed by theoretical calculations only. Generation of pharmaceutical stability data may therefore be required for specific cases for documentation and reliability purposes. Sensitive and validated laboratory methods are available in tertiary care hospitals, which may be useful for components of an AiO PN admixtures and concomitant therapy but have to be adapted for the specific in vitro investigation. Such evaluation tools may help to assess the possibility to admix a specific item into a defined AiO PN composition or to check an individual nutrient and/or drug interaction upon request from the clinic in a reasonable and relative short time period [2]. Light microscopy may for example be applied to assess oil-in-water (oil droplet sizing) emulsions. Even though the admixing of drugs to AiO PN admixtures is not recommended, it may be needed in some cases. Compatibility and stability assessment of such combinations may be performed by means of defined drug analytic methods for quantification, adapted from blood plasma or serum to PN matrix [6,50]. Simple test methods have to be elaborated and validated to be used for stability and compatibility assessment of individual admixes to AiO PN regimens upon request [2,16,50].

Table 3. Advices to the possible drug admixture to AiO PN admixture.

Advice Not to Admix	• lipophilic drugs with solubilizes such as cremophors, tweens, etc. • drugs with rapid chemical or physical instabilities • drugs with narrow therapeutic indices (cytotoxics, etc.) • macromolecular recombinant biotech drugs, (signaling proteins, monoclonal antibodies or fusion proteins) • synthetic non-biological complexes (nanomedicines) • drugs with short elimination half-lives and dosage intervals not adjusted to the PN administration period
Admixing May be Possible	• stability documentation is sufficiently available • no ingredients with potential incompatibilities (CAVE polyvalent cations) • large therapeutic index drugs (analgesics, sedatives, H_2-antagonists, etc.) • simple stability testing is possible (pH, emulsion characterization and visual inspection) • well-established, often used, and physico–chemically fully characterized small-molecular drugs

The following points should be considered as good practice using concomitant parenteral drug therapy in PN patients [57,67]:

- Check if the medication is really needed.
- Ask for pharmaceutical advice, ideally from the nutrition support team when therapy regimen are complicated or when drug admixing to PN admixture is considered.
- Admix compatible drugs to PN only just before administration in order to minimize interactions.
- Document procedure, creating a database to control and reference drug-PN admixing interventions.
- If possible collect samples for later analysis and evaluation.
- Use alternative infusion lines (inclusive of other catheter lumen) for drug administration whenever possible. In absence of a separate line, intermittent intravenous drug administration in saline or glucose solutions may be considered. Sufficient catheter rinsing before and after drug administration is mandatory. Special attention is needed for metabolic adverse effects when stopping PN administration because of intermittent drug administration. Insulin stimulation induced by glucose infusion may for example be reduced by lowering the PN administration rates over the last half hour before stopping.

10. Monitoring of Artificial Nutrition

Regular, defined and appropriate assessment may help to avoid respectively decrease the metabolic complications of artificial nutrition. This should include the determination of (specific) individual nutrients, the monitoring and the course of the underlying disease and laboratory testing in addition to the routine clinical assessment. Specific laboratory tests of artificial nutrition-associated parameters include ([5–7]: Hematological testing, lipid status, liver and kidney function (especially in PN), glucose, sodium, potassium, calcium, magnesium, phosphate, CRP, and iron status. Monitoring of anthropometrics such as body weight, body mass index (BMI) and hydration status should as well be performed to ensure the metabolic tolerance of artificial nutrition. Extended and frequent monitoring is required at the initiation of PN for up to two months. Monitoring of long-term, clinically stable PN patients is recommended every 3 to 6 months [6].

11. Home Artificial Nutrition

Some patients require a long-term artificial nutrition, if possible performed in a home setting when no other hospital treatment is needed. The convenient and mostly nocturnal administration enables patients to have a nearly "normal" everyday life and in many cases to keep on working. Patients receiving home artificial nutrition show enhanced quality of life and better social integration [68]. Home artificial nutrition complications rates are lower than in hospital setting, possibly because of the highly trained aseptic handling skills and to the more stable health patients' situation [7]. Nevertheless, it should undergo regular supervision by NSTs and a reliable reporting on critical incidences or health problems has to be in place. European data show that home EN incidence is around 400 per million and home PN incidence around 5 per million people per year. These differences are most likely due to different healthcare systems and resources [3,5,68,69]. To draw conclusions how to better care these home artificial nutrition patients, national registries are necessary to improve and to benchmark the different national experiences [2].

12. Conclusions

The provision of artificial nutrition is a necessary when oral/enteral feeding is insufficient or impossible. With the development of artificial nutrition, administration of EN and mainly PN became convenient and safer, even possible in a home setting. Well-controlled procedures and steady monitoring of the patients by an experienced NST are key issues in the successful management of artificial nutrition, from the prescription (medical care) to through the validation (pharmaceutical care) to the implementation (nursing care) of the therapy. Proper handling, compounding and concomitant drug administration are of the highest relevance for therapeutic success and patient's safety, in EN as well as in PN therapy.

Author Contributions: Conceptualization, E.R. and S.M.; writing—Original draft preparation, E.R., M.M.; writing—Review and editing, Z.S. and S.M.

References

1. Pironi, L.; Steiger, E.; Brandt, C.; Joly, F.; Wanten, G.; Chambrier, C.; Aimasso, U.; Sasdelli, A.S.; Zeraschi, S.; Kelly, D.; et al. Home parenteral nutrition provision modalities for chronic intestinal failure in adult patients: An international survey. *Clin. Nutr.* **2019**. [CrossRef] [PubMed]
2. Mühlebach, S. Diets and Diet Therapy: Parenteral Nutrition. In *Encyclopedia of Food Security and Sustainablility (FOSS)*; Ferranti, P., Berry, E., Anderson, J., Eds.; Elsevier: Amsterdam, The Netherlands, 2019; pp. 131–142. [CrossRef]
3. National Collaborating Centre for Acute Care. *Nutrition Support in Adults Oral Nutrition Support, Enteral Tube Feeding and Parenteral Nutrition*; National Collaborating Centre for Acute Care: London, UK, 2006.
4. Mühlebach, S.; Driscoll, H.; Hardy, G. Pharmaceutical Aspects of Parenteral Nutrition Support. In *Basics in Clinical Nutrition*, 4th ed.; Sobotka, L., Ed.; Galen: Prague, Czech Republic, 2011; pp. 373–400.

5. Aeberhard, C.; Mühlebach, S. Parenteral Nutrition—Basics and Good Practice. *Aktuel Ernahr.* **2017**, *42*, 53–76. [CrossRef]
6. Bischoff, S.C.; Arends, J.; Dörje, F.; Engeser, P.; Hanke, G.; Köchling, K.; Leischkeret, A.H.; Mühlebach, S.; Schneider, A.; Seipt, A.; et al. S3-Leitlinie der Deutschen Gesellschaft für Ernährungsmedizin (DGEM) in Zusammenarbeit mit der GESKES und der AKE. *Aktuel Ernahrungsmed* **2013**, *38*, e101–e154. [CrossRef]
7. Wanten, G.; Calder, P.C.; Forbes, A. Managing adult patients who need home parenteral nutrition. *BMJ* **2011**, *342*, d1447. [CrossRef] [PubMed]
8. Dudrick, S.J. Early developments and clinical applications of total parenteral nutrition. *J. Parenter. Enter. Nutr.* **2003**, *27*, 291–299. [CrossRef]
9. Brennan, G.T.; Ha, I.; Hogan, C.; Nguyen, E.; Jamal, M.M.; Bechtold, M.L.; Nguyen, D.L. Does preoperative enteral or parenteral nutrition reduce postoperative complications in Crohn's disease patients: A meta-analysis. *Eur. J. Gastroenterol. Hepatol.* **2018**, *30*, 997–1002. [CrossRef]
10. Dreznik, Y.; Horesh, N.; Gutman, M.; Gravetz, A.; Amiel, I.; Jacobi, H.; Zmora, O.; Rosin, D. Preoperative Nutritional Optimization for Crohn's Disease Patients Can Improve Surgical Outcome. *Dig. Surg.* **2018**, *35*, 442–447. [CrossRef]
11. Heidegger, C.P.; Berger, M.M.; Graf, S.; Zingg, W.; Darmon, P.; Costanza, M.C.; Thibault, R.; Pichard, C. Optimisation of energy provision with supplemental parenteral nutrition in critically ill patients: A randomised controlled clinical trial. *Lancet* **2013**, *381*, 385–393. [CrossRef]
12. Anderson, A.D.; Palmer, D.; MacFie, J. Peripheral parenteral nutrition. *Br. J. Surg.* **2003**, *90*, 1048–1054. [CrossRef]
13. Gura, K.M. Is there still a role for peripheral parenteral nutrition? *Nutr. Clin. Pract.* **2009**, *24*, 709–717. [CrossRef]
14. Omotani, S.; Tani, K.; Nagai, K.; Hatsuda, Y.; Mukai, J.; Myotoku, M. Water Soluble Vitamins Enhance the Growth of Microorganisms in Peripheral Parenteral Nutrition Solutions. *Int. J. Med. Sci.* **2017**, *14*, 1213–1219. [CrossRef] [PubMed]
15. Sugrue, D.; Jarrell, A.S.; Kruer, R.; Davis, S.; Johnson, D.; Tsui, E.; Snyder, S.; Crow, J. Appropriateness of peripheral parenteral nutrition use in adult patients at an academic medical center. *Clin. Nutr. ESPEN* **2018**, *23*, 117–121. [CrossRef] [PubMed]
16. Hvas, C.L.; Farrer, K.; Donaldson, E.; Blackett, B.; Lloyd, H.; Forde, C.; Garside, G.; Paine, P.; Lal, S. Quality and safety impact on the provision of parenteral nutrition through introduction of a nutrition support team. *Eur. J. Clin. Nutr.* **2014**, *68*, 1294–1299. [CrossRef] [PubMed]
17. Bozzetti, F.; Mariani, L.; Bertinet, D.B.; Chiavenna, G.; Crose, N.; De Cicco, M.; Gigli, G.; Micklewright, A.; Moreno Villares, J.M.; Orban, A.; et al. Central venous catheter complications in 447 patients on home parenteral nutrition: An analysis of over 100.000 catheter days. *Clin. Nutr.* **2002**, *21*, 475–485. [CrossRef] [PubMed]
18. Lopez-Briz, E.; Ruiz Garcia, V.; Cabello, J.B.; Bort-Marti, S.; Carbonell Sanchis, R.; Burls, A. Heparin versus 0.9% sodium chloride locking for prevention of occlusion in central venous catheters in adults. *Cochrane Database Syst. Rev.* **2018**, *7*, Cd008462. [CrossRef] [PubMed]
19. Raupp, P.; von Kries, R.; Schmidt, E.; Pfahl, H.G.; Gunther, O. Incompatibility between fat emulsion and calcium plus heparin in parenteral nutrition of premature babies. *Lancet* **1988**, *1*, 700. [CrossRef]
20. Wouters, Y.; Theilla, M.; Singer, P.; Tribler, S.; Jeppesen, P.B.; Pironi, L.; Vinter-Jensen, L.; Rasmussen, H.H.; Rahman, F.; Wanten, G.J.A. Randomised clinical trial: 2% taurolidine versus 0.9% saline locking in patients on home parenteral nutrition. *Aliment. Pharmacol. Ther.* **2018**, *48*, 410–422. [CrossRef]
21. Muehlebach, S.; Driscoll, D.; Aeberhard, C.; Stanga, Z. Stability and compatibility of parenteral nutrition (PN) admixtures. In *Basics in Clinical Nutrition*, 5th ed.; Sobotka, L., Ed.; Galen: Prague, Czech Republic, 2019; pp. 354–361.
22. McKinnon, B.T. FDA safety alert: Hazards of precipitation associated with parenteral nutrition. *Nutr. Clin. Pract.* **1996**, *11*, 59–65. [CrossRef]
23. Jauch, K.W.; Schregel, W.; Stanga, Z.; Bischoff, S.C.; Brass, P.; Hartl, W.; Muehlebach, S.; Pscheidl, E.; Thul, P.; Volk, O. Access technique and its problems in parenteral nutrition—Guidelines on Parenteral Nutrition, Chapter 9. *GMS Ger. Med. Sci.* **2009**, *7*, Doc19. [CrossRef]

24. Ayers, P.; Adams, S.; Boullata, J.; Gervasio, J.; Holcombe, B.; Kraft, M.D.; Marshall, N.; Neal, A.; Sacks, G.; Seres, D.S. ASPEN parenteral nutrition safety consensus recommendations. *J. Parenter. Enter. Nutr.* **2014**, *38*, 296–333. [CrossRef]
25. Pirlich, M.; Bodoky, G.; Kent-Smith, L. Complications of enteral nutrition. In *Basics in Clinical Nutrition*, 5th ed.; Sobotka, L., Ed.; Galen: Prague, Czech Republic, 2019; pp. 319–323.
26. Montejo, J.C. Enteral nutrition-related gastrointestinal complications in critically ill patients: A multicenter study. The Nutritional and Metabolic Working Group of the Spanish Society of Intensive Care Medicine and Coronary Units. *Crit. Care Med.* **1999**, *27*, 1447–1453. [CrossRef] [PubMed]
27. Staun, M.; Pironi, L.; Bozzetti, F.; Baxter, J.; Forbes, A.; Joly, F.; Jeppesen, P.; Moreno, J.; Hebuterne, X.; Pertkiewicz, M.; et al. ESPEN Guidelines on Parenteral Nutrition: Home parenteral nutrition (HPN) in adult patients. *Clin. Nutr.* **2009**, *28*, 467–479. [CrossRef] [PubMed]
28. Aubry, E.; Friedli, N.; Schuetz, P.; Stanga, Z. Refeeding syndrome in the frail elderly population: Prevention, diagnosis and management. *Clin. Exp. Gastroenterol.* **2018**, *11*, 255–264. [CrossRef] [PubMed]
29. Friedli, N.; Stanga, Z.; Culkin, A.; Crook, M.; Laviano, A.; Sobotka, L.; Kressig, R.W.; Kondrup, J.; Mueller, B.; Schuetz, P. Management and prevention of refeeding syndrome in medical inpatients: An evidence-based and consensus-supported algorithm. *Nutrition* **2018**, *47*, 13–20. [CrossRef] [PubMed]
30. Laesser, C.; Cumming, P.; Reber, E.; Stanga, Z.; Muka, T.; Bally, L. Management of Glucose Control in Noncritically Ill, Hospitalized Patients Receiving Parenteral and/or Enteral Nutrition: A Systematic Review. *J. Clin. Med.* **2019**, *8*, 935. [CrossRef] [PubMed]
31. Umpierrez, G.E.; Hellman, R.; Korytkowski, M.T.; Kosiborod, M.; Maynard, G.A.; Montori, V.M.; Seley, J.J.; Van den Berghe, G. Management of hyperglycemia in hospitalized patients in non-critical care setting: An endocrine society clinical practice guideline. *J. Clin. Endocrinol. Metab.* **2012**, *97*, 16–38. [CrossRef] [PubMed]
32. Muehlebach, S.; Driscoll, D.F.; Hardy, G. How to prepare parenteral nutrition (PN) admixtures, and the role and function of the pharmacis. In *Basics in Clinical Nutrition*, 5th ed.; Sobotka, L., Ed.; Galen: Prague, Czech Republic, 2019; pp. 345–353.
33. Gales, B.J.; Riley, D.G. Improved total parenteral nutrition therapy management by a nutritional support team. *Hosp. Pharm.* **1994**, *29*, 469–470.
34. Taxis, K.; Barber, N. Ethnographic study of incidence and severity of intravenous drug errors. *BMJ* **2003**, *326*, 684. [CrossRef]
35. American Diabetes Association. 15. Diabetes Care in the Hospital: Standards of Medical Care in Diabetes-2019. *Diabetes Care* **2019**, *42*, S173–S181. [CrossRef]
36. Anez-Bustillos, L.; Dao, D.T.; Baker, M.A.; Fell, G.L.; Puder, M.; Gura, K.M. Intravenous Fat Emulsion Formulations for the Adult and Pediatric Patient: Understanding the Differences. *Nutr. Clin. Pract.* **2016**, *31*, 596–609. [CrossRef]
37. Steger, P.J.; Muhlebach, S.F. Lipid peroxidation of i.v. lipid emulsions in TPN bags: The influence of tocopherols. *Nutrition* **1998**, *14*, 179–185. [CrossRef]
38. Steger, P.J.; Muhlebach, S.F. Lipid peroxidation of intravenous lipid emulsions and all-in-one admixtures in total parenteral nutrition bags: The influence of trace elements. *J. Parenter. Enter. Nutr.* **2000**, *24*, 37–41. [CrossRef] [PubMed]
39. Lobo, D.; Lewington, A.; Allison, S. Basic Concepts of Fluid and Electrolyte Therapy. Available online: https://www.researchgate.net/publication/249625074_Basic_Concepts_of_Fluid_and_Electrolyte_Balance (accessed on 1 January 2013).
40. Muhlebach, S. Practical aspects of multichamber bags for total parenteral nutrition. *Curr. Opin. Clin. Nutr. Metab. Care* **2005**, *8*, 291–295. [CrossRef] [PubMed]
41. Evering, V.H.; Andriessen, P.; Duijsters, C.E.; Brogtrop, J.; Derijks, L.J. The Effect of Individualized Versus Standardized Parenteral Nutrition on Body Weight in Very Preterm Infants. *J. Clin. Med. Res.* **2017**, *9*, 339–344. [CrossRef]
42. Yailian, A.L.; Serre, C.; Fayard, J.; Faucon, M.; Thomare, P.; Filali, S.; Pivot, C.; Vetele, F.; Pirot, F.; Olivier, E. Production and stability study of a hospital parenteral nutrition solution for neonates. *J. Pharm. Anal.* **2019**, *9*, 83–90. [CrossRef]
43. Mühlebach, S. Incompatibility reactions in drug therapy–preventable medication errors. *Eur. Hosp. Pharm. J. Pract.* **2007**, *13*, 30–31.

44. Driscoll, D. Examination of selection of light-scattering and light-obscuration acceptance criteria for lipid injectable emulsions. *Pharm. Forum.* **2004**, *30*, 2244–2253.
45. Schmutz, C.W. Zubereitung Parenteraler Ernährungsmischungen in der Spitalapotheke: Untersuchungen zur Pharmazeutischen Qualität und Stabilität. Ph.D. Thesis, Universität Basel, Basel, Switzerland, 1993.
46. Washington, C. The stability of intravenous fat emulsions in total parenteral nutrition mixtures. *Int. J. Pharm.* **1990**, *66*, 1–21. [CrossRef]
47. Davis, S. The stability of fat emulsions for intravenous administration. In *Advances in Clinical Nutrition*; Springer: Berlin, Germany, 1983; pp. 213–239.
48. Newton, D.W.; Driscoll, D.F. Calcium and phosphate compatibility: Revisited again. *Am. J. Health Syst. Pharm.* **2008**, *65*, 73–80. [CrossRef]
49. Gräflein, C. Parenterale Ernährung mit Stabilitätsgeprüften, Modularen Standardlösungen in der Neonatologie. Ph.D. Thesis, Philosophisch-Naturwissenschaftliche Fakultät der Universität Basel, Basel, Switzerland, 2004.
50. Aeberhard, C.; Steuer, C.; Saxer, C.; Huber, A.; Stanga, Z.; Muhlebach, S. Physicochemical stability and compatibility testing of levetiracetam in all-in-one parenteral nutrition admixtures in daily practice. *Eur. J. Pharm. Sci.* **2017**, *96*, 449–455. [CrossRef]
51. Pharmacopea, U. Globule size distribution in lipid injectable emulsions. *U. S. Pharm. Rockv. MD US Pharm.* **2011**, *1*, 297–299.
52. Ribeiro, D.O.; Pinto, D.C.; Lima, L.M.; Volpato, N.M.; Cabral, L.M.; de Sousa, V.P. Chemical stability study of vitamins thiamine, riboflavin, pyridoxine and ascorbic acid in parenteral nutrition for neonatal use. *Nutr. J.* **2011**, *10*, 47. [CrossRef] [PubMed]
53. Muhlebach, S.; Franken, C.; Stanga, Z. Practical handling of AIO admixtures—Guidelines on Parenteral Nutrition, Chapter 10. *GMS Ger. Med. Sci.* **2009**, *7*, Doc18. [CrossRef] [PubMed]
54. Allwood, M.C.; Martin, H.; Greenwood, M.; Maunder, M. Precipitation of trace elements in parenteral nutrition mixtures. *Clin. Nutr.* **1998**, *17*, 223–226. [CrossRef]
55. Laborie, S.; Lavoie, J.C.; Pineault, M.; Chessex, P. Contribution of multivitamins, air, and light in the generation of peroxides in adult and neonatal parenteral nutrition solutions. *Ann. Pharmacother.* **2000**, *34*, 440–445. [CrossRef]
56. Allwood, M.C.; Kearney, C. Compatibility and stability of additives in parenteral nutrition admixtures. *Nutrition* **1998**, *14*, 697–706. [CrossRef]
57. Muehlebach, S.; Aeberhard, C.; Stanga, Z. Drugs and Nutritional Admixtures. In *Basics in Clinical Nutrition*; Sobotka, L., Ed.; Galen: Prague, Czech Republic, 2019; p. 362.
58. Volkert, D.; Beck, A.M.; Cederholm, T.; Cruz-Jentoft, A.; Goisser, S.; Hooper, L.; Kiesswetter, E.; Maggio, M.; Raynaud-Simon, A.; Sieber, C.C.; et al. ESPEN guideline on clinical nutrition and hydration in geriatrics. *Clin. Nutr.* **2019**, *38*, 10–47. [CrossRef]
59. Prohaska, E.S.; King, A.R. Administration of antiretroviral medication via enteral tubes. *Am. J. Health Syst. Pharm.* **2012**, *69*, 2140–2146. [CrossRef]
60. Schier, J.G.; Howland, M.A.; Hoffman, R.S.; Nelson, L.S. Fatality from administration of labetalol and crushed extended-release nifedipine. *Ann. Pharmacother.* **2003**, *37*, 1420–1423. [CrossRef]
61. Subotic, U.; Hannmann, T.; Kiss, M.; Brade, J.; Breitkopf, K.; Loff, S. Extraction of the plasticizers diethylhexylphthalate and polyadipate from polyvinylchloride nasogastric tubes through gastric juice and feeding solution. *J. Pediatr. Gastroenterol. Nutr.* **2007**, *44*, 71–76. [CrossRef]
62. Stein, J.; Dormann, A. Sonden-und Applikationstechniken. In *Praxishandbuch Klinische Ernährung und Infusionstherapie*; Springer: Berlin, Germany, 2003; pp. 291–310.
63. Treleano, A.; Wolz, G.; Brandsch, R.; Welle, F. Investigation into the sorption of nitroglycerin and diazepam into PVC tubes and alternative tube materials during application. *Int. J. Pharm.* **2009**, *369*, 30–37. [CrossRef] [PubMed]
64. Shibata, N.; Ikuno, Y.; Tsubakimoto, Y.; Hoshino, N.; Minouchi, T.; Yoshio, K.; Inoue, T.; Taga, T.; Ando, A.; Hodohara, K.; et al. Adsorption and pharmacokinetics of cyclosporin A in relation to mode of infusion in bone marrow transplant patients. *Bone Marrow Transplant.* **2000**, *25*, 633–638. [CrossRef] [PubMed]
65. Griese-Mammen, N.; Hersberger, K.E.; Messerli, M.; Leikola, S.; Horvat, N.; van Mil, J.W.F.; Kos, M. PCNE definition of medication review: Reaching agreement. *Int. J. Clin. Pharm.* **2018**, *40*, 1199–1208. [CrossRef] [PubMed]

66. Muehlebach, S.; Aeberhard, C.; Stanga, Z. Pharmaceutical aspects in enteral feeding and drugs. In *Basics in Clinical Nutrition*; Sobotka, L., Ed.; Galen: Prague, Czech Republic, 2019; p. 314.
67. Mühlebach, S. Basics in clinical nutrition: Drugs and nutritional admixtures. *E-SPEN Eur. E-J. Clin. Nutr. Metab.* **2009**, *3*, e134–e136. [CrossRef]
68. Bischoff, S.C.; Austin, P.; Boeykens, K.; Chourdakis, M.; Cuerda, C.; Jonkers-Schuitema, C.; Lichota, M.; Nyulasi, I.; Schneider, S.M.; Stanga, Z.; et al. ESPEN guideline on home enteral nutrition. *Clin. Nutr.* **2019**. [CrossRef] [PubMed]
69. Van Gossum, A.; Bakker, H.; De Francesco, A.; Ladefoged, K.; Leon-Sanz, M.; Messing, B.; Pironi, L.; Pertkiewicz, M.; Shaffer, J.; Thul, P.; et al. Home parenteral nutrition in adults: A multicentre survey in Europe in 1993. *Clin. Nutr.* **1996**, *15*, 53–59. [CrossRef]

12

Metabolic and Nutritional Characteristics of Long-Stay Critically Ill Patients

Marina V. Viana [1], Olivier Pantet [1], Geraldine Bagnoud [1,2], Arianne Martinez [1], Eva Favre [1], Mélanie Charrière [1,2], Doris Favre [1,2], Philippe Eckert [1,†] and Mette M. Berger [1,*,†]

1 Service of Adult Intensive Care Medicine and Burns, Lausanne University Hospital (CHUV), 1011 Lausanne, Switzerland
2 Service of Endocrinology, Diabetes and Metabolism, Lausanne University Hospital, 1011 Lausanne, Switzerland
* Correspondence: Mette.Berger@chuv.ch
† These authors contributed equally as co-seniors to this paper.

Abstract: Background: insufficient feeding is frequent in the intensive care unit (ICU), which results in poor outcomes. Little is known about the nutrition pattern of patients requiring prolonged ICU stays. The aims of our study are to describe the demographic, metabolic, and nutritional specificities of chronically critically ill (CCI) patients defined by an ICU stay >2 weeks, and to identify an early risk factor. Methods: analysis of consecutive patients prospectively admitted to the CCI program, with the following variables: demographic characteristics, Nutrition Risk Screening (NRS-2002) score, total daily energy from nutritional and non-nutritional sources, protein and glucose intakes, all arterial blood glucose values, length of ICU and hospital stay, and outcome (ICU and 90-day survival). Two phases were considered for the analysis: the first 10 days, and the next 20 days of the ICU stay. Statistics: parametric and non-parametric tests. Results: 150 patients, aged 60 ± 15 years were prospectively included. Median (Q1, Q3) length of ICU stay was 31 (26, 46) days. The mortality was 18% at ICU discharge and 35.3% at 90 days. Non-survivors were older ($p = 0.024$), tended to have a higher SAPSII score ($p = 0.072$), with a significantly higher NRS score ($p = 0.033$). Enteral nutrition predominated, while combined feeding was minimally used. All patients received energy and protein below the ICU's protocol recommendation. The proportion of days with fasting was 10.8%, being significantly higher in non-survivors (2 versus 3 days; $p = 0.038$). Higher protein delivery was associated with an increase in prealbumin over time ($r^2 = 0.19$, $p = 0.027$). Conclusions: High NRS scores may identify patients at highest risk of poor outcome when exposed to underfeeding. Further studies are required to evaluate a nutrition strategy for patients with high NRS, addressing combined parenteral nutrition and protein delivery.

Keywords: chronic critical illness; protein; Nutrition Risk Screening (NRS-2002); age; nutrition; vasopressors; shock; glucose; diabetes; underfeeding

---

1. Introduction

The intensive care unit (ICU) patient population has evolved over the last two decades with the appearance of an increasing number of patients requiring very long ICU stays, lasting up to several months after surviving the initial acute insult [1]. A long stay is usually defined as the requirement of more than one week of mechanical ventilation (MV) and of ICU therapy, but different definitions have been used [2]. Chronic critical illness (CCI) is the most frequent designation for these patients, which is characterized by lengthy hospital stays, intense suffering, high mortality rates, and substantial resource consumption [3]. Genetic influence has also been shown to be increasingly present, particularly in pediatric ICUs [4]. Preexisting chronic comorbidities are strong, independent predictors of this condition [5]. In the ICU, mechanical ventilation, sepsis, Glasgow score < 15, inadequate calorie intake, and higher body mass index (BMI) have been identified as independent predictors of this condition [6].

Recently, a study including 185 chronic, critically ill patients showed that the preadmission nutritional status reflected by the Nutrition Risk Screening (NRS-2002) (hereafter NRS) [7] might be a good predictor of the outcome: a score ≥ 5 points seemed to be a cutoff predictor of mortality [8]. Entering the acute disease with deficits such as weight loss, being older, or malnourished, seems to constitute a metabolic handicap that threatens the patient's response capacity and survival. In 2013, the same group observed that inadequate nutrition (defined as the provision of less than 60% of needs) and organ failure (defined by the sequential organ failure assessment (SOFA) score) are mortality risk factors [6].

The optimal timing and amount of feeding has been much debated. Indeed, the intestine of the sickest patients is not always available to accommodate full feeding as shown by the French randomized controlled, multicenter, parallel group trial called NUTRIREA-2 including 2410 patients with septic shock [9]. Furthermore, many patients are at risk of the refeeding syndrome [10]. A recent Brazilian study showed in a cohort of 100 critically ill patients with a mean ICU stay of 19 days, that those 45 patients receiving a caloric intake ≥70% during the first 72 h of hospitalization did not present better outcomes in the short term (mechanical ventilation, length of ICU stay) or after 1 year (functional capacity, mortality) [11]. For both above reasons, i.e., risk of stressing the intestine and of relative overfeeding [12], the early full feeding strategy seems unable to promote a good outcome. In this context, the most recent European Society for Clinical Nutrition and Metabolism (ESPEN) guidelines propose increasing progressively (ramping up) the energy delivery whatever the feeding route over 3–4 days [13]. Furthermore, prescribed energy goals should be covered somewhere between day 4 and 7, and preferentially be determined by indirect calorimetry.

To better coordinate the treatment of the long stay patients admitted to our ICU, and to identify procedures that could be improved, the service initiated a dedicated program enrolling patients requiring more than 2 weeks of ICU treatment. The present study aims to describe the metabolic and nutritional specificities of these patients, to analyze those associated with poor outcome, and to identify a factor that might enable early detection of CCI risk.

2. Methods

With the approval of the Commission Cantonale d'Ethique sur la Recherche humaine (CER 2018-02018), consecutive patients admitted to the 35 bed multidisciplinary ICU of the Lausanne University Hospital were analyzed. The patients had been prospectively enrolled in the long-stay program of the ICU, a plan of action called PLS (Patients Long Séjour) created in January 2017 to improve the care of patients requiring more than 2 weeks of ICU therapy (clinical trial identifier: NCT03938961). The PLS program consisted of weekly interdisciplinary meetings addressing ventilation, nutrition, cognitive and functional issues, symptom management, psychological support, and complication prevention. The meetings ended with detailed evaluation and a plan of action.

2.1. Patients

The inclusion criteria were age >18 years, and inclusion in the PLS program with an ICU stay >2 weeks. The exclusion criteria were admission for major burns >20% body surface, traumatic brain injury, and patients who refused participation.

2.2. Study Variables

Data were extracted from the computerized information system (Metavision® iMDsoft, Tel Aviv, Israel, version 5.46.44) and included age, admission (dry weight) and discharge body weight, body mass index (BMI), NRS-2002 score [7], severity of disease (SAPSII), Sequential Organ Failure Assessment (SOFA) score on days 1, 2, 5, 10, 30, and discharge [14]), requirement of continuous renal replacement therapy (CRRT), admission for sepsis, presence of diabetes, daily intakes (energy, protein, glucose: raw data and per kg), all arterial blood glucose values, 24 h insulin dose, arterial blood lactate (maximal value), daily feeding route, pressure ulcers occurring during the ICU stay, discharge Medical Research Council force score (MRC), length of mechanical ventilation, ICU and hospital length of stay, ICU and 90-days mortality. Laboratory: blood prealbumin (determined weekly), C-reactive protein (CRP), and procalcitonin (mean of the ICU stay).

2.3. Nutrition Protocol

The ICU's protocol called NUTSIA (NUTrition aux Soins Intensifs Adultes) is based on the ESPEN guidelines [13]. Enteral nutrition is recommended as the first option when nutritional therapy is indicated (i.e., for patients for whom oral intake is not possible), and should be initiated within the first 3 days after hemodynamic stabilization. Parenteral nutrition (PN) may be used as combined feeding, or total PN from day 4 and earlier in selected malnutrition situations. Energy goals are 20 kcal/kg/day during the first week, to be increased or adapted thereafter—indirect calorimetry is recommended from day 7. The initial energy goal should be reached by day 4–5. Energy intakes include the energy from feeding products and oral intakes, and the energy resulting from glucose (drug dilution) and fat (sedative propofol), which are administered for non-nutritional purposes.

Feeding products were: Peptamen Intense (Nestlé, Switzerland), Promote Fiber plus (Abbott, Switzerland), Isosource Energy Fiber (Nestlé, Switzerland), Nutriflex Omega special (BBraun, Switzerland), and Pharmacy compounded PN in individual cases.

Energy balances were calculated as the daily difference between the total substrate intakes (nutritional and non-nutritional sources) and the prescribed value. The mean daily and the cumulated values were calculated for the first 10 days, and a cutoff of cumulated deficit −70 kcal/kg was considered critical [15,16]. For proteins, the daily delivery was compared to the recommended target of 1.2 g/kg/day. The cumulated deficit was calculated for the first 10 days and a cutoff of −300 g was considered critical.

Glucose control is handled by nurses, with a blood glucose (BG) goal of 6–8 mmol/L (6–10 mmol/L in diabetic patients) maintained using continuous insulin infusion. Blood glucose is presented as the daily mean value, and is measured on a point of care blood gas analyzer. Its variability is indicated as the daily standard error of the daily BG values. Daily total insulin was recorded.

The 2 dieticians (one full time position present on working days) attended to patients requiring >3 ICU days. These individuals are in charge of checking route of feeding, energy needs (indirect calorimetry), proteins delivery, and adapting the feeding solutions [17]. They attend the weekly PLS meetings.

2.4. Other Variables

Muscle strength upon discharge was assessed using the MRC score [18], where the patient's effort is graded on a *scale* of 0–5. Six muscle groups were bilaterally measured (abduction of the arm, flexion of the forearm, extension of the wrist, flexion of the hip, extension of the knee, and dorsal flexion of the foot). All muscle groups were scored between 0 and 5 (0, no visible/palpable contraction; 1, visible/palpable contraction without movement of the limb; 2, movements of the limb but not against gravity; 3, movements against gravity (almost full passive range of motion) but not against resistance; 4, movement against gravity and resistance, arbitrarily judged to be sub-maximal for gender and age; 5, normal). Therefore, the maximal score is 60 points.

2.5. Statistical Analysis

Data of the entire stay were extracted, but analysis was limited to the first 30 days. The data are presented as means ± standard deviation (SD), or median (interquartile Q1, Q3) depending on normal distribution, which was assessed through histograms and calculation of skewness and kurtosis. For non-parametric variables, the Kruskal-Wallis test was used. Two phases were considered for the analysis of the nutritional related variables: the first days (D1–D10), and the next 20 days of the ICU stay (D11–D30). The continuous variables in survivors versus non-survivors were compared using the one-way and two-way ANOVA, while the categorical variables were compared using Chi^2 tests. For non-parametric variables, Kruskal-Wallis rank sum test was used. Kaplan–Meier analysis and Cox regression were used to compare mortality. For the Kaplan–Meier analysis, the log rank test was used to compare the curves of each NRS group (3–4 and 5–6–7 points). The generalized linear model (GLM) was used to analyze response variables that were not normally distributed such as substrate administration or blood glucose over the 30 days. Statistical programs were JMP version 14.2 for Windows, (SAS Institute GMH, Böblingen, Germany), and R Version 3.5.3, 2019 (R Foundation for Statistical Computing, Vienna, Austria). Significance level was set at $p < 0.05$.

3. Results

3.1. Patients

The current study included prospectively 150 patients admitted between 1 February 2017 and 31 December 2018. During the same period, 589 patients were admitted who required ICU for >7 days, but the majority were discharged before entering the PLS program. Table 1 summarizes patient demographics and clinical outcomes, with the details of survivors/non-survivors at ICU discharge. Most patients (60.7%) were admitted for medical causes (17/91 with a surgical background), followed by emergency surgery, and elective surgery (52% were admitted for sepsis, and 48% needed continuous renal replacement during their stay).

Table 1. Demographics, severity of illness, laboratory and outcome variables according to ICU vital status.

	Overall	Non-Survivors	Survivors	*p*
N (%)	150	27 (18%)	123 (82%)	
Age (mean (SD))	60.2 (14.6)	66.0 (10.9)	59.0 (15.0)	0.024
Sex (Males, %)	116 (77.3)	24 (88.9)	92 (74.8)	0.184
Body weight admission (kg, mean (SD)) discharge	78.3 (18.4) 75.7 (17.8)	77.4 (18.8) 81.5 (18.5)	78.4 (18.4) 74.3 (17.5)	0.785 0.054
BMI (mean (SD))	26.47 (6.09)	26.15 (6.42)	26.54 (6.05)	0.761
SAPS2 (mean (SD))	52.9 (18.3)	58.7 (15.8)	51.7 (18.6)	0.072
SOFA on Day1 (median (Q1, Q3))	8 (5, 11)	11 (9, 14)	9 (6, 12)	0.134
NRS (median (Q1, Q3))	5 (3, 6)	5 (4, 6)	4 (3, 6)	0.033
Medical/Emergency surgery/elective surgery	91/40/19	20/6/1	71/34/18	0.141
Diabetes (%)	26 (17.3)	7 (25.9)	19 (15.4)	0.307
Renal failure requiring CRRT (*n*, % of *n*)	72 (48.0%)	22 (81.5%)	50 (40.5%)	<0.001
Sepsis on admission (*n*, % of *n*)	78 (52.0)	15 (55.6)	63 (51.2)	0.845
CRP (median (Q1, Q3)) mean of stay	125 (81,170)	153 (97, 183)	116(77, 166)	0.096
Procalcitonin (median (Q1, Q3)) mean of stay	1.4 (0.4, 4.6)	3.2 (1.6, 7.7)	1.0 (0.3, 3.7)	0.008
Glucose (daily means (median (Q1, Q3))	7.7 (7.2, 8.4)	7.8 (7.4, 8.2)	7.6 (7.1, 8.4)	0.408
Lactate (daily max (median (Q1, Q3))	1.7 (1.4, 2.1)	2.0 (1.7, 2.7)	1.6 (1.4, 2.1)	0.004
Pressure ulcers (n patients with)	72 (48%)	12	60	0.835
MRC on discharge (median (Q1, Q3) (*n* = 91))	34 (24,42)	31 (25, 43)	35 (25,42)	0.825
Length of Mech.Ventilation (days) (median (Q1, Q3))	16.1 (10.0, 21.6)	17.8 (13.2, 26.8)	15.7 (9.8, 20.3)	0.152
Total length of ICU stay (median (Q1, Q3))	31 (23, 46)	29 (18, 44)	31 (24, 46)	0.268
Hospital length of stay (median (Q1, Q3))	57 (39, 82)	30 (24, 47)	63 (44, 91)	<0.001

Abbreviations: SOFA = Sequential Organ Failure Assessment, SAPS = Simplified Acute Physiology Score, BMI = Body Mass Index, NRS = Nutrition risk screening, CRP = C-reactive protein, Q1 and Q3 = q quartiles 25, 75.

Gender was equally distributed, but the non-survivors were older ($p = 0.024$) and tended to have a higher SAPSII score ($p = 0.072$). The admission SOFA score did not differ significantly but its evolution was different over time, decreasing significantly in survivors ($p < 0.0001$) (Figure A1). The cardiac component of the score remained elevated for a longer period of time (i.e., at 3–4 points) in the non-survivors. A significantly higher NRS score ($p = 0.033$) was observed in non-survivors. The Kaplan–Meier analysis showed that the scores NRS 5–6–7 are associated with a higher 90-days mortality of 43.8% versus 25.7% with NRS scores 3 and 4, respectively (Figure 1). Admission weight (mean 78.3 kg) and BMI were similar, but the weight change over time differed significantly ($p < 0.0001$) depending on the outcome. By the end of the stay, survivors had lost weight, while non-survivors had gained weight due to a persistent positive fluid balance. While 28 patients (18%) died in the ICU, further 26 patients died within 90 days, resulting in a total of 56 (35.3%) deaths—age and NRS differences became even more pronounced by day 90 (age $p < 0.001$; NRS $p = 0.005$; Table A1). A Cox regression model with 90-days mortality as an outcome showed an increased risk of death in patients with NRS ≥ 5 (HR 2.2 (1.18–4.2), $p = 0.013$), but not for the SAPS2 score (HR 1.0 (0.99–1.0), $p = 0.235$). Diabetes mellitus was present in 17.3% of patients, but was not associated with any mortality difference.

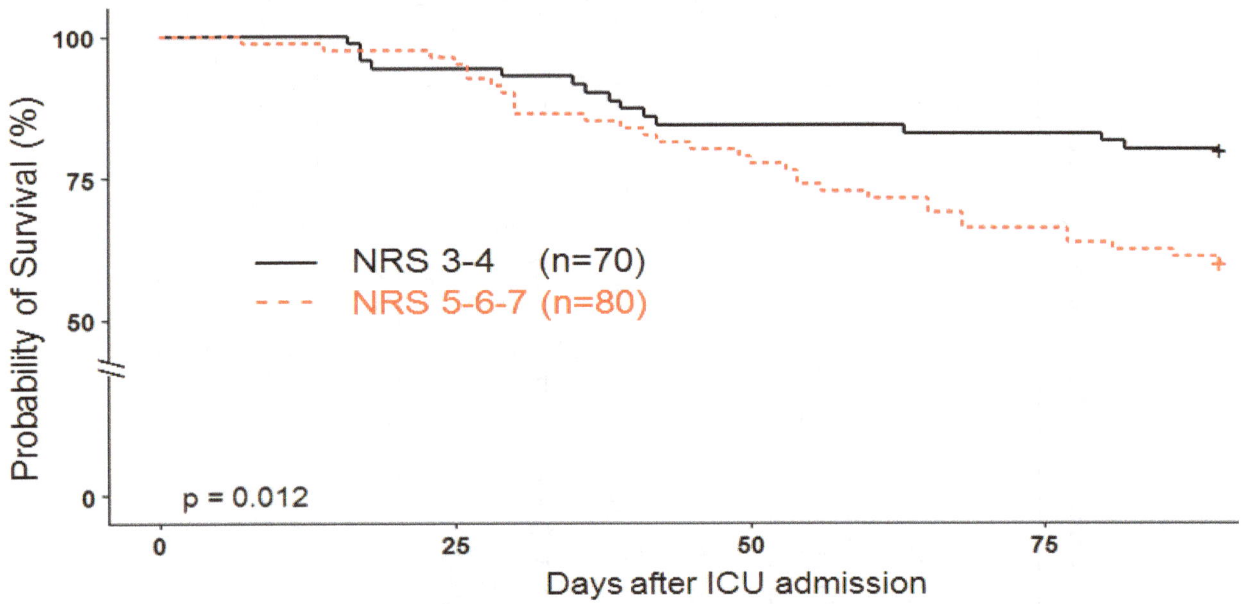

Figure 1. Kaplan–Meier analysis comparing elevated and low NRS scores. NRS: Nutrition Risk Screening and ICU: intensive care unit.

3.2. Nutrition

The proportion of days with intentional absence of feeding (fasting) was 10.8% of total days (Table 2 and Figure 2), being significantly higher in non-survivors ($p = 0.038$), with fasting contributing to the high day-to-day variability of intakes (Figure 3)—except for the number of fasting days (3 versus 2, $p = 0.043$). Table 2 shows that there was no difference between survivors and non-survivors. Fasting days were mostly observed during the first 5 days, but did occur throughout the 30 days. The feeding route was predominantly enteral, representing 55.7% of total days; combined enteral (EN) and parenteral (PN) feeding represented 8.1% and 14.1% of total days, respectively, and variable route combinations was used in 1% of total days.

Table 2. Nutrition characteristics according to ICU outcome (D = day).

	Overall	Non-Survivors	Survivors	p
N (%)	150	27 (18%)	123 (82%)	
Days of fasting: N per patient (median (Q1, Q3))	2.0 (1.0, 3.0)	3.0 (1.0, 4.0)	2.0 (1.0, 3.0)	0.043
Percentage of days (median (Q1, Q3))	5.4 (2.4, 10.0)	7.8 (4.3, 10.9)	4.9 (2.0, 9.3)	0.031
Prealbumin (delta of stay) (median (Q1, Q3)) g/L	0.07 (0.04, 0.12)	0.06 (0.02, 0.10)	0.07 (0.04, 0.13)	<0.001
Energy delivery D1–10 (median (Q1, Q3)) kcal/day (median (Q1, Q3)) kcal/kg/day	1161 (957, 1370) 15.8 (11.8, 18.9)	1121 (936, 1385) 16.4 (12.1, 17.9)	1161 (983, 1368) 15.7 (11.8, 19.1)	0.719 0.838
Energy delivery D11–30 (median (Q1, Q3)) kcal/day (median (Q1, Q3)) Kcal/kg/day	1559 (1368, 1762) 20.8 (17.9, 23.9)	1504 (1284, 1645) 20.2 (15.5, 21.9)	1581 (1387, 1772) 20.9 (18.1, 24.1)	0.104 0.151
Cumulated Energy balance D1–10 (median (Q1, Q3)) kcal/day (median (Q1, Q3)) kcal/kg/day	−5266 (−8365, −2697) −70 (−102, −37)	−5365 (−9208, −2852) −74 (−125, −38)	−5234 (−8043, −2651) −69 (−101, −36)	0.519 0.345
Cumulated Energy balance D1–30 (median (Q1, Q3)) kcal /day (median (Q1, Q3)) kcal /kg/day	−7700 (−11,607, −4702) −96.8 (−148.2, −59.7)	−7710 (−12,197, −5097) −92.4 (−151.1, −67.1)	−7677 (−11,350, −4554) −97.5 (−146.9, −58.4)	0.532 0.801
Protein delivery D1–10 (median (Q1, Q3)) g/day (median (Q1, Q3)) g/kg/day	53.7 (40.7, 64.3) 0.69 (0.52, 0.86)	54.0 (40.2, 61.9) 0.73 (0.57, 0.86)	53.4 (41.7, 65.7) 0.68 (0.50, 0.87)	0.673 0.768
Protein delivery D11–30 (median (Q1, Q3)) g/day (median (Q1, Q3)) g/kg/day	75.4 (62.0, 90.3) 1.0 (0.6, 1.4)	70.0 (49.4, 83.7) 0.95 (0.68, 1.1)	76.4 (63.3, 90.4) 1.0 (0.8, 1.2)	0.051 0.104
Cumulate protein balance D1–10(median (Q1, Q3)) g/day (median (Q1, Q3)) g/kg/day	−374 (−595, −223) −4.86 (−6.82, −3.36)	−352 (−538, −244) −4.63 (−6.18, −3.49)	−379 (−608, 216) −4.98 (−7.07, −3.34)	0.803 0.938
Cumulate protein balance D1–30 g/day (median (Q1, Q3)) g/kg/day	−603 (−1070, −304) −7.91 (−12.47, −4.13)	−531 (−1006, −355) −7.89 (−13.62, 4.74)	−611 (−1069, −299) −8.43 (−12.34, −4.11)	0.912 0.816

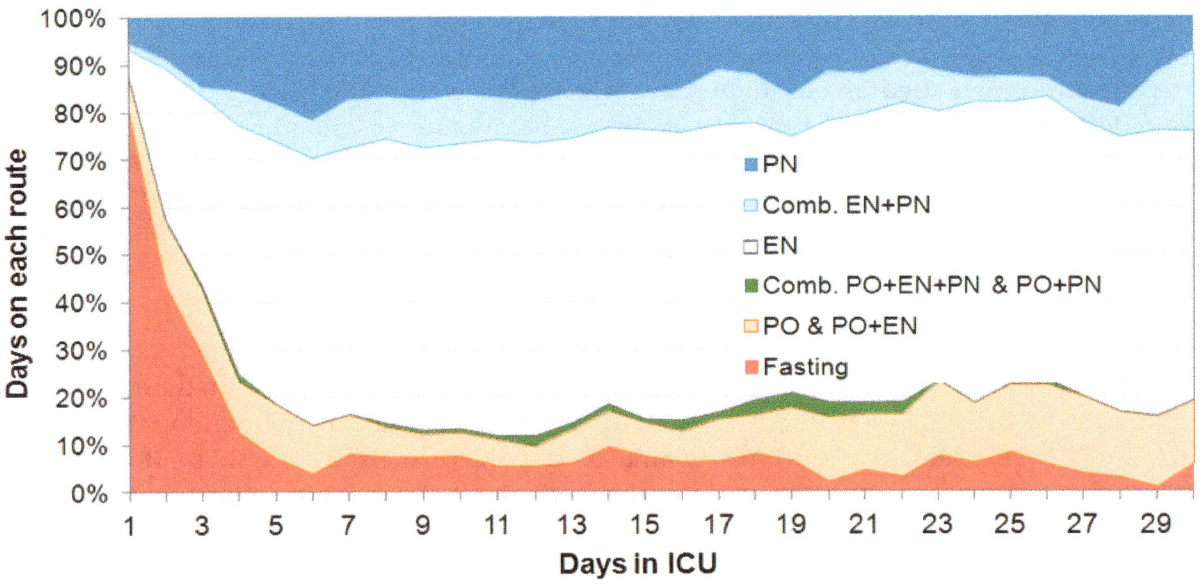

Figure 2. Evolution of the route of feeding over time presented as percentage of all patients over the first 30 days—there is a variable time of fasting during the first week. Enteral feeding was predominant, with a stable proportion of combined enteral–parenteral feeding (Comb EN + PN), or total parenteral nutrition (PN), and a variable proportion of the combinations oral–enteral, or oral–parenteral. Abbreviations: EN = enteral nutrition, PN = parenteral nutrition, Comb = combined, PO = oral.

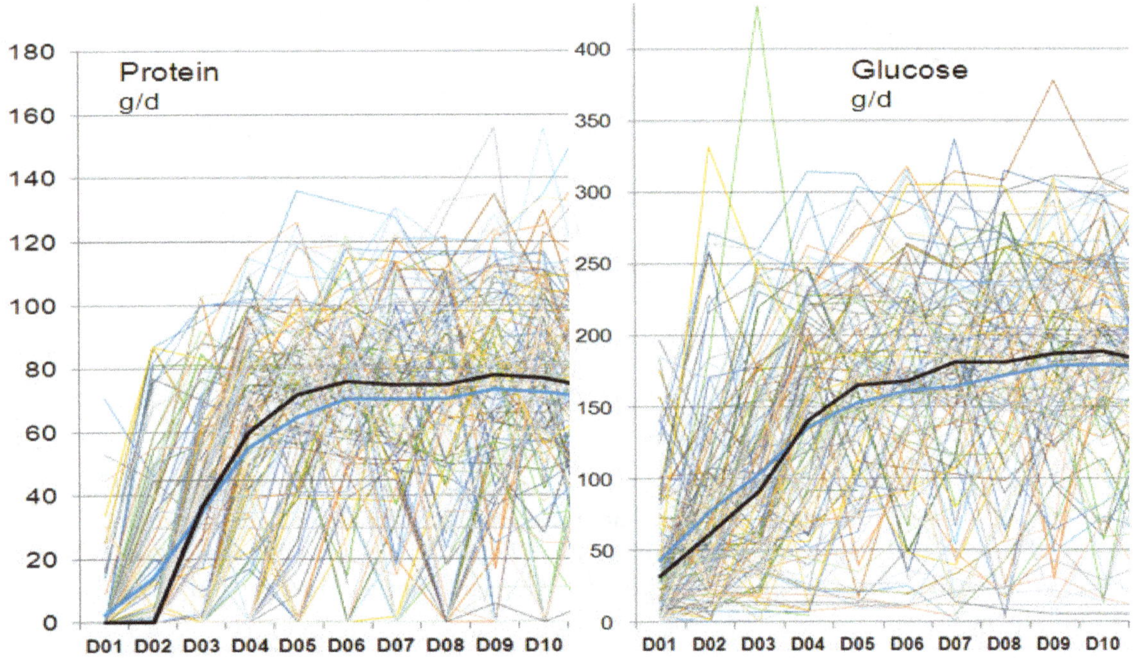

Figure 3. Individual delivery of protein and glucose by day during the first 10 days. Each line represents individual patient values. The erratic aspect aims at showing a phenomenon which is the extreme day to day variability and multiple interruptions that characterize the nutrition in the early phase. The thick dark lines show median (blue) and mean (black) values.

3.2.1. Energy

The mean prescribed energy during the first 10 days was 21.7 kcal/kg/day, and 23.4 kcal/kg/day thereafter (1750 kcal/day). The individual patients were characterized by a high variability of feeding, and total protein and glucose intakes (Figure 3). The progression of feeding occurred over the first 10 days (and not over 5 days as per protocol), i.e., before inclusion in the dedicated program (no difference between the two categories). Figure 4 shows the mean values for protein and energy, which were below the service's recommendations and below the prescribed values. Both groups were underfed, resulting in a median cumulated negative balance of −5266 kcal by day 10 (−70 kcal/kg). Nutrition delivery improved over time, but stagnated below the prescribed value.

Indirect calorimetry was available in 95 patients. The prescription was −236 kcal (range: −1391 to +483 kcal) below the measured energy expenditure. When this deficit is added to the daily energy deficit (difference between prescribed and delivered), the median deficit becomes −741 kcal/day (range: −2971 to −123 kcal per day) for the first 10 days.

3.2.2. Proteins

The delivery was lowest during the first 10 days (Figure 4), with a median of 64.3 g/day (0.70 g/kg/day), which is below the 1.2 g/kg/day service NUTSIA recommendation. By day 10, 80 patients (53.3%) exceeded −300 g of cumulated deficit. Protein intake thereafter increased to 1 g/kg/day remaining below recommendation, with a tendency to be lower in non-survivors.

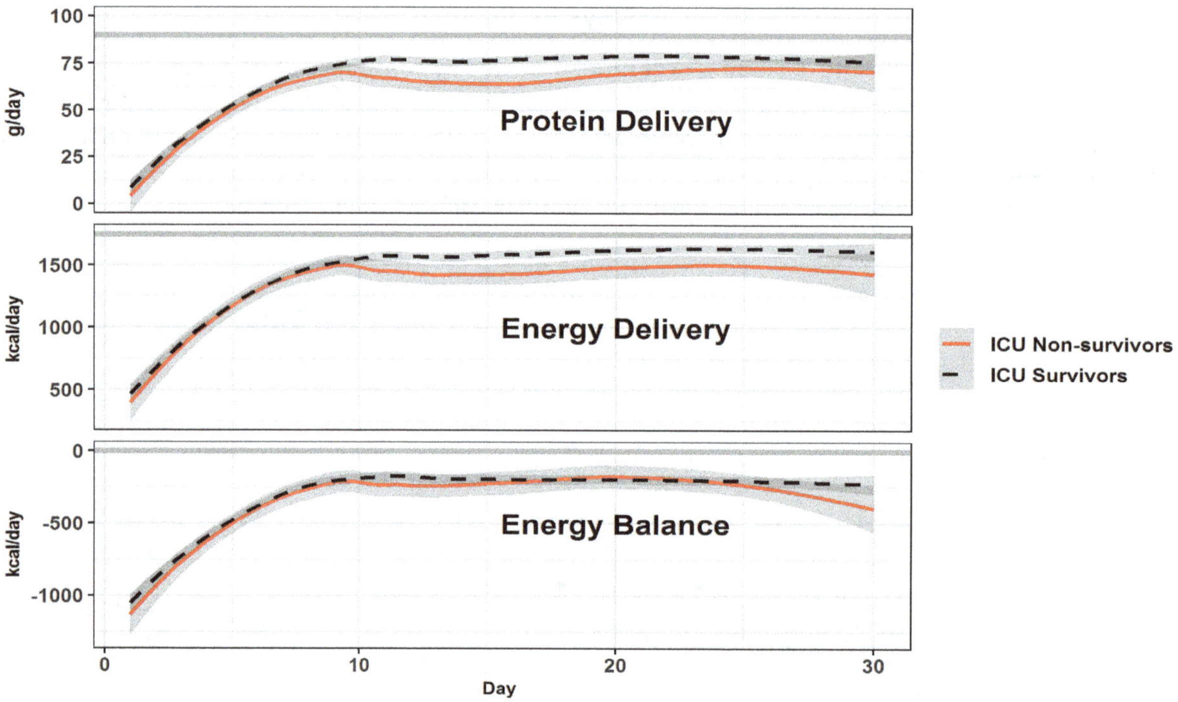

Figure 4. Mean protein and energy delivery with the resulting energy balance over the first 30 days according to ICU vital status (mean ± SD). The thick gray lines show protein target (1.2 g/kg/day), energy goal (prescribed value), and neutral energy balance. The differences in protein and energy delivery between survivors and non-survivors were significant after day 10 ($p < 0.001$). Energy balances were similarly negative.

Prealbumin, the lowest values were observed in patients with high NRS scores ($p = 0.067$). Prealbumin increased over time in the majority of patients in association with higher protein delivery ($r^2 = 0.19$; $p = 0.027$), and the increase (difference between first and last value of the ICU stay) was lower in non-survivors ($p < 0.001$).

3.2.3. Blood glucose

Altogether, 30,769 arterial blood glucose values were available for analysis (4–10 blood samples per day). Blood glucose and related variables differed between survivors and non-survivors (Figure 5), and over time. While glucose intakes were identical and low, non-survivors had higher BG values during the first 10 days, but not thereafter. Variability was higher, but not significant. Insulin needs were significantly higher and became again higher after day 20, while survivors' insulin needs declined, reaching below 30 u/day. Blood maximal lactate was also significantly higher during the first days in non-survivors.

The BG pattern differed in diabetic patients, being higher throughout the stay as per protocol, with higher variability and higher 24 h insulin requirements (Figure A2). This was particularly marked in surviving diabetic patients (Figure A3). Diabetic non-survivors were characterized by lower BG values and higher insulin needs during the first 5 days. Arterial lactate was elevated during the first 5 days in the majority of patients, being significantly higher in diabetic non-survivors.

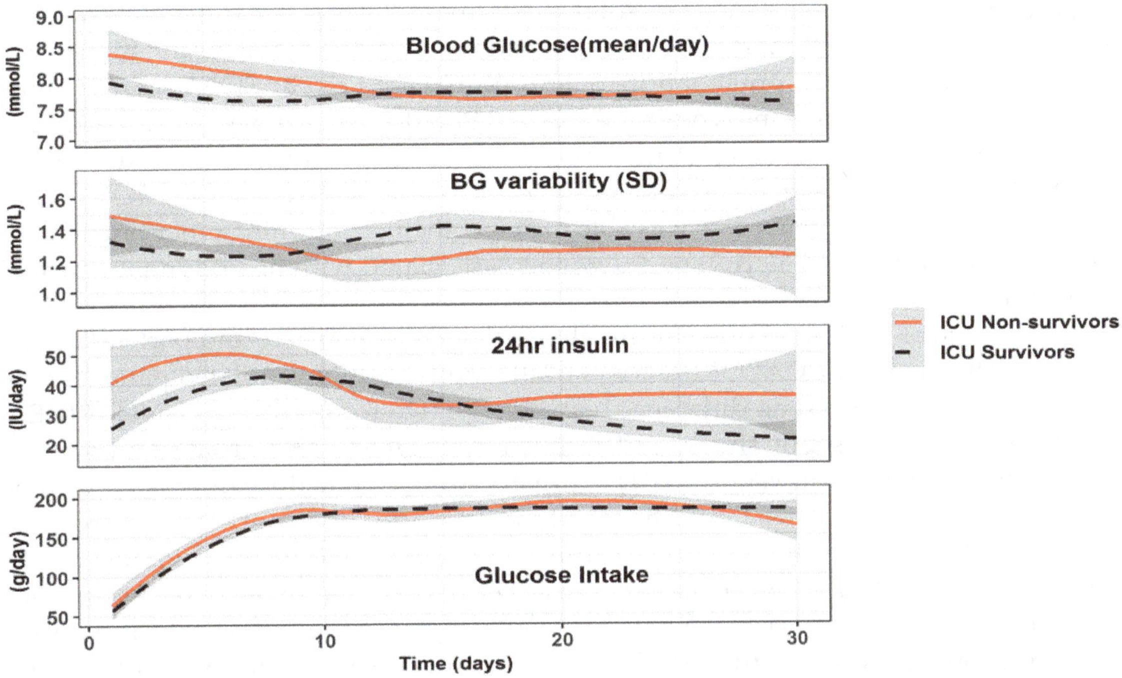

Figure 5. Evolution of mean blood glucose (mmol/L), Blood Glucose (BG) variability (standard error = SD of the individual daily values), 24 h insulin (total dose/24 h), and glucose intake (total in g/day). The figure shows that the 24 h Insulin delivery is not related to the glucose intake, which was similar in both groups (data are represented as mean ± SD).

3.3. MRC Discharge Score

MRC discharge score was available in 91 patients. The median value on discharge was low with 34 points. In those patients who did not suffer significant persistent renal failure on discharge (which results in elevated creatinine values), the median serum creatinine was 52 μmol/L (a low value in adult patients, and a surrogate for muscle mass).

4. Discussion

The main finding in our study is that CCI patients are not equal upon admission. Many patients begin their ICU journey without metabolic reserves reflected by a high NRS score. However, the impact is not immediate. During the first 10 days, the patients were exposed to very low and highly variable energy and protein intakes, and many were exposed to prolonged and repeated fasting. The acute underfeeding generated important energy and protein deficits, resulting in an additional malnutrition diagnosis in these critically ill patients. Combined EN and PN feeding was minimally used, despite being included in the service's protocol based on randomized trials [19,20]. In patients at risk of malnutrition upon admission, the underfeeding further erodes a previously altered metabolic status, resulting in a poor outcome. These results confirm recent observational data [16], where patients at low risk are likely to have a reasonable outcome despite several days of inadequate nutrition, while those at higher risk do not. The 2019 ESPEN recommendations [13] emphasize that no patient should be left longer than 72 h without initiating a balanced feeding. The majority of nutrition-related studies focus on the first days after admission, and have often included moderately sick or young patients that did not really benefit from artificial nutrition. By extracting the data of the entire stay, we observed that there was an early phase, and a later phase with a turning point around day 10. Thereafter, the patients were better fed, but the majority did not reach their prescribed goals.

The patient cohort was critically ill, as reflected by an elevated admission SAPSII score and an 18% ICU mortality, which was significantly higher than the general ICU patient's mortality (14.4%). The non-survivors were older, which belongs to the risk factors of CCI [1]. At the 90 days time point, a further 26 patients had died, increasing the total mortality to 35.3%. The initial SOFA score did not differ, but the score's evolution differed in survivors and non-survivors, remaining higher in the latter. The inclusion of the evolution of organ failure over time assessed by the SOFA score is an important strength of this study. Our data do not confirm those of a Brazilian cohort of 453 CCI patients, in which the initial SOFA score was a predictor of mortality [6]. One of the aims of the study was to find a variable facilitating the early detection of patients at critical illness risk. The total SOFA score did not predict the outcome, while the NRS score was able to detect them, confirming other Brazilian results [8]. A NRS score ≥ 5 should raise an alert, especially when associated with hemodynamic instability and high lactate values.

Timing and route of feeding in the critically ill has long been debated, and particularly the timing of PN initiation. The pragmatic CALORIES trial in 2400 mechanically ventilated patients randomized to EN or PN from day 1 showed no difference between the two routes [21]. The NUTRIREA-2 study included 2410 patients with septic shock, and showed that full early EN from day 1 was associated with more intestinal complications ($p < 0.001$) compared to the same dose of PN [9], with no benefit of EN on infectious complications. Providing early full feeding does not seem to prevent patients from becoming CCI, as shown by a Brazilian study including 100 critically ill patients. The study further shows that providing a caloric intake ≥70% in the first 72 h of admission did not improve short term or 1-year outcomes [11]. Among the possible explanations of these disappointing results, the early endogenous glucose production [20,22] in response to acute illness should be considered. This production covers approximately two thirds of energy expenditure during the first days of disease. In addition, enteral full feeding is not always tolerated, as shown by NUTRIREA-2 [9], and the risk of refeeding syndrome is a reality [10]. The dose of both feeding and vasopressors might be the explanation as shown by the secondary analysis of a large septic cohort which showed that EN providing close to recommended intakes of energy and proteins over the stay was associated with a better outcome [23]. A propensity-matched analysis, including 52,563 ventilated adult patients stratified by dose of noradrenalin [24], suggests that in patients on low- or medium-dose noradrenalin, early EN seems associated with a reduction in mortality but not in the patients requiring high-dose noradrenalin. The recommendation to provide early, but progressive feeding starting ideally during the first 48 h, while discouraging early full feeding whatever the route, formulated in the latest ESICM [25] and ESPEN [13] guidelines was built on such data.

The ICU's internal protocol recommends progressing to the goal by day 4–5 based on ESPEN recommendations, which was not achieved without any difference between survivors and non-survivors. The latter were characterized by a higher percentage of fasting days during the first days after admission (associated with hemodynamic instability), but also occurring at random thereafter. The reasons for the feeding interruptions are multiple in an ICU, and have not changed much over the last decades [26]. The elevated mean cardiovascular SOFA scores reflect a persistent hemodynamic instability, which is probably one of the reasons for withholding feeding, and for difficult EN progression. These poor results may need a change in our ICU feeding procedure. Volume based feeding needs consideration as recent studies show that it is safe, and effectively improves energy and protein delivery compared to traditional rate-based feeding [27].

An American study analyzed the discharge destinations of critically ill surgical patients according to the magnitude of their energy and protein deficit. The authors showed that nutrition was a major outcome determinant [16]. Yeh et al. used a cumulated deficit cutoff of −6000 kcal and of −300 g protein. The patients who remained below those cutoffs were three times more likely to be discharged home. The authors also observed a longer ICU stay and higher mortality in those patients exceeding these values. In the present cohort, the patients entered the PLS program only after 2 weeks. Large energy and protein deficits had built up, but did not differ between survivors and non-survivors, both being similarly underfed by day 10: 80 patients (53.3%) exceeded the −300 g protein deficit and 50 patients (33%) exceeded the −6000 kcal cutoff. Knowing that the indirect calorimetry values for energy expenditure were higher than prescription in the majority of patients, the real deficit is even greater. Malnutrition causes loss of lean body mass, which is a determinant of the outcome [28,29], with the early protein deficit being an important contributor to the loss. The positive response of prealbumin to higher protein delivery shows that increasing proteins delivery is a treatment option. Critical illness is characterized by a high degree of stress with an accelerated protein degradation that results in malnutrition, systemic inflammation, and organ dysfunction [30]. Supporting this hypothesis, Briassoulis et al. showed that in critically ill children, only 22.7% of patients without protein deficiencies versus 37% of those at risk or already deficient, developed multiple-organ system failure [31]. Further transferrin and prealbumin levels increased already after 5 days of early EN, and the patients with positive nitrogen balance had higher prealbumin levels [32]. In critically ill patients, this muscle loss occurs very rapidly as shown in the landmark study by Puthucheary et al. [33]. In patients with two or more organ failures, the mean loss of muscle measured by ultrasound of the thigh was 22% in 10 days. The present patients were in multiple organ failure as reflected by their high SOFA score. However, there is currently no standardized procedure to assess sarcopenia in long-stay catabolic patients [34], and only surrogates are available: low (33 points) muscle strength at discharge (MRC score) and the discharge creatinine values below those recorded at admission reflect the loss of muscle mass. These results highlight the importance of an early multidisciplinary awareness for metabolic and nutritional issues, i.e., waiting 2 weeks to address them is too long. The timing, dose, and route of feeding must be addressed more stringently and earlier, and the recommendations of the dieticians applied more diligently in the high risk patients already by day 3–4.

Among the factors associated with ICU weakness, hyperglycemia has been considered important, as insulin therapy might be an attenuating factor of muscle loss through its anabolic properties [35]. Hyperglycemia is associated with increased mortality in critically ill patients [36], an issue that appears to improve by tight glycemic control [37]. The debate regarding optimal glycemic control continues as diabetic patients are frequent and exhibit a different response to tight glucose control [38]. However, there is little data in patients with prolonged ICU stay. One study reported that tighter glycemic control was associated with improved outcomes in CCI patients with stress hyperglycemia, but not in CCI patients with diabetes [39]. In the present study, the initial BG values were elevated, independently of low glucose intake. BG normalized around day 10, and remained stable thereafter, being higher in the non-survivors despite similar glucose intakes. The observed changes in BG and insulin needs over time may be related to the decrease in lean body mass. The future non-survivors also required more insulin during the 2nd phase, possibly reflecting a metabolic derangement. Diabetic patients exhibited a different pattern compared to non-diabetics corresponding to the application of the internal protocol.

Limitations of the study: our current study is observational, including only 150 patients, but the patients were enrolled prospectively to the PLS program and the study was aimed at identifying early risk criteria. The strength of the data comes from the quality of data extraction from the computer system, resulting in longitudinal continuous daily data. Regarding fasting, the study was not designed to record the reasons for the feeding interruptions, so exact causes are missing but are unlikely to differ from other observations [26]. Furthermore, our study lacks a measure for the loss of lean body mass. Except for ultrasound, which was not available in our clinical setting, there is currently no standardized procedure to assess sarcopenia in CCI patients [34]. Whole body multi-frequency bioimpedance, phase angle, and ultrasound assessment of the cross-sectional area of the thigh might become clinically useful tools, as they are non-invasive and little costly. We therefore consider integrating them into the nutrition protocol.

In randomized trials, our group showed that, in case of insufficient enteral feeding during the first 3 days (i.e., <60% of 25 kcal/kg/day which is <15 kcal/kg/day), supplemental PN (SPN) guided by indirect calorimetry to cover the measured value from day 4, reduced nosocomial infections [19] and related costs [40]. Furthermore, our group recently showed that this reduction was explained by modifications of the immune response and attenuation of the inflammatory response [20], with a trend to less loss of muscle mass ($p = 0.07$). This combined strategy should probably be applied more frequently, especially in patients with NRS ≥ 5 who obviously are not covering their needs, and who have persistent high cardiac SOFA scores. The two above Swiss SPN studies also show that a two-phase approach may be the most respectful of physiological mechanisms. Critically ill patients are generally unstable during the first days, and their endogenous energy production is elevated [22], providing 200–300 g glucose per day. This endogenous glucose production has an elevated protein cost, and 120 g/day were shown to be catabolized for neoglucogenesis. Full feeding during this period is therefore associated with a risk of overfeeding [12]. The present study shows that the very simple NRS score is probably able to identify patients who will not tolerate a prolonged underfeeding. This two-step, more physiological approach and the absence of difference between the enteral and parenteral feeding was recently summarized [41]. It is also important to integrate that "nutrition is more than the sum of its parts" as described by Briassoulis et al. [42], who emphasized that focusing only and separately on proteins or energy is not sufficient. An integrated, individualized approach, including all substrates and micronutrients is needed [43].

5. Conclusions

The present study shows that high NRS scores upon admission may identify patients at higher risk of a poor outcome, and those who require individualized nutrition therapy [43]. Exposing these high-risk patients to underfeeding further deteriorates their response capacity, including immune defenses [40], possibly favoring the development of chronic critical illness. The NRS score is not a malnutrition score, but identifies those patients who are at risk of high mortality at an early stage, this risk increasing further with underfeeding. Having no reserves, these patients will cope worse, and continue eroding their lean body mass, contributing to the poor prognosis [28,29]. Our study also shows that the most unstable patients, who become chronic, are exposed to discontinuous feeding, partly explained by persistent shock and high blood lactate values which question the clinicians about intestinal integrity, and the feasibility of EN [25]. In our previous studies [15], and in others [16], the cutoff of −70 kcal/kg of cumulated energy deficit was associated with increasing complications. Preventing such a deficit to build up requires identifying the patients at risk by their elevated NRS and hemodynamic instability. This would enable the introduction of combined feeding by day 4–5, while checking the real needs by indirect calorimetry. This strategy should be tested prospectively.

Author Contributions: Conceptualization P.E., E.F., O.P., and M.M.B.; methodology M.M.B., M.V.V., and P.E.; validation, M.V.V., O.P., G.B., A.M., E.F., M.C., D.F., P.E., and M.M.B.; formal analysis, M.M.B. and M.V.V.; methodology, M.V.V., E.V., A.M., and M.M.B.; supervision, M.M.B.; validation, M.V.V., G.B., M.C., and D.F.; investigation, M.V.V., O.P., A.M., E.F., M.C., D.F., and G.B.; resources, P.E. and M.M.B.; data curation, G.B., M.V.V., M.M.B., M.C., and D.F.; writing—original draft preparation, M.M.B. and M.V.V.; writing—review and editing, M.V.V., O.P., G.B., A.M., E.F., M.C., D.F., P.E., and M.M.B.; project administration, M.M.B., P.E., and O.P.

Appendix A

Table A1. Demographics, severity of illness, laboratory, and outcome variables according to the 90-day outcome.

	Overall	Non-Survivors	Survivors	*p*
N (%)	150	53 (35.3%)	97 (64.7%)	
Age (mean (SD))	60.2 (14.6)	66.1 (12.3)	57.0 (14.9)	<0.001
Sex (Males, %)	116 (77.3)	45 (84.9)	71 (73.2)	0.093
BMI (mean (SD))	26.47 (6.09)	26.56 (5.9)	26.42 (6.23)	0.899
SAPS2 (mean (SD))	52.9 (18.3)	55.5 (16.9)	51.6 (18.9)	0.211
SOFA on Day1 (median (Q1, Q3))	8 (5,11)	11 (8, 13)	9 (6, 12)	0.056
NRS (median (Q1, Q3))	5 (3, 6)	5 (4, 6)	4 (3, 6)	0.005

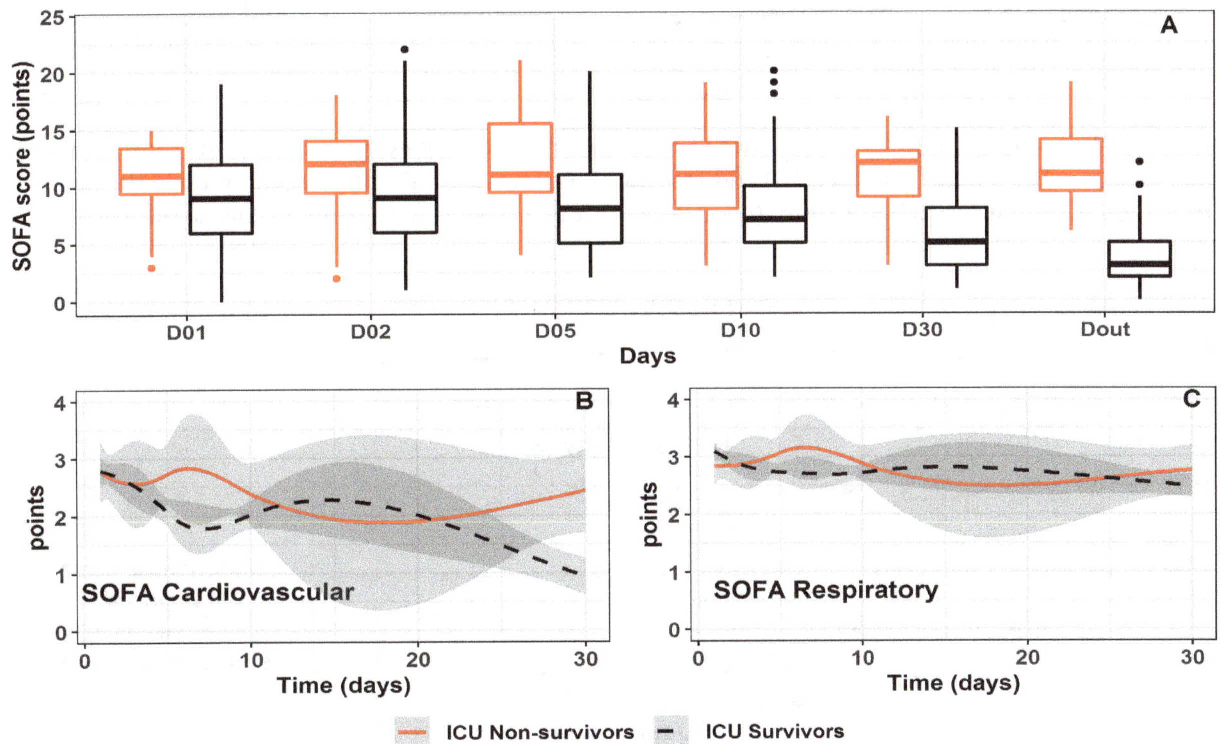

Figure A1. Evolution of the total SOFA score (**A**), and of its cardiac (**B**) and respiratory (**C**) components over time. The total SOFA score is shown as box plots (median is the line within the box, whiskers are 10th and 90th percentiles, the points above and below indicate outliers; "Dout" on time axis is the day of discharge). The boxes B and C show smooth curve uniting the days of available SOFA. The gray bands represent the 95% confidence intervals. Total SOFA changes over time were significantly different ($p < 0.0001$) between survivors and non-survivors, driven by the cardiovascular component of the score. The respiratory score did not differ between groups, remaining around three points for a long period: respiratory insufficiency was a frequent reason for prolonged ICU stay.

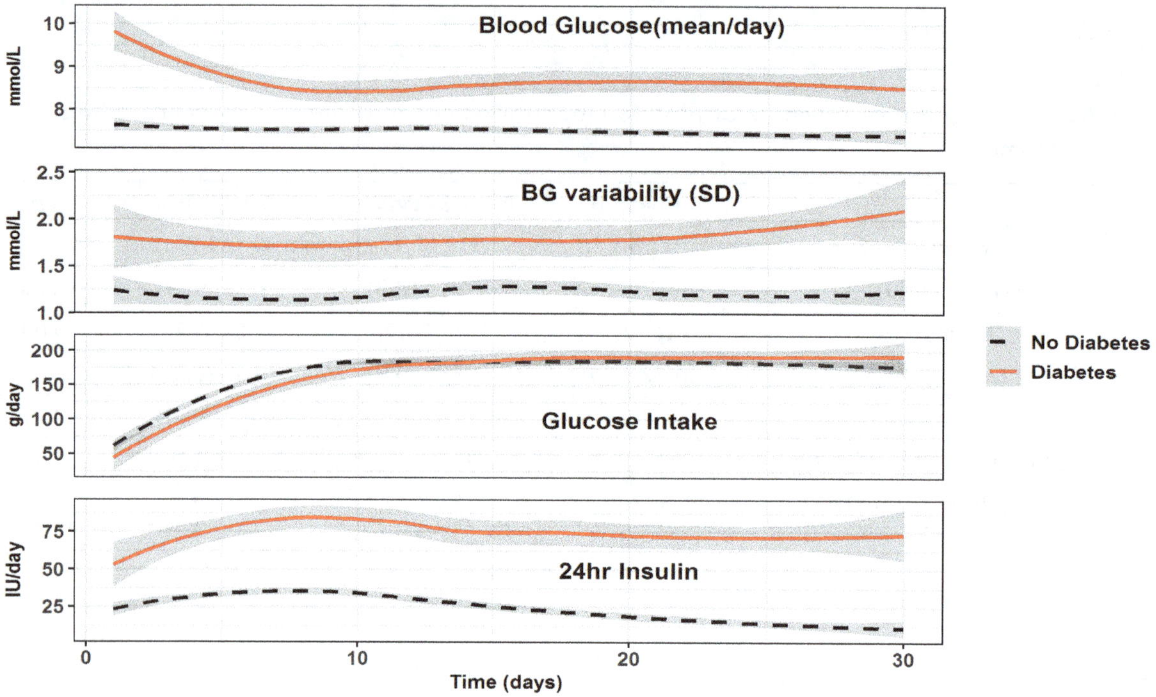

Figure A2. Evolution of glucose variables in the patients with diabetes ($n = 26$) versus those without diabetes ($n = 124$). Blood glucose (BG) and insulin needs were significantly higher in diabetic patients ($p < 0.0001$), as was the BG variability ($p < 0.001$) through the stay, with similar glucose intakes.

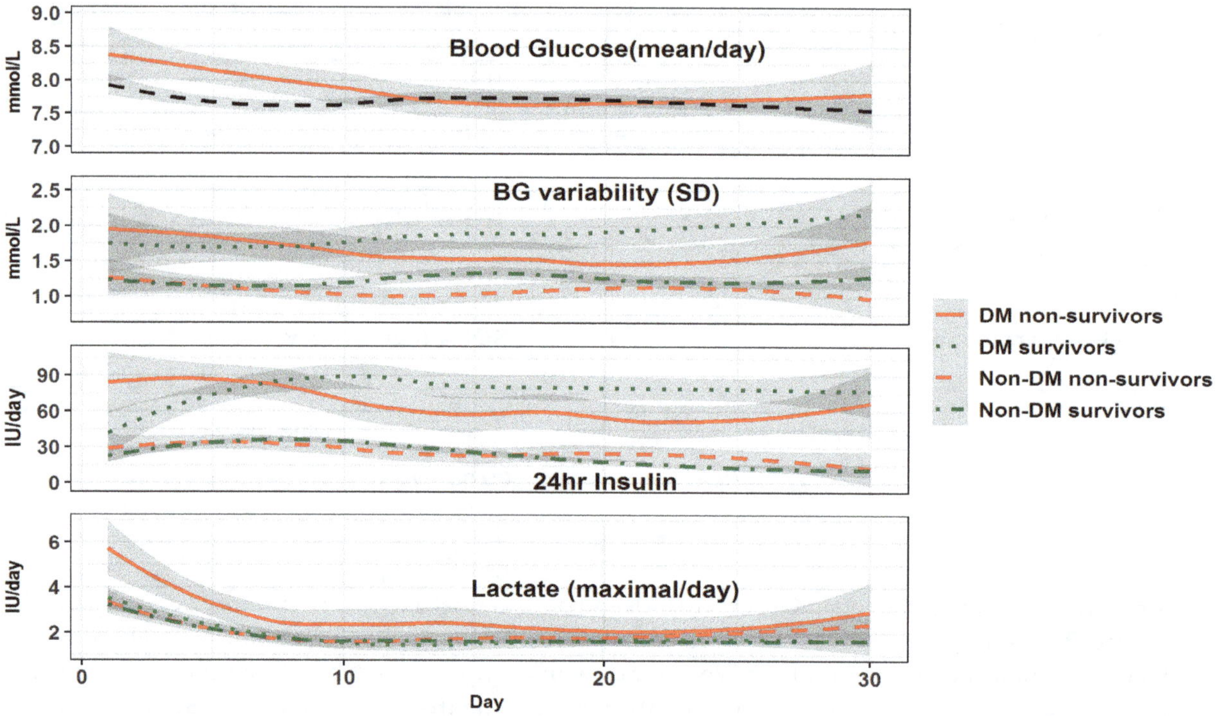

Figure A3. Glucose variables according to ICU outcome in patients with diabetes (DM) versus those without diabetes. Blood glucose (BG) was highest ($p < 0.001$) in DM-survivors compared to all, While the insulin needs did not differ in non-diabetic patients between survivors and non-survivors, the DM-non-survivors were characterized by significantly higher insulin needs during the first 6 days ($p < 0.001$), and lower needs than DM-survivors thereafter. Arterial lactate was elevated in all patients groups, and significantly higher in DM-non-survivors during the first 7 days ($p < 0.001$).

References

1. Nelson, J.E.; Cox, C.E.; Hope, A.A.; Carson, S.S. Chronic critical illness. *Am. J. Respir. Crit. Care Med.* **2010**, *182*, 446–454. [CrossRef] [PubMed]
2. Kahn, J.M.; Le, T.; Angus, D.C.; Cox, C.E.; Hough, C.L.; White, D.B.; Yende, S.; Carson, S.S.; ProVent Study Group Investigators. The epidemiology of chronic critical illness in the United States. *Crit. Care Med.* **2015**, *43*, 282–287. [CrossRef] [PubMed]
3. Loss, S.H.; Nunes, D.S.L.; Franzosi, O.S.; Salazar, G.S.; Teixeira, C.; Vieira, S.R.R. Chronic critical illness: Are we saving patients or creating victims? *Rev. Bras. Ter. Intensiva* **2017**, *29*, 87–95. [CrossRef] [PubMed]
4. Briassoulis, G.; Filippou, O.; Mavrikiou, M.; Natsi, L.; Ktistaki, M.; Hatzis, T. Current trends of clinical and genetic characteristics influencing the resource use and the nurse-patient balance in an intensive care setting. *J. Crit. Care* **2005**, *20*, 139–146. [CrossRef] [PubMed]
5. Frengley, J.D.; Sansone, G.R.; Kaner, R.J. Chronic Comorbid Illnesses Predict the Clinical Course of 866 Patients Requiring Prolonged Mechanical Ventilation in a Long-Term, Acute-Care Hospital. *J. Intensive Care Med.* **2018**, 0885066618783175. [CrossRef] [PubMed]
6. Loss, S.H.; Marchese, C.B.; Boniatti, M.M.; Wawrzeniak, I.C.; Oliveira, R.P.; Nunes, L.N.; Victorino, J.A. Prediction of chronic critical illness in a general intensive care unit. *Rev. Assoc. Med. Bras.* **2013**, *59*, 241–247. [CrossRef] [PubMed]
7. Kondrup, J.; Rasmussen, H.H.; Hamberg, O.; Stanga, Z. Nutritional risk screening (NRS 2002): A new method based on an analysis of controlled clinical trials. *Clin. Nutr.* **2003**, *22*, 321–336. [CrossRef]
8. Maciel, L.R.M.D.A.; Franzosi, O.S.; Nunes, D.S.L.; Loss, S.H.; Dos Reis, A.M.; Rubin, B.A.; Vieira, S.R.R. Nutritional Risk Screening 2002 Cut-Off to Identify High-Risk Is a Good Predictor of ICU Mortality in Critically Ill Patients. *Nutr. Clin. Pract.* **2019**, *34*, 137–141. [CrossRef]
9. Reignier, J.; Boisrame-Helms, J.; Brisard, L.; Lascarrou, J.B.; Ait Hssain, A.; Anguel, N.; Argaud, L.; Asehnoune, K.; Asfar, P.; Bellec, F.; et al. Enteral versus parenteral early nutrition in ventilated adults with shock: A randomised, controlled, multicentre, open-label, parallel-group study (NUTRIREA-2). *Lancet* **2018**, *391*, 133–143. [CrossRef]
10. Doig, G.S.; Simpson, F.; Heighes, P.T.; Bellomo, R.; Chesher, D.; Caterson, I.D.; Reade, M.C.; Harrigan, P.W.; Refeeding Syndrome Trial Investigators Group. Restricted versus continued standard caloric intake during the management of refeeding syndrome in critically ill adults: A randomised, parallel-group, multicentre, single-blind controlled trial. *Lancet Respir. Med.* **2015**, *3*, 943–952. [CrossRef]
11. Couto, C.F.L.; Dariano, A.; Texeira, C.; Silva, C.H.D.; Torbes, A.B.; Friedman, G. Adequacy of enteral nutritional support in intensive care units does not affect the short- and long-term prognosis of mechanically ventilated patients: A pilot study. *Rev. Bras. Ter. Intensiva* **2019**, *31*, 34–38. [CrossRef] [PubMed]
12. Oshima, T.; Berger, M.M.; De Waele, E.; Guttormsen, A.B.; Heidegger, C.P.; Hiesmayr, M.; Singer, P.; Wernerman, J.; Pichard, C. Indirect calorimetry in nutritional therapy. A position paper by the ICALIC study group. *Clin. Nutr.* **2017**, *36*, 651–662. [CrossRef] [PubMed]
13. Singer, P.; Reintam-Blaser, A.; Berger, M.M.; Alhazzani, W.; Calder, P.C.; Casaer, M.; Hiesmayr, M.J.; Mayer, K.; Montejo, J.M.; Pichard, C.; et al. ESPEN Guidelines: Nutrition in the ICU. *Clin. Nutr.* **2019**, *38*, 48–79. [CrossRef] [PubMed]
14. Vincent, J.L.; de Mendonca, A.; Cantraine, F.; Moreno, R.; Takala, J.; Suter, P.M.; Sprung, C.L.; Colardyn, F.; Blecher, S. Use of the SOFA score to assess the incidence of organ dysfunction/failure in intensive care units: Results of a multicenter, prospective study. Working group on "sepsis-related problems" of the European Society of Intensive Care Medicine. *Crit. Care Med.* **1998**, *26*, 1793–1800. [CrossRef] [PubMed]
15. Berger, M.M.; Pichard, C. Parenteral nutrition in the ICU: Lessons learned over the past few years. *Nutrition* **2019**, *59*, 188–194. [CrossRef]
16. Yeh, D.D.; Fuentes, E.; Quraishi, S.A.; Cropano, C.; Kaafarani, H.; Lee, J.; King, D.R.; DeMoya, M.; Fagenholz, P.; Butler, K.; et al. Adequate Nutrition May Get You Home: Effect of Caloric/Protein Deficits on the Discharge Destination of Critically Ill Surgical Patients. *J. Parenter. Enter. Nutr.* **2016**, *40*, 37–44. [CrossRef] [PubMed]
17. Soguel, L.; Revelly, J.P.; Schaller, M.D.; Longchamp, C.; Berger, M.M. Energy deficit and length of hospital stay can be reduced by a two-step quality improvement of nutrition therapy: The intensive care unit dietitian can make the difference. *Crit. Care Med.* **2012**, *40*, 412–419. [CrossRef]

18. Paternostro-Sluga, T.; Grim-Stieger, M.; Posch, M.; Schuhfried, O.; Vacariu, G.; Mittermaier, C.; Bittner, C.; Fialka-Moser, V. Reliability and validity of the Medical Research Council (MRC) scale and a modified scale for testing muscle strength in patients with radial palsy. *J. Rehabil. Med.* **2008**, *40*, 665–671. [CrossRef]
19. Heidegger, C.P.; Berger, M.M.; Graf, S.; Zingg, W.; Darmon, P.; Costanza, M.C.; Thibault, R.; Pichard, C. Optimisation of energy provision with supplemental parenteral nutrition in critically ill patients: A randomised controlled clinical trial. *Lancet* **2013**, *381*, 385–393. [CrossRef]
20. Berger, M.M.; Pantet, O.; Jacquelin-Ravel, N.; Charriere, M.; Schmidt, S.; Becce, F.; Audran, R.; Spertini, F.; Tappy, L.; Pichard, C. Supplemental parenteral nutrition improves immunity with unchanged carbohydrate and protein metabolism in critically ill patients: The SPN2 randomized tracer study. *Clin. Nutr.* **2018**. [CrossRef]
21. Harvey, S.E.; Parrott, F.; Harrison, D.A.; Bear, D.E.; Segaran, E.; Beale, R.; Bellingan, G.; Leonard, R.; Mythen, M.G.; Rowan, K.M.; et al. Trial of the route of early nutritional support in critically ill adults—Calories Trial. *N. Engl. J. Med.* **2014**, *371*, 1673–1684. [CrossRef] [PubMed]
22. Tappy, L.; Schwarz, J.M.; Schneiter, P.; Cayeux, C.; Revelly, J.P.; Fagerquist, C.K.; Jéquier, E.; Chioléro, R. Effects of isoenergetic glucose-based or lipid-based parenteral nutrition on glucose metabolism, *de novo* lipogenesis, and respiratory gas exchanges in critically ill patients. *Crit. Care Med.* **1998**, *26*, 860–867. [CrossRef] [PubMed]
23. Elke, G.; Wang, M.; Weiler, N.; Day, A.G.; Heyland, D.K. Close to recommended caloric and protein intake by enteral nutrition is associated with better clinical outcome of critically ill septic patients: Secondary analysis of a large international nutrition database. *Crit. Care* **2014**, *18*, R29. [CrossRef] [PubMed]
24. Ohbe, H.; Jo, T.; Matsui, H.; Fushimi, K.; Yasunaga, H. Differences in effect of early enteral nutrition on mortality among ventilated adults with shock requiring low-, medium-, and high-dose noradrenaline: A propensity-matched analysis. *Clin. Nutr.* **2019**. [CrossRef] [PubMed]
25. Reintam Blaser, A.; Starkopf, J.; Alhazzani, W.; Berger, M.M.; Casaer, M.P.; Deane, A.M.; Fruhwald, S.; Hiesmayr, M.; Ichai, C.; Jakob, S.M.; et al. Early enteral nutrition in critically ill patients: ESICM clinical practice guidelines. *Intensive Care Med.* **2017**, *43*, 380–398. [CrossRef] [PubMed]
26. Heyland, D.K.; Cook, D.J.; Winder, B.; Brylowski, L.; Van de Mark, H.; Guyatt, G.H. Enteral nutrition in the critically ill patient: A prospective survey. *Crit. Care Med.* **1995**, *23*, 1055–1060. [CrossRef] [PubMed]
27. Brierley-Hobson, S.; Clarke, G.; O'Keeffe, V. Safety and efficacy of volume-based feeding in critically ill, mechanically ventilated adults using the 'Protein & Energy Requirements Fed for Every Critically ill patient every Time' (PERFECT) protocol: A before-and-after study. *Crit. Care* **2019**, *23*, 105. [CrossRef]
28. Friedman, J.; Lussiez, A.; Sullivan, J.; Wang, S.; Englesbe, M. Implications of sarcopenia in major surgery. *Nutr. Clin. Pract.* **2015**, *30*, 175–179. [CrossRef]
29. Moisey, L.L.; Mourtzakis, M.; Cotton, B.A.; Premji, T.; Heyland, D.K.; Wade, C.E.; Bulger, E.; Kozar, R.A.; Nutrition and Rehabilitation Investigators Consortium (NUTRIC). Skeletal muscle predicts ventilator-free days, ICU-free days, and mortality in elderly ICU patients. *Crit. Care* **2013**, *17*, R206. [CrossRef] [PubMed]
30. Bouharras El Idrissi, H.; Molina Lopez, J.; Perez Moreno, I.; Florea, D.I.; Lobo Tamer, G.; Herrera-Quintana, L.; Perez De La Cruz, A.; Rodriguez Elvira, M.; Planells Del Pozo, E.M. Imbalances in protein metabolism in critical care patient with systemic inflammatory response syndrome at admission in intensive care unit. *Nutr. Hosp.* **2015**, *32*, 2848–2854. [CrossRef]
31. Briassoulis, G.; Zavras, N.; Hatzis, T. Malnutrition, nutritional indices, and early enteral feeding in critically ill children. *Nutrition* **2001**, *17*, 548–557. [PubMed]
32. Briassoulis, G.; Tsorva, A.; Zavras, N.; Hatzis, T. Influence of an aggressive early enteral nutrition protocol on nitrogen balance in critically ill children. *J. Nutr. Biochem.* **2002**, *13*, 560. [PubMed]
33. Puthucheary, Z.A.; Rawal, J.; McPhail, M.; Connolly, B.; Ratnayake, G.; Chan, P.; Hopkinson, N.S.; Padhke, R.; Dew, T.; Sidhu, P.S.; et al. Acute skeletal muscle wasting in critical illness. *JAMA* **2013**, *310*, 1591–1600. [CrossRef] [PubMed]
34. Hernandez-Socorro, C.R.; Saavedra, P.; Lopez-Fernandez, J.C.; Ruiz-Santana, S. Assessment of Muscle Wasting in Long-Stay ICU Patients Using a New Ultrasound Protocol. *Nutrients* **2018**, *10*, 1849. [CrossRef]
35. Hermans, G.; De Jonghe, B.; Bruyninckx, F.; Van den Berghe, G. Interventions for preventing critical illness polyneuropathy and critical illness myopathy. *Cochrane Database Syst. Rev.* **2014**. [CrossRef] [PubMed]

36. Krinsley, J.S.; Chase, J.G.; Gunst, J.; Martensson, J.; Schultz, M.J.; Taccone, F.S.; Wernerman, J.; Bohe, J.; De Block, C.; Desaive, T.; et al. Continuous glucose monitoring in the ICU: Clinical considerations and consensus. *Crit. Care* **2017**, *21*, 197. [CrossRef] [PubMed]
37. Mesotten, D.; Preiser, J.C.; Kosiborod, M. Glucose management in critically ill adults and children. *Lancet Diabetes Endocrinol.* **2015**, *3*, 723–733. [CrossRef]
38. Krinsley, J.S.; Maurer, P.; Holewinski, S.; Hayes, R.; McComsey, D.; Umpierrez, G.E.; Nasraway, S.A. Glucose Control, Diabetes Status, and Mortality in Critically Ill Patients: The Continuum From Intensive Care Unit Admission to Hospital Discharge. *Mayo Clin. Proc.* **2017**, *92*, 1019–1029. [CrossRef]
39. Schulman, R.C.; Moshier, E.L.; Rho, L.; Casey, M.F.; Godbold, J.H.; Mechanick, J.I. Association of glycemic control parameters with clinical outcomes in chronic critical illness. *Endocr. Pract.* **2014**, *20*, 884–893. [CrossRef]
40. Pradelli, L.; Graf, S.; Pichard, C.; Berger, M.M. Supplemental parenteral nutrition in intensive care patients: A cost saving strategy. *Clin. Nutr.* **2018**, *37*, 573–579. [CrossRef]
41. Arabi, Y.M.; Al-Dorzi, H.M. Trophic or full nutritional support? *Curr. Opin. Crit. Care* **2018**, *24*, 262–268. [CrossRef]
42. Briassoulis, G.; Briassoulis, P.; Ilia, I. Nutrition Is More Than the Sum of Its Parts. *Pediatr. Crit. Care Med.* **2018**, *19*, 1087–1089. [CrossRef]
43. Berger, M.M.; Pichard, C. Feeding should be individualized in the critically ill patients. *Curr. Opin. Crit. Care* **2019**, *25*, 307–313. [CrossRef]

13

Decreased Bioelectrical Impedance Phase Angle in Hospitalized Children and Adolescents with Newly Diagnosed Type 1 Diabetes

Paweł Więch [1,*], Dariusz Bazaliński [1], Izabela Sałacińska [1], Monika Binkowska-Bury [1], Bartosz Korczowski [2], Artur Mazur [2], Maria Kózka [3] and Mariusz Dąbrowski [1,4]

1 Institute of Nursing and Health Sciences, Faculty of Medicine, University of Rzeszów, 35-959 Rzeszów, Poland; darek.bazalinski@wp.pl (D.B.); izabela.salacinska@wp.pl (I.S.); monika.binkowska@yahoo.com (M.B.-B.); mariusz.dabrowski58@gmail.com (M.D.)
2 Pediatric Department, Clinical Provincial Hospital No. 2 in Rzeszów, Faculty of Medicine, University of Rzeszów, 35-301 Rzeszów, Poland; korczowski@op.pl (B.K.); drmazur@poczta.onet.pl (A.M.)
3 Department of Clinical Nursing, Faculty of Health Sciences, Collegium Medicum, Jagiellonian University, 31-501 Kraków, Poland; makozka@cm-uj.krakow.pl
4 Diabetic Outpatient Clinic, Medical Center "Beta-Med", 35-073 Rzeszów, Poland; mariusz.dabrowski58@gmail.com
* Correspondence: p.k.wiech@gmail.com

Abstract: The aim of this study was to assess the body composition and nutritional status of hospitalized pediatric patients with newly diagnosed type 1 diabetes by using bioelectrical impedance analysis (BIA) with phase angle (PA) calculation. PA is considered to be a useful and very sensitive indicator of the nutritional and functional status, and it has not yet been evaluated in such a population. Sixty-three pediatric patients aged 4 to 18 years, with newly diagnosed type 1 diabetes, were included in the study. The control group consisted of 63 healthy children and adolescents strictly matched by gender and age in a 1:1 case: control manner. In both groups, BIA with PA calculation was performed. Diabetic patients, in comparison to control subjects, had a highly significantly lower PA of 4.85 $\pm$ 0.86 vs. 5.62 $\pm$ 0.81, $p < 0.001$. They also demonstrated a lower percentage of body cell mass (BCM%), 46.89 $\pm$ 5.67% vs. 51.40 $\pm$ 4.19%, p < 0.001; a lower body cell mass index (BCMI), 6.57 $\pm$ 1.80% vs. 7.37 $\pm$ 1.72%, $p = 0.004$; and a lower percentage of muscle mass (MM%), 44.61 $\pm$ 6.58% vs. 49.40 $\pm$ 7.59%, $p < 0.001$, compared to non-diabetic controls. The significantly lower PA value in diabetic patients indicate their worse nutritional and functional status compared to healthy subjects. To assess the predictive and prognostic value of this finding in this population, further prospective studies involving larger sample of patients are required.

Keywords: type 1 diabetes mellitus; bioelectrical impedance analysis; phase angle; children; adolescents

1. Introduction

Application of bioelectrical impedance analysis (BIA) to assess the body composition dates back to late 1980s [1]. Although differences between results obtained by BIA and Dual-Energy X-Ray Absorptiometry (DXA) are observed both in adult and in pediatric populations, BIA is considered as an easy to use, reliable, safe, non-invasive, and non-expensive method of the assessment of body composition, and it has been widely used in a number of epidemiological studies [2–5].

Bioelectrical impedance phase angle (PA) is considered to be a more sensitive and more accurate indicator of the nutritional and functional status than BIA alone, because PA better reflects the degree of cellular health and indicates early water shift from intracellular to extracellular compartment in subjects with malnutrition [6–8].

The reference values of PA in healthy subjects differ depending on age, sex, and body mass index (BMI) [9–11]. The PA values in adults are different compared with children and adolescents. Growing up is associated with increasing phase angles, a situation that is probably due to an increase in cell mass with age, especially in periods of childhood and adolescence [9]. This trend was observed by Redondo-Del-Río et al. for both genders (4–5 years: 5.2 vs. 12–13 years: 5.7–5.8 vs. 15–16 years: 6.1–6.5) [10].

Norman et al. summarized in their review the prognostic value of PA in dialysis subjects, patients with cancer, liver cirrhosis, heart failure, systemic sclerosis, human immunodeficiency virus (HIV) positive, geriatric, and surgical patients. In all cases lower PA values were associated with increased mortality and lower survival rates [12]. PA also correlates with function, disease severity, and prognosis in people with stable chronic obstructive pulmonary disease (COPD) [13]. Low PA at hospital admission appeared also to be associated with malnutrition and nutritional risk [14]. In the study by Zhang et al., patients with a better nutrition state demonstrated relatively higher PA than the patients with severe malnutrition, which suggests that PA has the potential to be a quantitative index in assessing nutrition state, while current assessing methods such as the Subjective Global Assessment (SGA) contain many subjective factors [7]. Thus, PA can be considered not only as an indicator of nutritional status but also as an important prognostic factor of malnutrition risk and clinical outcome, especially in chronic diseases leading to malnutrition and cachexia. The European Society for Clinical Nutrition and Metabolism (ESPEN) strongly recommends PA as a reliable prognostic nutritional measure [15]. Currently, it is expected that nutrition state assessment based on PA will be established and implemented in clinical trials [7].

The primary objective of our study was to assess the PA value in hospitalized children and adolescents with newly diagnosed type 1 diabetes compared to healthy controls. To our knowledge, it is the first study in such a group, as through searching Embase, Web of Science, PubMed, and Scopus databases by use of the terms "type 1 diabetes mellitus" and "children"; combined with "body composition" or/and "phase angle"; "bioelectrical impedance analysis", "type 1 diabetes mellitus", and "children"; and combined with "nutritional status" and "phase angle", we found only two full-text papers assessing the PA in diabetic patients, but both of them were conducted in adult populations [16,17].The search was limited to articles published in English from 1990 to 30 July 2018. The secondary objective was to analyze body composition in this group of patients.

2. Experimental Section

2.1. Ethics

The study was approved by the institutional Bioethics Committee at the University of Rzeszów (Resolution No. 5/02/2012) and by all appropriate administrative bodies. The study was conducted in accordance with ethical standards laid down in an appropriate version of the Declaration of Helsinki and in Polish national regulations.

2.2. Subjects

This pair-matched, case control study was carried out between March 2012 and August 2014. Sixty-three children and adolescents (28 girls, 44.4%) with type 1 diabetes hospitalized in the Clinical Department of Pediatrics with the Pediatric Neurology Unit at the Clinical Regional Hospital No. 2 in Rzeszow comprised the study group. The flow chart demonstrating the selection of the study and control groups is presented in Figure 1, while characteristics of both groups are presented in Table 1.

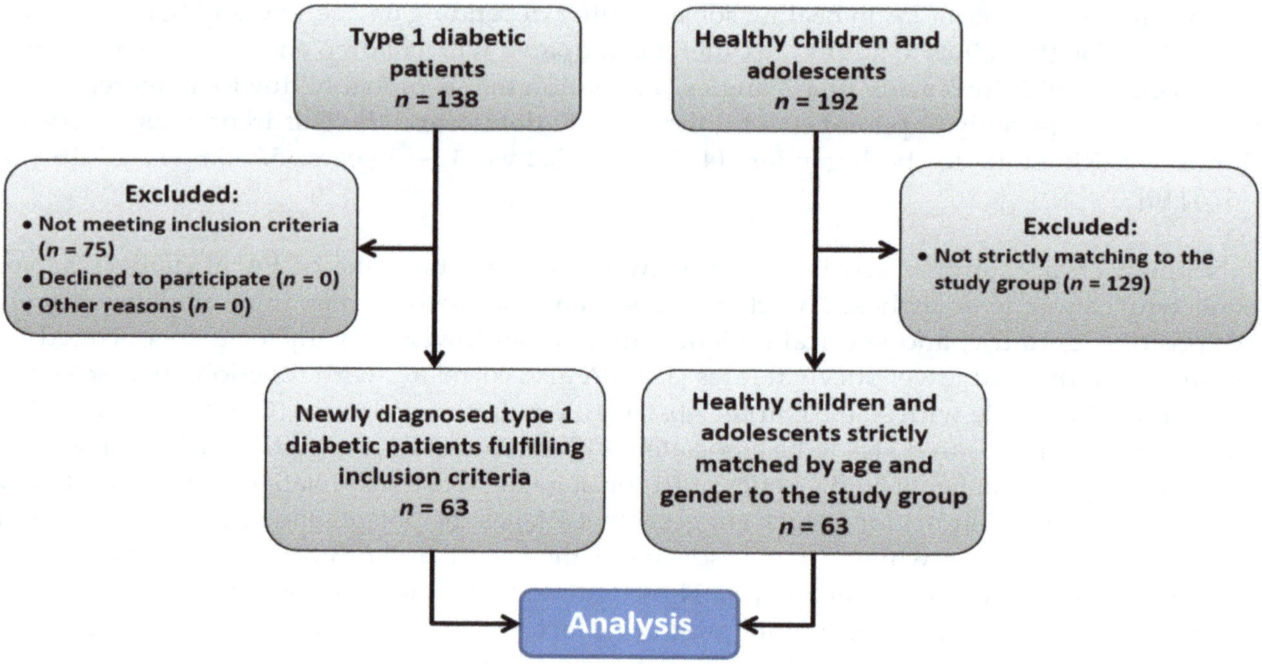

Figure 1. Flow chart of the selection of study participants.

Table 1. Demographic and anthropometric parameters of the study participants.

Parameter	Type 1 Diabetes Group	Control Group	p-Value
Age (years)	10.78 ± 3.72	10.80 ± 3.73	0.967
Girls	10.93 ± 3.55	10.96 ± 3.56	0.947
Boys	10.66 ± 3.90	10.66 ± 3.90	1.000
Body weight (kg)	42.15 ± 21.08	39.93 ± 14.97	0.907
Girls	38.71 ± 16.69	38.53 ± 11.92	0.962
Percentile * (n):			
<3	2	1	0.613
3–10	4	1	
10–90	20	23	
90–97	1	1	
>97	1	2	
Boys	44.89 ± 23.91	41.05 ± 17.11	0.720
Percentile * (n):			
<3	0	1	0.400
3–10	4	2	
10–90	24	26	
90–97	3	5	
>97	4	1	
Height (cm)	145.80 ± 22.16	144.12 ± 19.63	0.653
Girls	143.93 ± 19.64	143.66 ± 18.60	0.958
Low-to-age *	1	1	0.354
Normal *	27	25	
High-to-age *	0	2	
Boys	147.30 ± 24.17	144.49 ± 20.68	0.602
Low-to-age *	0	0	0.673
Normal *	31	33	
High-to-age *	4	2	

Table 1. *Cont.*

Parameter	Type 1 Diabetes Group	Control Group	*p*-Value
BMI (kg/m^2)	18.56 ± 4.57	18.52 ± 3.30	0.460
Girls	17.76 ± 3.40	18.26 ± 3.08	0.244
Underweight *	10	5	0.371
Normal weight *	15	19	
Overweight *	3	3	
Obesity *	0	1	
Boys	19.21 ± 4.94	18.72 ± 3.49	0.939
Underweight *	1	1	0.573
Normal weight *	27	24	
Overweight *	6	10	
Obesity *	1	0	

SD—standard deviation; BMI—body mass index. Values are presented as mean ± SD. * According to Polish normative values [18].

The inclusion criteria were as follows: newly diagnosed type 1 diabetes; age 4 to 18 years; no other autoimmune or chronic diseases having impact on height, weight, or nutritional status; and written informed consent signed by parents or legal guardians and also by adolescents aged over 16 years. The control group consisted of the same number of children and adolescents taken from primary, junior high, and high schools from urban and rural areas. The inclusion criteria for this group were the same, with the exception of having type 1 diabetes. The diabetic and healthy subjects were strictly matched by gender and age (to the nearest possible date of birth) in a 1:1 case:control manner.

2.3. Assessments

Body height was measured to the nearest 0.1 cm using a portable stadiometer (Seca 213). The measurements were performed under standard conditions in an upright position and barefoot. Body mass was assessed with an accuracy of 0.1 kg using a personal scale (Seca 799). Body mass index (BMI) was calculated as weight (kg)/height $(m)^2$. To avoid bias associated with dehydration at the time of diabetes diagnosis, in the first step, acid–base and water–electrolyte balance in the study group were normalized. In the treatment of hyperglycemia, a continuous intravenous insulin infusion was used in the first several hours after admission. After glucose metabolism control was achieved, children and adolescents were switched to subcutaneous multiple daily injections of insulin using the basal/bolus method. The assessment of body composition and nutritional status in diabetic subjects was performed between the 5th and 7th days after admission after when stable metabolic state was achieved. BIA was performed using an AKERN BIA 101 analyzer (Akern SRL, Pontassieve, Florence, Italy). PA was calculated from the following equation:

$$\mathrm{PA} = \left(\frac{X_C}{R}\right) \times \left(\frac{180^\circ}{\pi}\right) \quad (1)$$

(Xc—reactance, R—resistance)

The equations used by the software to assess the specific parameters are restricted property of the company, but to a significant degree, they are based on computed algorithms developed by Sun S. et al. [19] and Horlick et al. [20]. According to widely accepted and available methodologies [21], participants were in a fasting state and, before measurement (24 h), they did not practice physical exercises. Before the BIA measurement, they were asked to empty the bladder completely and to remove all clothing and metal elements. The measurements were carried out between 07:00 and 12:00 in a fasting state, in the supine position, with abducted upper (30°) and lower (45°) extremities, and after at least 5 min of rest. A tetrapolar system with a contralateral mode was used (amplitude of measured current: 800 uA; sinusoidal; 50 kHz). To ensure reliability and repeatability of the results obtained, two measurements, one after another, were performed. All the measurements were performed by the same person. The accuracy of the equipment was checked before the measurements with a 500 ohm resistor supplied by the manufacturer. The disposable electrodes (Biatrodes, Pontassieve, FI, Italy; the individual impedance of a single electrode: 25–30 Ω; compliance with the Medical Directive 93/42/EEC; accordance with ISO 10993-1:2003) were placed on the dorsal surface of the right upper limb (over the wrist) and the right lower limb (on the ankle) while the minimum distance between the two electrodes was 5 cm. The results were transferred and analyzed by specialized software (Bodygram1_31 by AKERN).

In all children and adolescents, weight and height was measured and BMI was calculated. The obtained results were compared to Polish normative values charts according to age and gender [18]. Weight was divided into five categories according to percentiles: <3 low-to-age weight, 3–10 alert level, 10–90 normal weight, 90–97 alert level, and >97 high-to-age weight. Height was divided into three percentile categories: >97 high-to-age height, 3–97 normal range, and <3 low-to-age height. BMI was divided into four categories: underweight, normal weight, overweight, and obese, according to normative charts for age and gender. BIA analysis included: fat mass (FM), fat free mass (FFM) muscle mass (MM) (kg and %), total body water (TBW), intra- and extracellular water (ICW and ECW; liters and %), body cell mass (BCM; kg and %), and body cell mass index (BCMI). Upon resistance and reactance results, phase angle was calculated. In addition, fat mass index (FMI) and fat free mass index (FFMI) were calculated.

Phase angle results were compared between diabetic and control groups as a whole and separately for each gender. In addition, we analyzed PA values in relation to the reference values for age, gender, and BMI obtained by Bosy-Westphal et al. in the study conducted in Germany, the neighboring country, which can be considered applicable for our population [9].

2.4. Statistical Analysis

Statistical analysis of the data was performed using SigmaPlot for Windows, version 12.5 (Systat Software Inc., San Jose, CA, USA). The continuous data are presented as mean ± SD (standard deviation). Differences between study and control groups were analyzed using a two-tailed Student's t-test for independent samples after performing a Shapiro-Wilk normality test and a constant variance test. In the case of normality and constant variance test failure, the Mann-Whitney rank sum test was performed. The categorical data were compared using the $\chi 2$ test. The linear correlation between PA and HbA1c was assessed using the Pearson product moment correlation test after checking the normality of distribution by the Shapiro-Wilk test. A p-value of <0.05 was considered statistically significant.

3. Results

The phase angle value in diabetic patients was highly significantly lower compared to healthy subjects. Among components of the PA equation, only reactance appeared to be significantly different between the study and control groups (Table 2) regardless of gender (Table 3). Resistance, although higher in diabetic subjects, did not reach statistical significance. Although the muscle mass and body cell mass measured in kg were not significantly different between the diabetic and control groups, MM%, BCM%, and BCMI were also significantly lower in diabetic subjects (Table 2). The differences remained significant when these variables were also analyzed separately for each gender (Table 3).

Table 2. Bioelectrical Impedance Analysis results in study participants.

Parameter	Type 1 Diabetes Group (N = 63)	Control group (N = 63)	p-Value
	Mean ± SD	Mean ± SD	
Fat mass (kg)	10.84 ± 8.33	9.07 ± 5.20	0.481
Fat mass (% of body mass)	23.96 ± 9.50	22.49 ± 9.44	0.386
Fat mass index (kg/m^2)	4.66 ± 2.78	4.24 ± 2.33	0.364
Fat free mass (kg)	31.31 ± 14.49	30.86 ± 12.26	0.840
Fat free mass (% of body mass)	76.04 ± 9.50	77.51 ± 9.44	0.386
Fat free mass index (kg/m^2)	13.81 ± 2.74	14.20 ± 2.26	0.218
Muscle mass (kg)	18.87 ± 10.01	20.03 ± 9.17	0.341
Muscle mass (% of body mass)	44.61 ± 6.58	49.40 ± 7.59	<0.001
Total body water (L)	24.48 ± 10.61	24.28 ± 9.10	0.903
Total body water (% of body mass)	59.95 ± 8.62	61.36 ± 8.56	0.359
Extracellular water (L)	11.10 ± 4.44	10.57 ± 3.85	0.707
Extracellular water (% of body mass)	46.89 ± 7.34	44.05 ± 3.67	0.064
Intracellular water (L)	13.70 ± 6.49	13.76 ± 5.44	0.946
Intracellular water (% of body mass)	53.11 ± 7.34	55.95 ± 3.67	0.064
Body cell mass (kg)	15.14 ± 8.27	16.23 ± 7.57	0.308
Body cell mass (% of body mass)	46.89 ± 5.67	51.40 ± 4.19	<0.001
Body cell mass index (kg/m^2)	6.57 ± 1.80	7.37 ± 1.72	0.004
Resistance (ohm)	684.92 ± 99.29	659.98 ± 94.10	0.150
Reactance (ohm)	57.62 ± 10.41	63.83 ± 6.93	<0.001
Phase angle (−)	4.85 ± 0.86	5.62 ± 0.81	<0.001

A tetrapolar system with a contralateral mode; amplitude of a measured current of 800 uA, sinusoidal, 50kHz. Significant differences are in bold and indicate significant values ($p < 0.05$). Values are presented as mean ± SD.

Table 3. BIA results in study participants according to gender.

Parameter	Girls		p-Value	Boys		p-Value
	Diabetes (N = 28)	Control (N = 28)		Diabetes (N = 35)	Control (N = 35)	
Fat mass (kg)	9.98 ± 6.53	9.77 ± 4.53	0.891	11.53 ± 9.57	8.50 ± 5.67	0.215
Fat mass (% of body mass)	23.65 ± 9.72	25.12 ± 8.56	0.555	24.21 ± 9.46	20.38 ± 9.47	0.072
Fat mass index (kg/m^2)	4.37 ± 2.40	4.71 ± 2.39	0.611	4.90 ± 3.06	3.86 ± 2.25	0.079
Fat free mass (kg)	28.74 ± 11.00	28.76 ± 9.52	0.994	33.37 ± 16.63	32.55 ± 13.98	0.930
Fat free mass (% of body mass)	76.35 ± 9.72	74.88 ± 8.86	0.555	75.79 ± 9.46	79.62 ± 9.47	0.072
Fat free mass index (kg/m^2)	13.18 ± 2.52	13.46 ± 1.78	0.628	14.32 ± 2.84	14.78 ± 2.45	0.247
Muscle mass (kg)	16.79 ± 7.25	18.29 ± 6.59	0.421	20.53 ± 11.60	21.42 ± 10.70	0.597
Muscle mass (% of body mass)	43.62 ± 5.70	47.20 ± 6.17	0.028	45.41 ± 7.19	51.15 ± 8.23	0.003
Total body water (L)	22.25 ± 7.82	22.35 ± 6.92	0.958	26.25 ± 12.23	25.81 ± 10.37	0.893
Total body water (% of body mass)	59.75 ± 9.02	58.55 ± 7.54	0.590	60.11 ± 8.42	63.61 ± 8.77	0.093
Extracellular water (L)	10.48 ± 3.64	9.85 ± 3.12	0.629	11.59 ± 4.98	11.15 ± 4.30	0.930
Extracellular water (% of body mass)	48.31 ± 8.70	44.25 ± 3.08	0.119	45.76 ± 5.92	43.89 ± 4.12	0.131
Intracellular water (L)	12.13 ± 4.99	12.65 ± 4.05	0.793	14.95 ± 7.31	14.65 ± 6.25	0.995
Intracellular water (% of body mass)	51.69 ± 8.70	55.75 ± 3.08	0.119	54.24 ± 5.92	56.11 ± 4.12	0.131
Body cell mass (kg)	13.39 ± 5.99	14.79 ± 5.38	0.362	16.55 ± 9.57	17.37 ± 8.86	0.565
Body cell mass (% of body mass)	45.60 ± 6.30	50.90 ± 3.05	<0.001	47.91 ± 4.96	51.79 ± 4.93	0.002
Body cell mass index (kg/m^2)	6.11 ± 1.50	6.91 ± 1.27	0.037	6.93 ± 1.95	7.73 ± 1.96	0.039
Resistance (ohm)	712.75 ± 102.10	700.57 ± 79.01	0.620	662.66 ± 92.47	627.51 ± 93.53	0.119
Reactance (ohm)	58.07 ± 12.66	66.71 ± 5.14	0.003	57.26 ± 8.38	61.51 ± 7.36	0.027
Phase angle (−)	4.66 ± 0.84	5.49 ± 0.56	<0.001	5.00 ± 0.85	5.72 ± 0.97	0.001

A tetrapolar system with a contralateral mode; amplitude of a measured current of 800 uA, sinusoidal, 50kHz. Significant differences ($p < 0.05$) indicated in bold. Values are presented as mean ± SD.

We also found significant differences between the study and control group for both genders in the analysis of PA values in relation to the reference values for a healthy population obtained by Bosy-Westphal et al. in the study conducted in Germany, the neighboring country [9]. In our study, among girls with diabetes, only 14 (50.0%) had a PA value equal or higher than the 10th percentile expected for gender, age and BMI, while among healthy girls such number was 27 (96.4%), $p < 0.001$ for the difference. Among boys these numbers were 20 (57.1%) and 30 (85.7%) respectively and this difference was also statistically significant, $p = 0.017$. The more detailed results are presented in the Table 4.

Table 4. Number of subjects with PA value according to age, gender and BMI in relation to reference values.

Age Range (years)	Phase Angle Percentiles	Girls		Boys	
		Diabetes	Control	Diabetes	Control
All (n)		28	28	35	35
	≥10th percentile	14	27	20	30
	<10th percentile	14	1	15	5
	<5th percentile	13	1	11	1
4–9 (n)		10	10	13	13
	≥10th percentile	3	10	7	10
	<10th percentile	7	0	6	3
	<5th percentile	7	0	5	0
10–13 (n)		13	13	16	16
	≥10th percentile	9	13	10	14
	<10th percentile	4	0	6	2
	<5th percentile	3	0	5	1
14–18 (n)		5	5	6	6
	≥10th percentile	2	4	3	6
	<10th percentile	3	1	3	0
	<5th percentile	3	1	1	0

Phase angle (PA) value ≥10th percentile, <10th percentile and <5th percentile according to age, gender and body mass index (BMI) in relation to reference values from Bosy-Westphal et al. [9].

The mean HbA1c value in children and adolescents with newly diagnosed type 1 diabetes was 11.37% ± 2.26% (100.7 ± 24.7 mmol/mol). Girls had a mean HbA1c value significantly higher compared to boys, 12.22% ± 1.89% (110.1 ± 20.7 mmol/mol) vs. 10.71% ± 2.32% (93.4 ± 25.3 mmol/mol), respectively, $p = 0.012$. A trend towards negative linear correlation between the PA value and the HbA1c value in diabetic patients was observe; however, it did not attain a statistical significance ($r = -0.220$, $p = 0.085$).

In a subgroup of patients (four with newly diagnosed diabetes and nine with longer-lasting diabetes), we performed a follow-up after 13 to 21 (mean of 15.5) months of treatment. We found a significant improvement in the mean PA value and BCMI (from 5.52 ± 0.77 to 5.84 ± 0.67, $p = 0.003$, and from 6.85 ± 1.99 to 8.04 ± 2.15, $p < 0.001$, respectively). However, at baseline, six patients had a PA value above the mean value expected for age, gender, and BMI, while at follow-up, this number decreased to five. The percentage of FM, FFM, TBW, ECW, ICW, and MM did not change significantly compared to baseline.

No significant differences between the study and control groups regarding mean weight, height, and BMI were found, nor when individual results were analyzed in relation to Polish normative values.

4. Discussion

The primary objective of our study was to assess PA values in children and adolescents with newly diagnosed type 1 diabetes in comparison to healthy subjects, which has not yet been studied. The PA value is calculated from resistance (R) and reactance (Xc) values and reflects the nutritional and functional status. In the human body, resistance is related to tissue hydration while reactance occurs due to the cell membrane capacitance (i.e., the ability of the non-conducting object to save electrical charges) [8]. Data regarding PA assessment in the diabetic population are scarce. In the study by Buscemi et al. conducted in both type 1 and type 2 diabetic subjects, PA values appeared to be significantly lower in young adult type 1 diabetic male patients compared to control subjects, while in women, this difference was insignificant [16]. Dittmar et al. revealed significantly lower PA among men and women with type 2 diabetes compared to control subjects. They also found inverse relationships between the PA value and HbA1c levels and concluded that lower PA values at 50 and 100 kHz might indicate catabolism and long duration of the disease in type 2 diabetic patients [17]. No other studies assessing PA values in patients with diabetes were found in the PubMed, Scopus, or EMBASE databases.

Obviously, body composition of children and adolescents with type 1 diabetes significantly changes over the course of the disease, and, in many of them, an excess of fat mass develops, which was observed in different studies. Davis et al. observed a significantly lower FM% and similar lean mass in children with type 1 diabetes at the time of diagnosis compared to the non-diabetic group. After insulin introduction, sharp increases in fat mass and an insignificant loss of lean body mass during the first six weeks of treatment in diabetic group was revealed. The authors explained this phenomenon as a consequence of severe insulin deficiency and a catabolic state at the time of type 1 diabetes diagnosis [22]. In contrast to this study, in our observations, neither fat mass nor percentage of body fat in children and adolescents with newly diagnosed type 1 diabetes were significantly different compared to the control group, though we found a significantly lower percentage of muscle mass. We did not observe significant changes in body composition during the follow-up in the study group; however, the follow-up period was not long enough to find more pronounced changes. Interestingly, in the Greek study in children and adolescents with short-lasting type 1 diabetes (3.7 ± 2.0 years), FFMI was significantly higher compared to non-diabetic subjects, while FM% and FMI were not significantly different between the groups [23]. Patients with type 1 diabetes gain more weight than their peers, mainly due to the increase in fat mass, which was documented in the study by Szadkowska et al. In their observation, the prevalence of overweight and obesity among young adults (up to 40 years) with type 1 diabetes and an age at diabetes onset <20 years was significantly higher compared to the control group, and diabetic patients were characterized by higher fat mass [24]. Such unfavorable changes in body composition might have a negative impact on health in the future. Excessive weight gain in diabetic patients was associated with elevated waist circumference and blood pressure, lower insulin sensitivity, dyslipidemia, and with more extensive atherosclerosis in further observations [25,26].

It is well known that type 1 diabetes is associated with an elevated risk of complications, and poor metabolic control correlates with microangiopathy, macroangiopathy, and diabetic neuropathy [26,27]. Uncontrolled type 1 diabetes also has an impact on bone and muscle, i.e., lean body mass; moreover, it also impairs their function [28,29]. Coleman et al. indicate that decreased muscle mass and impaired muscle function has a significant impact on insulin sensitivity, glucose and lipids disposal, and on basal metabolic rate, which makes it difficult to achieve a stable metabolic control of type 1 diabetes. Thus, physical activity, which leads to an improvement in muscle mass and function, can also be helpful in the improvement of metabolic control and in delaying or even preventing the development of diabetic complications [30].

Poor metabolic control in childhood and adolescence and bad glycemic legacy (metabolic memory) is associated with an elevated risk of future complications in adulthood and can also lead to premature death, mainly due to cardiovascular disease. Thus, good diabetes care in early years can improve this prognosis [26,31].

Phase angle has not yet been analyzed prospectively in type 1 diabetic patients. The significant increases in PA values during the follow-up observed in our study can be simply explained by the growth of children and adolescents, because number of subjects with PA exceeding mean for age, gender, and BMI did not increase; on the contrary, it even decreased during observation. This may indicate the persistence of worse nutritional and functional status in this population.

The main limitation of our study was the relatively small number of participants, which did not allow us to find other differences between diabetic and control groups. Furthermore, only thirteen patients with diabetes were followed-up. Nevertheless, our study presents some new data and interesting findings which may indicate the directions of future research.

5. Conclusions

Low values of phase angle and altered body composition in newly diagnosed type 1 diabetic patients indicate their worse nutritional and functional status. However, although phase angle is a predictor of unfavorable clinical outcome in people with a number of chronic diseases, the predictive and prognostic value of our findings in patients with type 1 diabetes needs to be determined in further long-term prospective studies to establish its role in this population.

Author Contributions: Study concept and design: P.W., B.K., M.D.; funding acquisition: P.W., D.B., M.B.-B., A.M.; data acquisition: P.W., D.B., I.S.; statistical analysis: M.D.; analysis and interpretation of data: M.D., P.W.; supervision: B.K., A.M., M.B.-B; M.K.; manuscript drafting: M.D., P.W.; critical revision of the work for important intellectual content: P.W., D.B., I.S., M.B.-B., B.K., M.K., A.M., M.D.

Acknowledgments: The abstract based on these data was accepted for the American Diabetes Association 78th Scientific Sessions held in Orlando, FL in June 2018. The raw data used in this paper are deposited in the University of Rzeszów Repository: https://repozytorium.ur.edu.pl/ under the title of the manuscript or under the name of any of the authors.

References

1. Baumgartner, R.N.; Chumlea, W.C.; Roche, A.F. Estimation of body composition from bioelectric impedance of body segments. *Am. J. Clin. Nutr.* **1989**, *50*, 221–226. [CrossRef] [PubMed]
2. Shafer, K.J.; Siders, W.A.; Johnson, L.K.; Lukaski, H.C. Validity of segmental multiple-frequency bioelectrical impedance analysis to estimate body composition of adults across a range of body mass indexes. *Nutrition* **2009**, *25*, 25–32. [CrossRef]
3. Stoklossa, C.A.J.; Forhan, M.; Padwal, R.S.; Gonzalez, M.C.; Prado, C.M. Practical considerations for body composition assessment of adults with class II/III obesity using Bioelectrical Impedance Analysis or Dual-Energy, X.-Ray Absorptiometry. *Curr. Obes. Rep.* **2016**, *5*, 389–396. [CrossRef] [PubMed]
4. Wan, C.S.; Ward, L.C.; Halim, J.; Gow, M.L.; Ho, M.; Briody, J.N.; Leung, K.; Cowell, C.T.; Garnett, S.P. Bioelectrical impedance analysis to estimate body composition, and change in adiposity, in overweight and obese adolescents: Comparison with dual-energy x-ray absorptiometry. *BMC Pediatr.* **2014**, *14*, 249. [CrossRef] [PubMed]
5. Böhm, A.; Heitmann, B.L. The use of bioelectrical impedance analysis for body composition in epidemiological studies. *Eur. J. Clin. Nutr.* **2013**, *67*, S79. [CrossRef] [PubMed]
6. Selberg, O.; Selberg, D. Norms and correlates of bioimpedance phase angle in healthy human subjects, hospitalized patients, and patients with liver cirrhosis. *Eur. J. Appl. Physiol.* **2002**, *86*, 509–516. [CrossRef] [PubMed]
7. Zhang, G.; Huo, X.; Wu, C.; Zhang, C.; Duan, Z. A bioelectrical impedance phase angle measuring system for assessment of nutritional status. *Biomed. Mater. Eng.* **2014**, *24*, 3657–3664. [CrossRef] [PubMed]
8. Khalil, S.F.; Mohktar, M.S.; Ibrahim, F. The theory and fundamentals of bioimpedance analysis in clinical status monitoring and diagnosis of diseases. *Sensors* **2014**, *14*, 10895–10928. [CrossRef] [PubMed]

9. Bosy-Westphal, A.; Danielzik, S.; Dörhöfer, R.P.; Later, W.; Wiese, S.; Müller, M.J. Phase angle from bioelectrical impedance analysis: Population reference values by age, sex, and body mass index. *JPEN J. Parenter. Enteral. Nutr.* **2006**, *30*, 309–316. [CrossRef]
10. Redondo-del-Río, M.P.; Camina-Martín, M.A.; Marugan-de-Miguelsanz, J.M.; de- Mateo-Silleras, B. Bioelectrical impedance vector reference values for assessing body composition in a Spanish child and adolescent population. *Am. J. Hum. Biol.* **2017**, *29*, e22978. [CrossRef] [PubMed]
11. Kuchnia, A.J.; Teigen, L.M.; Cole, A.J.; Mulasi, U.; Gonzalez, M.C.; Heymsfield, S.B.; Vock, D.M.; Earthman, C.P. Phase angle and impedance ratio: Reference cut-points from the United States National Health and Nutrition Examination Survey 1999-2004 from bioimpedance spectroscopy data. *JPEN J. Parenter. Enteral. Nutr.* **2017**, *41*, 1310–1315. [CrossRef] [PubMed]
12. Norman, K.; Stobäus, N.; Pirlich, M.; Bosy-Westphal, A. Bioelectrical phase angle and impedance vector analysis–clinical relevance and applicability of impedance parameters. *Clin. Nutr.* **2012**, *31*, 854–861. [CrossRef] [PubMed]
13. Maddocks, M.; Kon, S.S.; Jones, S.E.; Canavan, J.L.; Nolan, C.M.; Higginson, I.J.; Gao, W.; Polkey, M.I.; Man, W.D. Bioelectrical impedance phase angle relates to function, disease severity and prognosis in stable chronic obstructive pulmonary disease. *Clin. Nutr.* **2015**, *34*, 1245–1250. [CrossRef] [PubMed]
14. Kyle, U.G.; Genton, L.; Pichard, C. Low phase angle determined by bioelectrical impedance analysis is associated with malnutrition and nutritional risk at hospital admission. *Clin. Nutr.* **2013**, *32*, 294–299. [CrossRef] [PubMed]
15. Cederholm, T.; Barazzoni, R.; Austin, P.; Ballmer, P.; Biolo, G.; Bischoff, S.C.; Compher, C.; Correia, I.; Higashiguchi, T.; Holst, M.; et al. ESPEN guidelines on definitions and terminology of clinical nutrition. *Clin. Nutr.* **2017**, *36*, 49–64. [CrossRef] [PubMed]
16. Buscemi, S.; Blunda, G.; Maneri, R.; Verga, S. Bioelectrical characteristics of type 1 and type 2 diabetic subjects with reference to body water compartments. *Acta. Diabetol.* **1998**, *35*, 220–223. [CrossRef]
17. Dittmar, M.; Reber, H.; Kahaly, G.J. Bioimpedance phase angle indicates catabolism in Type 2 diabetes. *Diabet. Med.* **2015**, *32*, 1177–1185. [CrossRef]
18. Kułaga, Z.; Różdżyńska-Świątkowska, A.; Grajda, A.; Gurzkowska, B.; Wojtyło, M.; Góźdź, M.; Świąder-Leśniak, A.; Litwin, M. Percentile charts for growth and nutritional status assessment in Polish children and adolescents from birth to 18 year of age. *Standard. Med. Ped.* **2015**, *12*, 119–135.
19. Sun, S.S.; Chumlea, W.C.; Heymsfield, S.B.; Lukaski, H.C.; Schoeller, D.; Friedl, K.; Kuczmarski, R.J.; Flegal, K.M.; Johnson, C.L.; Hubbard, V.S. Development of bioelectrical impedance analysis prediction equations for body composition with the use of a multicomponent model for use in epidemiologic surveys. *Am. J. Clin. Nutr.* **2003**, *77*, 331–340. [CrossRef]
20. Horlick, M.; Arpadi, S.M.; Bethel, J.; Wang, J.; Moye, J. Jr.; Cuff, P.; Pierson, R.N.Jr.; Kotler, D. Bioelectrical impedance analysis models for prediction of total body water and fat-free mass in healthy and HIV-infected children and adolescents. *Am. J. Clin. Nutr.* **2002**, *76*, 991–999. [CrossRef]
21. Kyle, U.G.; Bosaeus, I.; De Lorenzo, A.D.; Deurenberg, P.; Elia, M.; Gómez, J.M.; Heitmann, B.L.; Kent-Smith, L.; Melchior, J.C.; Pirlich, M.; et al. Bioelectrical impedance analysis—part I: Review of principles and methods. *Clin. Nutr.* **2004**, *23*, 1226–1243. [CrossRef] [PubMed]
22. Davis, N.L.; Bursell, J.D.; Evans, W.D.; Warner, J.T.; Gregory, J.W. Body composition in children with type 1 diabetes in the first year after diagnosis: Relationship to glycaemic control and cardiovascular risk. *Arch. Dis. Child.* **2012**, *97*, 312–315. [CrossRef] [PubMed]
23. Galli-Tsinopoulou, A.; Grammatikopoulou, M.G.; Stylianou, C.; Kokka, P.; Emmanouilidou, E. A preliminary case-control study on nutritional status, body composition, and glycemic control of Greek children and adolescents with type 1 diabetes. *J. Diabetes.* **2009**, *1*, 36–42. [CrossRef] [PubMed]
24. Szadkowska, A.; Madej, A.; Ziółkowska, K.; Szymańska, M.; Jeziorny, K.; Mianowska, B.; Pietrzak, I. Gender and Age—Dependent effect of type 1 diabetes on obesity and altered body composition in young adults. *Ann. Agric. Environ. Med.* **2015**, *22*, 124–128. [CrossRef] [PubMed]
25. DCCT Research Group. Weight gain associated with intensive therapy in the Diabetes Control and Complications Trial. *Diabetes Care* **1988**, *11*, 567–573. [CrossRef]
26. Purnell, J.Q.; Zinman, B.; Brunzell, J.D.; DCCT/EDIC Research Group. The effect of excess weight gain with intensive diabetes mellitus treatment on cardiovascular disease risk factors and atherosclerosis in type 1 diabetes mellitus: Results from the Diabetes Control and Complications Trial/Epidemiology of Diabetes

Interventions and Complications Study (DCCT/EDIC) study. *Circulation.* **2013**, *127*, 180–187. [CrossRef] [PubMed]

27. Gubitosi-Klug, R.A.; DCCT/EDIC Research Group. The Diabetes Control and Complications Trial/Epidemiology of Diabetes Interventions and Complications Study at 30 years: Summary and future directions. *Diabetes Care.* **2014**, *37*, 44–49. [CrossRef]
28. Wierzbicka, E.; Swiercz, A.; Pludowski, P.; Jaworski, M.; Szalecki, M. Skeletal Status, Body Composition, and Glycaemic Control in Adolescents with Type 1 Diabetes Mellitus. *J. Diabetes Res.* **2018**, *2018*, 8121634. [CrossRef]
29. Maratova, K.; Soucek, O.; Matyskova, J.; Hlavka, Z.; Petruzelkova, L.; Obermannova, B.; Pruhova, S.; Kolouskova, S.; Sumnik, Z. Muscle functions and bone strength are impaired in adolescents with type 1 diabetes. *Bone* **2018**, *106*, 22–27. [CrossRef]
30. Coleman, S.K.; Rebalka, I.A.; D'Souza, D.M.; Hawke, T.J. Skeletal muscle as a therapeutic target for delaying type 1 diabetic complications. *World J. Diabetes* **2015**, *6*, 1323–1336. [CrossRef]
31. Mameli, C.; Mazzantini, S.; Nasr, M.B.; Fiorina, P.; Scaramuzza, A.E.; Zuccotti, G.V. Explaining the increased mortality in type 1 diabetes. *World J. Diabetes* **2015**, *6*, 889–895. [CrossRef] [PubMed]

14

Nutrition in Gastrointestinal Disease: Liver, Pancreatic and Inflammatory Bowel Disease

Lena J. Storck [1,*], Reinhard Imoberdorf [1] and Peter E. Ballmer [1,2]

1 Kantonsspital Winterthur, Department of Medicine, 8401 Winterthur, Switzerland
2 Zürcher RehaZentrum Davos, 7272 Davos Clavadel, Switzerland
* Correspondence: lena.storck@ksw.ch

Abstract: Liver, pancreatic, and inflammatory bowel diseases are often associated with nutritional difficulties and necessitate an adequate nutritional therapy in order to support the medical treatment. As most patients with non-alcoholic fatty liver disease are overweight or obese, guidelines recommend weight loss and physical activity to improve liver enzymes and avoid liver cirrhosis. In contrast, patients with alcoholic steatohepatitis or liver cirrhosis have a substantial risk for protein depletion, trace elements deficiency, and thus malnutrition. Patients with chronic pancreatitis and patients with inflammatory bowel disease have a similar risk for malnutrition. Therefore, it clearly is important to screen these patients for malnutrition with established tools and initiate adequate nutritional therapy. If energy and protein intake are insufficient with regular meals, oral nutritional supplements or artificial nutrition, i.e., tube feeding or parenteral nutrition, should be used to avoid or treat malnutrition. However, the oral route should be preferred over enteral or parenteral nutrition. Acute liver failure and acute pancreatitis are emergencies, which require close monitoring for the treatment of metabolic disturbances. In most patients, energy and protein requirements are increased. In acute pancreatitis, the former recommendation of fasting is obsolete. Each disease is discussed in this manuscript and special recommendations are given according to the pathophysiology and clinical routine.

Keywords: monitoring; malnutrition; micronutrient deficiency; inflammation; oral nutritional supplements; artificial nutrition

---

1. Introduction

Gastrointestinal diseases are often associated with nutritional deficiencies. The complications range from digestive problems to nutrient absorption disorders and necessitate an adequate nutritional therapy in order to support the medical treatment. In this article, we focus on diseases of three important organs: Liver, pancreas, and intestine.

The liver is the main metabolic organ of the human organism because of its multiple functions; e.g., the liver controls the glucose homeostasis by regulation of glycogen synthesis, glycogenolysis, and gluconeogenesis. In addition, important body proteins and lipids are metabolized and synthesized in liver cells. Next to these metabolic pathways, the liver has an exocrine function by secretion of bile acids and detoxification of ammonia by urea production and glutamine synthesis. Taken these extensive functions into account, it is obvious that liver diseases and thus restrictions in liver functions have far-reaching consequences also for clinical nutrition. An important and by dietary habits increasing liver disease is non-alcoholic fatty liver disease (NAFLD), when the fat content of hepatocytes increases [1,2]. NAFLD aggregates benign hepatosteatosis, progressive and inflammatory non-alcoholic steatohepatitis (NASH) [3]. Insulin resistance, hyperinsulinemia, elevated plasma free fatty acids, fatty liver, hepatocyte injury, liver inflammation, oxidative stress, mitochondrial dysfunction, imbalanced pro-inflammatory cytokines, and fibrosis characterize NAFLD [4]. The other main cause for the development of steatosis is alcohol abuse. Chronic high alcohol consumption causes reduced fatty-acid oxidation as well as increased triglyceride synthesis and deposition, and thereby supports the development of alcoholic steatohepatitis (ASH). Usually, steatohepatitis can be reversible if the relevant noxious agent is eliminated. Inadequate or lack of treatment over many years increases the risk for the development of a liver cirrhosis. Thus, 15–20% of patients with NAFLD will develop liver cirrhosis [5]. Next to these liver diseases that develop over many years, acute liver failure may occur usually as a medical emergency.

Another important organ, which can develop inflammatory processes, is the pancreas. This organ plays a central role in digestion due to its exocrine and endocrine function. A total of 98% of pancreatic tissue is part of the exocrine function, whereby pancreatic enzymes are secreted for food digestion. The endocrine part is located in the Langerhans cells, secreting insulin and glucagon for regulation of glucose homeostasis. Acute pancreatitis is a severe disease, causing self-digestion of the pancreas due to prematurely activated digestive enzymes. Patients with chronic pancreatitis have recurrent inflammatory episodes that replace the pancreatic parenchyma by fibrous connective tissue resulting in a progressive loss of exocrine and endocrine function. Characteristic complications and symptoms are pain, pseudocysts, and pancreatic duct stenosis [6].

The largest digestive organ is the intestine, which regulates the absorption of nutrients. Two important diseases of the intestine are Crohn's disease (CD) and ulcerative colitis (UC) that are characterized by periods of remission and inflammatory flare-ups [7]. In CD, the small and large intestine as well as the mouth, esophagus, stomach, and the anus can be affected with typical ulcerations that occur discontinuously. In contrast, UC mostly affects the colon and rectum and usually shows a continuous pattern of the mucosa. Despite multiple differences, these two diseases share similar symptoms such as abdominal pain, diarrhea, and malnutrition. Hence, these diseases were grouped in the term inflammatory bowel disease (IBD) [7,8].

Nutritional care is clearly important in the treatment of patients with IBD, pancreas or liver disease. Nutritional management includes prevention and/or treatment of malnutrition and micronutrient deficiencies as well as specific recommendations for each condition.

2. Liver Diseases

2.1. Non-Alcoholic Fatty Liver Disease (NAFLD)

So far, there are no approved pharmacological therapies for NAFLD [3]. One reason is that the pathophysiology of NAFLD is not yet fully understood despite enormous advance in this field of research. Since overnutrition is the key problem of NAFLD and most of the patients are overweight or obese, weight loss is an obvious therapeutic possibility, hence, intensive lifestyle interventions are well studied [4,5]. The guideline on clinical nutrition in liver disease recommend a 7–10% weight loss to improve steatosis and liver enzymes [3,9]. To improve fibrosis, a weight loss of more than 10% is necessary [10]. Lifestyle interventions including diet and physical activity should be the first-line treatment and only if all efforts fail, bariatric surgery should be proposed [11,12].

In addition, the composition of the diet may also have an effect on liver fat. Low-carbohydrate diet may be helpful with weight loss, but over a long time, a low-carbohydrate diet stimulated NAFLD pathogenesis in an animal model [4]. It is speculated that the carbohydrate's composition is crucial [4]. For example, fructose can easily induce metabolic complications in the liver and in contrast, fiber might be helpful to maintain blood glucose and thus prevent NAFLD. Furthermore, a fat-rich diet induces hepatic steatosis, but only saturated fatty acids are detrimental for the liver metabolism. Monounsaturated fatty acids might be beneficial and polyunsaturated fatty acids might even be a treatment option for NAFLD [4].

The evidence suggest that increased oxidative stress and changes in several molecular factors like pro- and anti-inflammatory cytokines are mainly involved in the progression of NAFLD [13]. Therefore, antioxidants like vitamin C or polyphenols (e.g., resveratrol, curcumin, quercetin, anthocyanin, green tea polyphenols) might have beneficial effects to improve NAFLD [4]. Kitade et al. (2017) showed that the dietary administration of the carotenoids β-crypoxanthin and astaxanthin not only prevents but also reverses NASH progression in mice by regulating M1/M2 macrophage/Kupffer cell polarization [13]. NAFLD induced by diets high in sucrose/fructose or fat can be prevented or improved by soy protein (β-Conglycinin) by decreasing the expression and function of the two nuclear receptors SREBP-1c and PPAR $\gamma 2$. Fish oil with ω-3 fatty acids inhibits SREBP-1c activity, but controversially increases PPAR $\gamma 2$ expression [13,14]. In summary, research results for the effects of micronutrients on NAFLD showed positive effects on some factors in liver metabolism. However, it remains unclear whether the use of antioxidants and ω-3 fatty acids improve liver disease, thus, further investigations are needed and no recommendation can be given [4]. In contrast and only in non-diabetic adults, vitamin E (800 IU α-tocopherol daily) can improve liver enzymes and histologic pathology [11,15].

The Mediterranean Diet, which is characterized by a high content of antioxidants and fiber, a balanced lipid profile and a low content of simple sugar, seems to be the optimal diet for the management of NAFLD. This diet is a natural multi-ingredient supplement that may exert its related health benefits by the synergistic and/or complementary action of each food compound [16]. A Mediterranean diet low in carbohydrates mobilizes more liver fat compared to a low fat diet with a similar weight loss [17].

2.2. *Alcoholic Steatohepatitis (ASH), Liver Cirrhosis, and Acute Liver Failure*

The nutritional recommendations for patients with ASH and liver cirrhosis are fundamentally different compared to the recommendations for patients with NAFLD, because these patients have a high risk for protein depletion, trace elements deficiency, and malnutrition. Twenty percent of patients with a compensated and 60% of patients with a decompensated liver disease are malnourished [18–20].

Therefore, screening for malnutrition is highly recommended on a regular basis in patients with ASH and liver cirrhosis, but the nutritional assessment can be difficult in patients with cirrhosis especially if there is associated fluid retention and/or obesity. Patients with cirrhosis may have a combination of loss of skeletal muscle and gain of adipose tissue, culminating in the condition of "sarcopenic obesity". In addition, patients had a loss or deficiency of several other nutrients such as vitamin D and zinc [21]. The Nutritional Risk Screening-2002 and the Malnutrition Universal Screening Tool are validated and well-known tools to screen patients at risk for malnutrition [22]. Specifically in patients with liver disease, the Royal Free Hospital Nutrition Prioritizing Tool (RFH-NPT) was developed and when compared to Nutritional Risk Screening, it was more sensitive to identify malnourished liver patients. Next to the important variables unplanned weight loss and reduced dietary intake, the RFH-NPT has additional score points for complications like fluid overload and diuretics [23,24]. In addition, the presence or absence of sarcopenia may be assessed with radiological methods, because sarcopenia is a strong predictor of mortality and morbidity in patients with liver disease [25,26]. Next to radiological methods, handgrip strength is a simple, objective, and practical method to assess sarcopenia [21].

In case of malnutrition, patients need extensive nutritional counseling and therapy. The treatment is a challenge as the nutritional problems are multifactorial [11]. Usually, the resting energy expenditure is increased [27,28] and patients are required to consume 35–40 kcal/kg body weight [23]. Non-malnourished patients should eat 1.2 g protein/kg body weight per day to cover the protein needs, whereas the optimal intake of malnourished and/or sarcopenic patients is 1.5 g protein/kg body weight [11,23]. If energy and protein intake are not adequate with regular meals, oral nutritional supplements (ONS), or artificial nutrition (tube feeding or parenteral) should be used to avoid or treat malnutrition. However, the oral route should be preferred over enteral or parenteral nutrition. The standard formulas should be used, preferably formulas with high energy density (≥1.5 kcal/mL). In case of tube feeding, a percutaneous endoscopic gastrostomy placement is not recommended and can only be used in exceptional cases because of a higher risk of complications, e.g., infections, ascites, or oesophageal varices [22].

Patients with ASH or liver cirrhosis have poor hepatic glycogen stores due to the impaired synthetic capacity of hepatic cells, hence, an overnight fast in these patients is equivalent to a nearly 72 hours fast in healthy persons. As a result, metabolism shifts to fatty acids as a dominant substrate for oxidation. Some tissues dependent on glucose will need neoglucogenesis from amino acids as fatty acids cannot be used for this process. This leads to mobilization of amino acids from the skeletal muscles so that the adequate amount of glucose can be produced. Repeated and frequent fasting results in recurrent proteolysis resulting in muscle loss in human cirrhotic patients [21,29]. Therefore, fasting periods should be avoided and patients with severe liver disease, who have to fast for more than twelve hours, should receive intravenous glucose (2–3 g/kg body weight). When the fasting period lasts longer than 72 hours, total parenteral nutrition may be required [11]. At home, periods of starvation should also be kept short and, therefore, the consumption of three to five meals a day and a late evening snack are recommended [30]. One complication of severe liver disease is hepatic encephalopathy, a disorder of the central nervous system with a wide spectrum, ranging from psychomotor impairments to coma [31]. In case of hepatic encephalopathy, protein intake should no longer be restricted in cirrhotic patients as it increases protein catabolism and thus promotes malnutrition [32]. Advanced cirrhosis patients could benefit from branched-chain amino acids (0.25 g/kg body weight) in order to improve event-free survival and quality of life [33].

Acute liver failure may occur as a medical emergency. In multi-organ failure, a severe derangement of the whole metabolism can occur in these patients due to loss of hepatocellular functions. The metabolic condition is characterized by impaired hepatic glucose production and lactate clearance as well as protein catabolism associated with hyperaminoacidemia and hyperammonemia [11,34,35]. In general, patients with acute liver failure should be treated in the same way as other critically ill patients. Therefore, the patients need to be monitored regularly and if necessary, macronutrients, vitamins, and trace elements should be supplemented [11]. On the one hand, the energy requirement of patients with acute liver disease is increased [36], but on the other hand, a hypercaloric diet induces hyperglycemia and hyperlipidemia. Therefore, it is important to achieve an iso-energetic diet in order to avoid malnutrition and complications. For metabolic monitoring, the following target values should be aimed at: Blood glucose 8–10 mmol/L, serum lactate <5 mmol/L, triglycerides <3 mmol/L, and ammonia <100 mmol/L. The protein requirement is set at 0.8–1.2 g/kg body weight [11]. A summary of nutritional recommendations in liver disease are presented in Figure 1.

Non-alcoholic fatty liver disease

- Obese patients: 7-10% weight loss with intensive lifestyle interventions including physical activity
- Normal weight patients: Increasing physical activity

Alcoholic steatohepatitis and liver cirrhosis

- High risk for malnutrition: Regular screening and assessment using oral nutritional supplements or artificial nutrition
- 35-40 kcal/kg body weight and 1.2-1.5g protein/kg body weight
- Avoid periods of starvation
- Encephalopathy: Protein restriction obsolete
- 0.25g branched-chain amino acids/kg body weight

Acute liver failure

- Analog to other critically ill patients
- Iso-energetic nutrition intake
- Close monitoring and needs-based supplementation

Figure 1. Summary of nutritional recommendations in liver disease.

3. Pancreatic Diseases

3.1. Acute Pancreatitis

The degree of the inflammatory response of the pancreas plays an important role for the assessment of clinical nutrition. Normally, patients with a mild or moderately severe pancreatitis do not need a specific nutritional? intervention, but every patient with acute pancreatitis should be screened for malnutrition with the regular tools and in case of malnutrition, receive an adequate nutritional therapy [37]. The energy and protein requirements are usually not increased and the patients are allowed to eat normal food independently of lipase and amylase activity [37,38]. In contrast to former medical opinions, fasting after an inflammatory episode has no positive effect on the clinical course or prognosis of acute pancreatitis. During the course of pancreatitis, exocrine secretion is blocked and therefore a stimulation of the exocrine function by food intake or artificial nutrition is not expected [6,37]. For those patients who can tolerate an oral diet, an initial low-fat solid diet is preferred [39,40]. This early approach to oral feeding may reduce the length of hospital stay in these patients [41].

In contrast, patients with severe necrotizing pancreatitis need an adequate clinical nutritional? strategy. Initial short-time fasting could be beneficial for patients with ileus or nausea and vomiting, but within 24–48 hours, enteral nutrition should be started. Early enteral nutrition has a more preventive then a nutritive effect, because early enteral nutrition decreased mortality and complications [42–44]. Parenteral nutrition instead could result in an intestinal villous atrophy within a few days, which then facilitates bacterial translocation and may result in severe infections. The administration of enteral nutrition counteracts translocation, and therefore enteral nutrition should be administered whenever possible to prevent intestinal atrophy [6,45].

Due to inflammation and pain, patients with severe acute pancreatitis have an increased energy and protein requirement [46]. Energy requirement is set at 25–30 kcal/kg body weight, glucose intake at 2–4 g/kg body weight, and protein at 1.2–1.5 g/kg body weight. Infusion rate for lipids should be 0.8–1.5 g/kg body weight and the infusion should be monitored regularly since triglycerides in plasma should be <12 mmol/L. Trace elements are supplemented in normal concentrations and high-dose vitamin supplements are not required [37]. In addition, administration of pre- and probiotics as well as immunonutrition cannot be recommended since studies so far have not shown a clear beneficial effect [47,48]. To reach the nutritional goal, enteral nutrition can be completed with oral food intake or parenteral nutrition if necessary. In case of total parenteral nutrition over a long time period, administration of 0.2–0.5 g glutamine/kg body weight could protect against infections and reduce mortality [49]. In addition, monitoring of volume substitution is very important and can decrease mortality [6]. An early return to normal food intake should be pursued [6]. After an episode of acute pancreatitis, approximately 20% of the patients develop the common complications diabetes and exocrine pancreatic insufficiency [50]. Therefore, patients should be regularly screened for these complications in order to prevent nutritional status.

3.2. Chronic Pancreatitis

Patients with chronic pancreatitis have a high risk for malnutrition due to maldigestion from pancreatic exocrine insufficiency in combination with inflammation and increased energy metabolism. Pancreatic exocrine insufficiency is the main pancreatic cause of malnutrition in these patients [51]. In addition, due to diarrhea and steatorrhea, patients with chronic pancreatitis often have a deficiency of the fat-soluble vitamins A, D, E, and K. Malnutrition is associated with an increased complication rate and increased mortality [52]. Therefore, malnutrition should be avoided using nutritional counseling and if necessary artificial nutrition. Energy requirement is set at 25–30 kcal/kg body weight and protein requirement at 1.5 g protein/kg body weight. Since alcohol is an important cause for chronic pancreatitis, patients should avoid alcohol completely [6,37,53].

In the case of pancreatic exocrine insufficiency, patients should be supplemented with pancreas enzymes. The exocrine insufficiency is diagnosed if the patients have either steatorrhea (>15 g/day fecal fats) or suffer from manifest maldigestion, respective malabsorption. For a first indication, patients can be asked whether they see undigested food in their feces or if the feces are difficult to wash away. Further examination could be a pancreatic function test and the evaluation of maldigestion-related symptoms like diarrhea or flatulence, poor nutritional status, and fecal elastase-1 concentration [51,52]. In patients with an exocrine insufficiency, low levels of circulation fat-soluble vitamins, proteins like albumin, lipoproteins, apolipoproteins, and mineral trace elements like magnesium, zinc, or calcium, can occur [54–57]. Since most of these abnormalities are related to pancreatic exocrine insufficiency, a laboratory analysis might be helpful in order to diagnose the insufficiency. However, other factors like toxic habits or deficient food intake may play a relevant role, too [51]. Pancreas enzymes should be taken during the meals and the dosage is based on lipase activity. A range of 20.000 to 40.000 lipase units per main meal should be administered as an initial dose and 10.000 to 20.000 units for the digestion of smaller in-between snacks [6,58]. It is not necessary to avoid high fat intake if the exocrine pancreas function is compensated [37]. The replacement therapy should promote digestion, but a complete normalization of digestion is usually not achieved. However, there are several options for a failure of normalization. First, the pH value in the stomach inactivates the pancreatic enzymes. Therefore, the addition of a proton-pump inhibitor before breakfast and dinner is recommended in cases of an unsatisfactory clinical response to the standard dose of pancreatic enzymes [59]. Second, the enzyme dose should be increased if needed to normalize digestion and the nutritional status of the patients. If these two strategies fail, another cause for maldigestion like bacterial overgrowth should be evaluated [51]. A summary of nutritional recommendations in pancreatic disease is shown in Figure 2.

Acute pancreatitis

- Mild: Normal energy requirements and oral food intake
- Severe: Enteral nutrition should be started within 24-48 hours, energy and protein requirement are increased, combination with parenteral nutrition possible, early return to oral food intake should be pursued

Chronic pancreatitis

- High risk for malnutrition: Regular screening and assessment using oral nutritional supplements or artificial nutrition
- 25-30 kcal/kg body weight and 1.2-1.5g protein/kg body weight
- In case of steatorrhea or maldigestion: Supplementation of pancreas enzymes

Figure 2. Summary of nutritional recommendations in pancreatic disease.

4. Inflammatory Bowel Diseases (IBD)

IBD is a heterogeneous and multifactorial disorder resulting from a complex interplay between genetic variation, intestinal microbiota, the host immune system, and environmental factors such as diet, drugs, breastfeeding, and smoking [60–62]. The relationship between dietary nutrients and intestinal homeostasis is complex and influenced by several interactions between host immune system, the intestinal barrier, and the gut microbiota [60,63]. Patients with IBD have a high risk for malnutrition, which may be the result of reduced oral intake, increased nutrient requirement, increased gastrointestinal losses of nutrients, and occasionally from drug–nutrient interactions [7,64]. In pediatric patients, malnutrition is the main cause for growth retardation [65,66]. In CD, malnutrition is a great problem compared to UC because any part of the gastrointestinal tract can be affected. Therefore, the risk for malnutrition remains even when the disease is quiescent. UC is normally restricted to the colon and hence shows few malabsorptive problems except in active disease [64]. Due to the high risk, patients with IBD should be screened for malnutrition using the established tools at the time of diagnosis and thereafter on a regular basis [67,68]. Malnourished patients should receive an adequate nutritional therapy because otherwise it worsens the prognosis, complication rates, mortality, and quality of life [67,69,70]. The energy requirement of patients with IBD are normally not increased as well as the protein requirement in remission. In contrast, protein requirement is increased in active IBD and therefore, the protein intake should be 1.2–1.5 g/kg body weight [67,71,72].

In addition, patients with IBD have a high risk for micronutrient deficiencies due to losses from diarrhea and/or inadequate dietary intake. The most common micronutrient deficiencies are iron, calcium, selenium, zinc, and magnesium depletion. Vitamin deficiencies include all vitamins and in particular B_{12}, folic acid, and vitamins A, D, and K [73,74]. For example, selenium, zinc, and magnesium depletions are caused by an inadequate dietary intake and chronic loss because of diarrhea. Symptoms associated with deficiencies include bone health impairment, fatigue, poor wound healing, and cartilage degeneration [73,74]. An example for the influence of medication is cholestyramine that can interfere with absorption of fat-soluble vitamins, iron, and B_{12} vitamin. Main side effect is steatorrhea due to impair absorption of fats [75]. Therefore, laboratory values of patients should be checked on a regular basis and possible deficits should be appropriately corrected.

The most frequent extraintestinal manifestation of IBD is iron-deficiency and anemia, which occurs more frequently in CD and which should be supplemented with iron. Anemia is usually associated with other important symptoms like fatigue, sleeping disorders, restless legs syndrome, or attention deficit [75]. Patients with mild anemia can receive oral iron, when they are tolerant for oral iron and when the disease is inactive. Intravenous iron should be considered in patients with active IBD, with previous intolerance to oral iron, with hemoglobin below 100 g/L, and in patients who need erythropoiesis-stimulating agents [67,76,77]. Furthermore, patients may have deficiencies of calcium, vitamin D, folate, vitamin B_{12}, and zinc [64]. When more than 20 cm of the distal ileum is resected, vitamin B_{12} must be administered to patients [67].

Low levels of calcium and vitamin D are common in patients with IBD, especially in those with duodenal and jejunal disease [61,73,74]. Calcium deficiency is linked to vitamin D deficiency, which is related to inadequate daily intake, inflammation status, diarrhea, and glucocorticoid therapy. The prevalence among IBD patients is up to 70% in CD patients and up to 40% in UC patients. Nonetheless, it is not established if the vitamin D deficiency is a cause or a consequence of IBD. However, there are suggestions that in genetically predisposed individuals, vitamin D deficiency may be a contributing factor in the development of IBD [78]. Beneficial effects of vitamin D in IBD are supported by pre-clinical studies mainly in mouse models, where the active form of vitamin D has shown to regulate gastrointestinal microbiota function and promote anti-inflammatory response [61].

When oral nutritional intake is insufficient during active disease, ONS are the first step. If oral feeding is not sufficient, tube feeding is superior to parenteral feeding. Parenteral nutrition is indicated in IBD (i) when oral or tube feeding is not sufficiently possible, (ii) when there is an obstructed bowel, where there is no possibility of placement of a feeding tube beyond the obstruction or where this has failed, or (iii) when other complications occur such as an anastomotic leakage or a high-output intestinal fistula [67]. During active disease, specific formulations or substrates, e.g., glutamine, ω-3 fatty acids are not recommended, neither is the use of probiotics. Probiotic therapy using Escherichia coli Nissle 1917 or VSL#3 can be considered for use in patients with mild to moderate UC for the induction of remission [79].

Enteral exclusive nutrition has been extensively used for induction of remission in pediatric CD, in which avoidance of steroids is critical for childhood growth. Several recent pediatric studies have demonstrated and confirmed that enteral exclusive nutrition can induce remission in 60–86% of children [80–82] and is associated with higher remission rates, better growth, and longer steroids-free periods [60]. However, the benefit was lost when partial enteral nutrition was used with access to a free diet [83]. Nonetheless, a recent study has shown that partial enteral nutrition can be effective for induction of remission in children and young adults in combination with a diet, which is based on components hypothesized to affect the microbiome or intestinal permeability [84]. In remission, ONS or artificial nutrition are only recommended if malnutrition cannot be treated sufficiently by dietary counseling. In addition, specific diets or supplementations with ω-3 fatty acids are not recommended for maintenance of remission. A systematic review has not supported the hypothesis that supplementation of ω-3 fatty acids can induce and maintain remission in IBD [85]. However, several studies have demonstrated that different genotypes can be associated with the variable response to nutritional intervention with ω-3 fatty acids [86]. Probiotic therapy can be considered in UC but not CD for maintenance of remission [67]. In addition, clinical trials show that curcumin supplementation might be effective for the induction and maintenance of remission in UC patients [87,88]. Curcumin suppresses cytokine production by macrophages and intestinal epithelial cells via the inhibition of NF-kB activation [89,90] and thus mitigates induced colitis in mouse models [91,92]. A summary of nutritional recommendations in IBD is presented in Figure 3.

Inflammatory bowel disease

- Regular screening for malnutrition and micronutrient deficiency
- Energy and protein requirement are stable in remission, but increased in active disease
- Supplementation of iron in case of anemia
- If oral feeding is not sufficient then tube feeding is superior to parenteral feeding

Figure 3. Summary of nutritional recommendations in inflammatory bowel disease.

5. Future Perspectives

Clinical nutrition is clearly important in the treatment of patients with liver, pancreatic, and inflammatory bowel disease. However, there are many gaps of knowledge in the pathophysiology of these diseases despite an enormous research effort and thus the effects from clinical nutrition cannot be at a maximum so far.

A major gap in knowledge is associated with the evolution of NAFLD in children and adolescents. Weight loss is important for histological improvement and the benefits of weight loss will extend beyond those expected from drug treatment of high-risk NASH. It is postulated that only public health strategies will have the opportunity to improve the burden of obesity-related diseases in the future [93]. In addition, due to our aging population, it is expected that the burden of liver disease due to cirrhosis from NASH will increase over the next two decades unless effective preventive and therapeutic interventions are implemented as part of a public health strategy [93].

Furthermore, knowledge about the human microbiome constantly increases. Trillions of microbial cells, which form a symbiotic relationship with the host, play a crucial role in the development of diseases, when the balance of the microbiome becomes disrupted [94]. Increase intestinal permeability and dysbiosis are common characteristics linking the liver to a number of gastrointestinal diseases [95]. For example, alcohol consumption and endogenous alcohol production by gut bacteria in obese individuals can disrupt the tight junctions of the intestinal epithelial barrier, resulting in increased gut permeability. The bacterial endotoxin in the portal circulation leads to liver inflammation and fibrosis through activation of toll-like receptor 4 [95]. Although several mechanisms by which the microbiome might affect liver disease have been proposed, more work is needed to fully understand these relationship [93].

IBD is also associated with a dysbiotic microbiome. However, it is unclear if this dysbiosis plays a role in the pathophysiology or is a result of the disease. Due to the importance of the microbiome in IBD, therapies manipulating the microbiome have gained popularity. While there are some promising trials demonstrating the efficacy of antibiotic combinations in treating IBD, more controlled trials are required [94]. In addition, a more precise understanding of the complex interrelation between dietary nutrients, host immunity, and the microbiome is necessary to increase the effectiveness of dietary interventions used to treat IBD [63]. Moreover, an in-depth knowledge of the genetic background is important for personalized nutritional management, which might lead to a maximum efficacy in therapy [63].

New trials in acute pancreatitis showed that approximately one-third of patients will develop prediabetes or diabetes within five years of an index episode of acute pancreatitis and 24–40% of the patients develop an exocrine pancreatic insufficiency, but the mechanisms and risk factors remain to be specified [96–99]. Furthermore, further evidence is required to determine the optimal panel of laboratory markers for nutritional evaluation in chronic pancreatitis, and the utility, reliability, and accuracy of these markers in diagnosing pancreatic exocrine insufficiency [51].

Author Contributions: L.J.S., R.I. and P.E.B. contributed to the conceptualization of the manuscript. L.J.S. wrote the original draft. R.I. and P.E.B. reviewed and edited the original draft. All authors contributed to the final version of the manuscript.

References

1. Mantovani, A.; Byrne, C.D.; Bonora, E.; Targher, G. Nonalcoholic fatty liver disease and risk of incident type 2 diabetes: A meta-analysis. *Diabetes Care* **2018**, *41*, 372–382. [CrossRef] [PubMed]
2. Loomba, R.; Abraham, M.; Unalp, A.; Wilson, L.; Lavine, J.; Doo, E.; Bass, N.M. Nonalcoholic steatohepatitis clinical research, N. association between diabetes, family history of diabetes, and risk of nonalcoholic steatohepatitis and fibrosis. *Hepatology* **2012**, *56*, 943–951. [CrossRef] [PubMed]
3. European association for the study of the liver, european association for the study of diabetes, european association for the study of obesity. EASL-EASD-EASO clinical practice guidelines for the management of non-alcoholic fatty liver disease. *Obes. Facts* **2016**, *9*, 65–90. [CrossRef] [PubMed]
4. Ullah, R.; Rauf, N.; Nabi, G.; Ullah, H.; Shen, Y.; Zhou, Y.D.; Fu, J. Role of nutrition in the pathogenesis and prevention of non-alcoholic fatty liver disease: Recent updates. *Int. J. Biol. Sci.* **2019**, *15*, 265–276. [CrossRef] [PubMed]
5. Vernon, G.; Baranova, A.; Younossi, Z.M. Systematic review: The epidemiology and natural history of non-alcoholic fatty liver disease and non-alcoholic steatohepatitis in adults. *Aliment. Pharm.* **2011**, *34*, 274–285. [CrossRef] [PubMed]
6. Hoffmeister, A.; Mayerle, J.; Beglinger, C.; Büchler, M.; Bufler, P.; Dathe, K.; Fölsch, U.; Friess, H.; Izbicki, J.; Kahl, S.; et al. S3-Leitlinie chronische pankreatitis: Definition, ätiologie, diagnostik, konservative, interventionell endoskopische und operative therapie der chronischen pankreatitis. leitlinie der Deutschen Gesellschaft für Verdauungs- und Stoffwechselkrankheiten (DGVS). *Zeitschrift für Gastroenterol.* **2012**, *50*, 1176–1224.
7. Hanauer, S.B. Inflammatory Bowel Disease: Epidemiology, Pathogenesis, and Therapeutic Opportunities. *Inflamm. Bowel Dis.* **2006**, *12*, S3–S9. [CrossRef]
8. Wedrychowicz, A.; Zajac, A.; Tomasik, P. Advances in nutritional therapy in inflammatory bowel diseases: Review. *World J. Gastroenterol.* **2016**, *22*, 1045–1066. [CrossRef]
9. Promrat, K.; Kleiner, D.E.; Niemeier, H.M.; Jackvony, E.; Kearns, M.; Wands, J.R.; Fava, J.L.; Wing, R.R. Randomized controlled trial testing the effects of weight loss on nonalcoholic steatohepatitis. *Hepatology* **2010**, *51*, 121–129. [CrossRef]
10. Vilar-Gomez, E.; Martinez-Perez, Y.; Calzadilla-Bertot, L.; Torres-Gonzalez, A.; Gra-Oramas, B.; Gonzalez-Fabian, L.; Friedman, S.L.; Diago, M.; Romero-Gomez, M. Weight loss through lifestyle modification significantly reduces features of nonalcoholic steatohepatitis. *Gastroenterology* **2015**, *149*, 367–378. [CrossRef]
11. Plauth, M.; Bernal, W.; Dasarathy, S.; Merli, M.; Plank, L.D.; Schutz, T.; Bischoff, S.C. ESPEN guideline on clinical nutrition in liver disease. *Clin. Nutr.* **2019**, *38*, 485–521. [CrossRef] [PubMed]
12. Mummadi, R.R.; Kasturi, K.S.; Chennareddygari, S.; Sood, G.K. Effect of bariatric surgery on nonalcoholic fatty liver disease: Systematic review and meta-analysis. *Clin. Gastroenterol. Hepatol.* **2008**, *6*, 1396–1402. [CrossRef] [PubMed]
13. Kitade, H.; Chen, G.; Ni, Y.; Ota, T. Nonalcoholic fatty liver disease and insulin resistance: New insights and potential new treatments. *Nutrients* **2017**, *9*, 387. [CrossRef] [PubMed]
14. Yamazaki, T.; Li, D.; Ikaga, R. Effective food ingredients for fatty liver: Soy protein beta-conglycinin and fish oil. *Int. J. Mol. Sci.* **2018**, *19*, 4107. [CrossRef] [PubMed]

15. Del Ben, M.; Polimeni, L.; Baratta, F.; Pastori, D.; Angelico, F. The role of nutraceuticals for the treatment of non-alcoholic fatty liver disease. *Br. J. Clin. Pharm.* **2017**, *83*, 88–95. [CrossRef] [PubMed]
16. Suarez, M.; Boque, N.; Del Bas, J.M.; Mayneris-Perxachs, J.; Arola, L.; Caimari, A. Mediterranean diet and multi-ingredient-based interventions for the management of non-alcoholic fatty liver disease. *Nutrients* **2017**, *9*, 1052. [CrossRef]
17. Gepner, Y.; Shelef, I.; Schwarzfuchs, D.; Zelicha, H.; Tene, L.; Yaskolka Meir, A.; Tsaban, G.; Cohen, N.; Bril, N.; Rein, M.; et al. Effect of distinct lifestyle Interventions on mobilization of fat storage pools: Central magnetic resonance imaging randomized controlled trial. *Circulation* **2018**, *137*, 1143–1157. [CrossRef]
18. Mendenhall, C.L.; Anderson, S.; Weesner, R.E.; Goldberg, S.J.; Crolic, K.A. Protein-calorie malnutrition associated with alcoholic hepatitis. *Am. J. Med.* **1984**, *76*, 211–222. [CrossRef]
19. Merli, M.; Riggio, O.; Dally, L. Italian Multicenter Cooperative Project on nutrition in liver cirrhosis. Nutritional status in cirrhosis. *J. Hepatol.* **1994**, *21*, 317–325.
20. Lautz, H.U.; Selberg, O.; Körber, J.; Bürger, M.; Müller, M.J. Protein-calorie malnutrition in liver cirrhosis. *Clin. Investig.* **1992**, *70*, 478–486. [CrossRef]
21. Anand, A.C. Nutrition and muscle in cirrhosis. *J. Clin. Exp. Hepatol.* **2017**, *7*, 340–357. [CrossRef] [PubMed]
22. Kondrup, J.; Allison, S.P.; Elia, M.; Vellas, B.; Plauth, M. ESPEN guidelines for nutrition screening 2002. *Clin. Nutr.* **2003**, *22*, 415–421. [CrossRef]
23. Amodio, P.; Bemeur, C.; Butterworth, R.; Cordoba, J.; Kato, A.; Montagnese, S.; Uribe, M.; Vilstrup, H.; Morgan, M.Y. The nutritional management of hepatic encephalopathy in patients with cirrhosis: International society for hepatic encephalopathy and nitrogen metabolism consensus. *Hepatology* **2013**, *58*, 325–336. [CrossRef] [PubMed]
24. Borhofen, S.M.; Gerner, C.; Lehmann, J.; Fimmers, R.; Gortzen, J.; Hey, B.; Geiser, F.; Strassburg, C.P.; Trebicka, J. The royal free hospital-nutritional prioritizing tool is an independent predictor of deterioration of liver function and survival in cirrhosis. *Dig. Dis. Sci.* **2016**, *61*, 1735–1743. [CrossRef] [PubMed]
25. Carey, E.J.; Lai, J.C.; Wang, C.W.; Dasarathy, S.; Lobach, I.; Montano-Loza, A.J.; Dunn, M.A.; Fitness, L.E. Exercise in liver transplantation, C. A multicenter study to define sarcopenia in patients with end-stage liver disease. *Liver Transpl.* **2017**, *23*, 625–633. [CrossRef] [PubMed]
26. Montano-Loza, A.J.; Meza-Junco, J.; Prado, C.M.; Lieffers, J.R.; Baracos, V.E.; Bain, V.G.; Sawyer, M.B. Muscle wasting is associated with mortality in patients with cirrhosis. *Clin. Gastroenterol. Hepatol.* **2012**, *10*, 166–173. [CrossRef] [PubMed]
27. Jhangiani, S.S.; Agarwal, N.; Holmes, R.; Cayten, C.G.; Pitchumoni, C.S. Energy expenditure in chronic alcoholics with and without liver disease. *Am. J. Clin. Nutr.* **1986**, *44*, 323–329. [CrossRef]
28. Schneeweiss, B.; Pammer, J.; Ratheiser, K.; Schneider, B.; Maldl, C.; Kramer, L.; Kranz, A.; Ferenci, P.; Druml, W.; Grimm, G.; et al. Energy metabolism in acute hepatic failure. *Gastroenterology* **1993**, *105*, 1515–1521. [CrossRef]
29. Tsien, C.D.; McCullough, A.J.; Dasarathy, S. Late evening snack: Exploiting a period of anabolic opportunity in cirrhosis. *J. Gastroenterol. Hepatol.* **2012**, *27*, 430–441. [CrossRef]
30. Plank, L.D.; Gane, E.J.; Peng, S.; Muthu, C.; Mathur, S.; Gillanders, L.; McIlroy, K.; Donaghy, A.J.; McCall, J.L. Nocturnal nutritional supplementation improves total body protein status of patients with liver cirrhosis: A randomized 12-month trial. *Hepatology* **2008**, *48*, 557–566. [CrossRef]
31. Ferenci, P.; Lockwood, A.; Mullen, K.; Tarter, R.; Weissenborn, K.; Blei, A.T. Hepatic encephalopathy–definition, nomenclature, diagnosis, and quantification: Final report of the working party at the 11th World Congresses of Gastroenterology, Vienna, 1998. *Hepatology* **2002**, *35*, 716–721. [CrossRef] [PubMed]
32. Cordoba, J.; Lopez-Hellin, J.; Planas, M.; Sabin, P.; Sanpedro, F.; Castro, F.; Esteban, R.; Guardia, J. Normal protein diet for episodic hepatic encephalopathy: Results of a randomized study. *J. Hepatol.* **2004**, *41*, 38–43. [CrossRef] [PubMed]
33. Ney, M.; Vandermeer, B.; van Zanten, S.J.; Ma, M.M.; Gramlich, L.; Tandon, P. Meta-analysis: Oral or enteral nutritional supplementation in cirrhosis. *Aliment. Pharm.* **2013**, *37*, 672–679. [CrossRef] [PubMed]
34. Clemmesen, J.O.; Kondrup, J.; Ott, P. Splanchnic and leg exchange of amino acids and ammonia in acute liver failure. *Gastroenterology* **2000**, *118*, 1131–1139. [CrossRef]
35. Rosen, H.M.; Yoshimura, N.; Hodgman, J.M.; Fischer, J.E. Plasma amino acid patterns in hepatic encepathalopathy of differing etiology. *Gastroenterology* **1977**, *72*, 483–487. [PubMed]

36. Walsh, T.S.; Wigmore, S.J.; Hopton, P.; Richardson, R.; Lee, A. Energy expenditure in acetaminophen-induced fulminant hepatic failure. *Crit. Care. Med.* **2000**, *28*, 649–654. [CrossRef] [PubMed]
37. Ockenga, J.; Löser, C.; Kraft, M.; Madl, C. S3-Leitlinie der Deutschen Gesellschaft für Ernährungsmedizin (DGEM) in Zusammenarbeit mit der GESKES, der AKE und der DGVS. *Aktuelle Ernährungsmedizin* **2014**, *39*, e43–e56. [CrossRef]
38. Meier, R.; Ockenga, J.; Pertkiewicz, M.; Pap, A.; Milinic, N.; Macfie, J.; Dgem; Loser, C.; Keim, V. ESPEN guidelines on enteral nutrition: Pancreas. *Clin. Nutr.* **2006**, *25*, 275–284. [CrossRef]
39. Larino-Noia, J.; Lindkvist, B.; Iglesias-Garcia, J.; Seijo-Rios, S.; Iglesias-Canle, J.; Dominguez-Munoz, J.E. Early and/or immediately full caloric diet versus standard refeeding in mild acute pancreatitis: A randomized open-label trial. *Pancreatology* **2014**, *14*, 167–173. [CrossRef]
40. Vaughn, V.M.; Shuster, D.; Rogers, M.A.M.; Mann, J.; Conte, M.L.; Saint, S.; Chopra, V. Early versus delayed feeding in patients with acute pancreatitis: A systematic review. *Ann. Intern. Med.* **2017**, *166*, 883–892. [CrossRef]
41. Aaronson, N.K.; Ahmedzai, S.; Bergman, B.; Bullinger, M.; Cull, A.; Duez, N.J.; Filiberti, A.; Flechtner, H.; Fleishman, S.B.; de Haes, J.C.J.M. The european organization for research and treatment of cancer qlq-c30: A quality-of-life instrument for use in international clinical trials in oncology. *J. Natl. Cancer Inst.* **1993**, *85*, 365–376. [CrossRef] [PubMed]
42. Marik, P.E.; Zaloga, G.P. Meta-analysis of parenteral nutrition versus enteral nutrition in patients with acute pancreatitis. *BMJ* **2004**, *328*, 1407. [CrossRef] [PubMed]
43. McClave, S.A.; Chang, W.K.; Dhaliwal, R.; Heyland, D.K. Nutrition support in acute pancreatitis: A systematic review of the literature. *J. Parenter. Enter. Nutr.* **2006**, *30*, 143–156. [CrossRef] [PubMed]
44. Al-Omran, M.; Albalawi, Z.H.; Tashkandi, M.F.; Al-Ansary, L.A. Enteral versus parenteral nutrition for acute pancreatitis. *Cochrane Database Syst. Rev.* **2010**, CD002837. [CrossRef] [PubMed]
45. Imrie, C.W.; Carter, C.R.; McKay, C.J. Enteral and parenteral nutrition in acute pancreatitis. *Best Pract. Res. Clin. Gastroenterol.* **2002**, *16*, 391–397. [CrossRef] [PubMed]
46. Shaw, J.H.F.; Wolfe, R.R. Glucose, fatty acid, and urea kinetics in patients with severe pancreatitis—The response to substrate infusion and total parenteral nutrition. *Ann. Surg.* **1986**, *204*, 665–672. [CrossRef] [PubMed]
47. Sun, S.; Yang, K.; He, X.; Tian, J.; Ma, B.; Jiang, L. Probiotics in patients with severe acute pancreatitis: A meta-analysis. *Langenbecks Arch. Surg.* **2009**, *394*, 171–177. [CrossRef]
48. Petrov, M.S.; Atduev, V.A.; Zagainov, V.E. Advanced enteral therapy in acute pancreatitis: Is there a room for immunonutrition? A meta-analysis. *Int. J. Surg.* **2008**, *6*, 119–124.
49. Asrani, V.; Chang, W.K.; Dong, Z.; Hardy, G.; Windsor, J.A.; Petrov, M.S. Glutamine supplementation in acute pancreatitis: A meta-analysis of randomized controlled trials. *Pancreatology* **2013**, *13*, 468–474. [CrossRef]
50. Lee, P.J.; Papachristou, G.I. New insights into acute pancreatitis. *Nat. Rev. Gastroenterol. Hepatol.* **2019**. [Epub ahead of print]. [CrossRef]
51. Dominguez-Munoz, J.E.; Phillips, M. Nutritional therapy in chronic pancreatitis. *Gastroenterol. Clin. North. Am.* **2018**, *47*, 95–106. [CrossRef] [PubMed]
52. Ockenga, J. Importance of nutritional management in diseases with exocrine pancreatic insufficiency. *HPB* **2009**, *11* (Suppl. S3), 11–15. [CrossRef] [PubMed]
53. Lévy, P.; Mathurin, P.; Roqueplo, A.; Rueff, B.; Bernades, P. A Multidimensional case-control study of dietary, alcohol, and tobacco habits in alcoholic men with chronic pancreatitis. *Pancreas* **1995**, *10*, 231–238. [CrossRef] [PubMed]
54. Duggan, S.N.; Smyth, N.D.; O'Sullivan, M.; Feehan, S.; Ridgway, P.F.; Conlon, K.C. The prevalence of malnutrition and fat-soluble vitamin deficiencies in chronic pancreatitis. *Nutr. Clin. Pr.* **2014**, *29*, 348–354. [CrossRef] [PubMed]
55. Lindkvist, B.; Dominguez-Munoz, J.E.; Luaces-Regueira, M.; Castineiras-Alvarino, M.; Nieto-Garcia, L.; Iglesias-Garcia, J. Serum nutritional markers for prediction of pancreatic exocrine insufficiency in chronic pancreatitis. *Pancreatology* **2012**, *12*, 305–310. [CrossRef] [PubMed]
56. Lindkvist, B.; Phillips, M.E.; Dominguez-Munoz, J.E. Clinical, anthropometric and laboratory nutritional markers of pancreatic exocrine insufficiency: Prevalence and diagnostic use. *Pancreatology* **2015**, *15*, 589–597. [CrossRef] [PubMed]

57. Montalto, G.; Soresi, M.; Carroccio, A.; Scafidi, E.; Barbagallo, C.M.; Ippolito, S.; Notarbartolo, A. Lipoproteins and chronic pancreatitis. *Pancreas* **1994**, *9*, 137–138. [CrossRef]
58. Dominguez-Munoz, J.E. Pancreatic exocrine insufficiency: Diagnosis and treatment. *J. Gastroenterol. Hepatol.* **2011**, *26* (Suppl. S2), 12–16. [CrossRef]
59. Lohr, J.M.; Dominguez-Munoz, E.; Rosendahl, J.; Besselink, M.; Mayerle, J.; Lerch, M.M.; Haas, S.; Akisik, F.; Kartalis, N.; Iglesias-Garcia, J.; et al. United european gastroenterology evidence-based guidelines for the diagnosis and therapy of chronic pancreatitis (HaPanEU). *United Eur. Gastroenterol. J.* **2017**, *5*, 153–199. [CrossRef]
60. Saez-Gonzalez, E.; Mateos, B.; Lopez-Munoz, P.; Iborra, M.; Moret, I.; Nos, P.; Beltran, B. Bases for the adequate development of nutritional recommendations for patients with inflammatory bowel disease. *Nutrients* **2019**, *11*, 1062. [CrossRef]
61. Fletcher, J.; Cooper, S.C.; Ghosh, S.; Hewison, M. The role of vitamin D in inflammatory bowel disease: Mechanism to management. *Nutrients* **2019**, *11*, 1019. [CrossRef] [PubMed]
62. De Souza, H.S.; Fiocchi, C. Immunopathogenesis of IBD: Current state of the art. *Nat. Rev. Gastroenterol. Hepatol.* **2016**, *13*, 13–27. [CrossRef] [PubMed]
63. Sugihara, K.; Morhardt, T.L.; Kamada, N. The role of dietary nutrients in inflammatory bowel disease. *Front. Immunol.* **2018**, *9*, 3183. [CrossRef] [PubMed]
64. Goh, J.; O'Morain, C.A. Review article: Nutrition and adult inflammatory bowel disease. *Aliment. Pharm.* **2003**, *17*, 307–320.
65. Hill, R.J.; Cleghorn, G.J.; Withers, G.D.; Lewindon, P.J.; Ee, L.C.; Connor, F.; Davies, P.S. Resting energy expenditure in children with inflammatory bowel disease. *J. Pediatr. Gastroenterol. Nutr.* **2007**, *45*, 342–346. [CrossRef] [PubMed]
66. Wiskin, A.E.; Wootton, S.A.; Culliford, D.J.; Afzal, N.A.; Jackson, A.A.; Beattie, R.M. Impact of disease activity on resting energy expenditure in children with inflammatory bowel disease. *Clin. Nutr.* **2009**, *28*, 652–656. [CrossRef]
67. Forbes, A.; Escher, J.; Hebuterne, X.; Klek, S.; Krznaric, Z.; Schneider, S.; Shamir, R.; Stardelova, K.; Wierdsma, N.; Wiskin, A.E.; et al. ESPEN guideline: Clinical nutrition in inflammatory bowel disease. *Clin. Nutr.* **2017**, *36*, 321–347. [CrossRef]
68. Sandhu, A.; Mosli, M.; Yan, B.; Wu, T.; Gregor, J.; Chande, N.; Ponich, T.; Beaton, M.; Rahman, A. Self-screening for malnutrition risk in outpatient inflammatory bowel disease patients using the malnutrition universal screening tool (MUST). *J. Parenter Enter. Nutr.* **2016**, *40*, 507–510. [CrossRef]
69. Gajendran, M.; Umapathy, C.; Loganathan, P.; Hashash, J.G.; Koutroubakis, I.E.; Binion, D.G. Analysis of hospital-based emergency department visits for inflammatory bowel disease in the USA. *Dig. Dis. Sci.* **2016**, *61*, 389–399. [CrossRef]
70. Ananthakrishnan, A.N.; McGinley, E.L. Infection-related hospitalizations are associated with increased mortality in patients with inflammatory bowel diseases. *J. Crohns. Colitis.* **2013**, *7*, 107–112. [CrossRef]
71. O'Keefe, S.J.D.; Ogden, J.; Rund, J.; Potter, P. Steroids and bowel rest versus elemental diet in the treatment of patients with Crohn's disease: The effects on protein metabolism and immune function. *J. Parenter. Enter. Nutr.* **1989**, *13*, 455–460. [CrossRef] [PubMed]
72. Royall, D.; Greenberg, G.R.; Allard, J.P.; Baker, J.P.; Jeejeebhoy, K.N. Total enteral nutrition support improves body composition of patients with active Crohn's disease. *J. Parenter. Enter. Nutr.* **1995**, *19*, 95–99. [CrossRef] [PubMed]
73. Weisshof, R.; Chermesh, I. Micronutrient deficiencies in inflammatory bowel disease. *Curr. Opin. Clin. Nutr. Metab. Care.* **2015**, *18*, 576–581. [CrossRef] [PubMed]
74. Hwang, C.; Ross, V.; Mahadevan, U. Micronutrient deficiencies in inflammatory bowel disease: From A to zinc. *Inflamm. Bowel Dis.* **2012**, *18*, 1961–1981. [CrossRef] [PubMed]
75. Scaldaferri, F.; Pizzoferrato, M.; Lopetuso, L.R.; Musca, T.; Ingravalle, F.; Sicignano, L.L.; Mentella, M.; Miggiano, G.; Mele, M.C.; Gaetani, E.; et al. Nutrition and IBD: Malnutrition and/or sarcopenia? A practical guide. *Gastroenterol. Res. Pr.* **2017**, *2017*, 1–11. [CrossRef]
76. Bergamaschi, G.; Di Sabatino, A.; Albertini, R.; Ardizzone, S.; Biancheri, P.; Bonetti, E.; Cassinotti, A.; Cazzola, P.; Markopoulos, K.; Massari, A.; et al. Prevalence and pathogenesis of anemia in inflammatory bowel disease. Influence of anti-tumor necrosis factor-alpha treatment. *Haematologica* **2010**, *95*, 199–205. [CrossRef] [PubMed]

77. Reinisch, W.; Staun, M.; Bhandari, S.; Munoz, M. State of the iron: How to diagnose and efficiently treat iron deficiency anemia in inflammatory bowel disease. *J. Crohns Colitis* **2013**, *7*, 429–440. [CrossRef]
78. Cantorna, M.T. Vitamin D and its role in immunology: Multiple sclerosis, and inflammatory bowel disease. *Prog. Biophys. Mol. Biol.* **2006**, *92*, 60–64. [CrossRef]
79. Fujiya, M.; Ueno, N.; Kohgo, Y. Probiotic treatments for induction and maintenance of remission in inflammatory bowel diseases: A meta-analysis of randomized controlled trials. *Clin. J. Gastroenterol.* **2014**, *7*, 1–13. [CrossRef]
80. Connors, J.; Basseri, S.; Grant, A.; Giffin, N.; Mahdi, G.; Noble, A.; Rashid, M.; Otley, A.; van Limbergen, J. Exclusive enteral nutrition therapy in paediatric Crohn's disease results in long-term avoidance of corticosteroids: results of a propensity-score matched cohort analysis. *J. Crohns Colitis* **2017**, *11*, 1063–1070. [CrossRef]
81. Levine, A.; Turner, D.; Pfeffer Gik, T.; Amil Dias, J.; Veres, G.; Shaoul, R.; Staiano, A.; Escher, J.; Kolho, K.L.; Paerregaard, A.; et al. Comparison of outcomes parameters for induction of remission in new onset pediatric Crohn's disease: Evaluation of the porto IBD group "growth relapse and outcomes with therapy" (GROWTH CD) study. *Inflamm. Bowel Dis.* **2014**, *20*, 278–285. [CrossRef] [PubMed]
82. Cohen-Dolev, N.; Sladek, M.; Hussey, S.; Turner, D.; Veres, G.; Koletzko, S.; Martin de Carpi, J.; Staiano, A.; Shaoul, R.; Lionetti, P.; et al. Differences in outcomes over time with exclusive enteral nutrition compared with steroids in children with mild to moderate Crohn's disease: Results from the GROWTH CD study. *J. Crohns Colitis* **2018**, *12*, 306–312. [CrossRef] [PubMed]
83. Levine, A.; Wine, E. Effects of enteral nutrition on Crohn's disease: Clues to the impact of diet on disease pathogenesis. *Inflamm. Bowel Dis.* **2013**, *19*, 1322–1329. [CrossRef] [PubMed]
84. Sigall-Boneh, R.; Pfeffer-Gik, T.; Segal, I.; Zangen, T.; Boaz, M.; Levine, A. Partial enteral nutrition with a Crohn's disease exclusion diet is effective for induction of remission in children and young adults with Crohn's disease. *Inflamm. Bowel Dis.* **2014**, *20*, 1353–1360. [CrossRef] [PubMed]
85. Turner, D.; Shah, P.S.; Steinhart, A.H.; Zlotkin, S.; Griffiths, A.M. Maintenance of remission in inflammatory bowel disease using omega-3 fatty acids (fish oil): A systematic review and meta-analyses. *Inflamm. Bowel Dis.* **2011**, *17*, 336–345. [CrossRef] [PubMed]
86. Paradis, A.M.; Fontaine-Bisson, B.; Bosse, Y.; Robitaille, J.; Lemieux, S.; Jacques, H.; Lamarche, B.; Tchernof, A.; Couture, P.; Vohl, M.C. The peroxisome proliferator-activated receptor alpha Leu162Val polymorphism influences the metabolic response to a dietary intervention altering fatty acid proportions in healthy men. *Am. J. Clin. Nutr.* **2005**, *81*, 523–530. [CrossRef] [PubMed]
87. Hanai, H.; Iida, T.; Takeuchi, K.; Watanabe, F.; Maruyama, Y.; Andoh, A.; Tsujikawa, T.; Fujiyama, Y.; Mitsuyama, K.; Sata, M.; et al. Curcumin maintenance therapy for ulcerative colitis: Randomized, multicenter, double-blind, placebo-controlled trial. *Clin. Gastroenterol. Hepatol.* **2006**, *4*, 1502–1506. [CrossRef] [PubMed]
88. Lang, A.; Salomon, N.; Wu, J.C.; Kopylov, U.; Lahat, A.; Har-Noy, O.; Ching, J.Y.; Cheong, P.K.; Avidan, B.; Gamus, D.; et al. Curcumin in combination with mesalamine induces remission in patients with mild-to-moderate ulcerative colitis in a randomized controlled trial. *Clin. Gastroenterol. Hepatol.* **2015**, *13*, 1444–1449.e1441. [CrossRef]
89. Wang, J.; Ghosh, S.S.; Ghosh, S. Curcumin improves intestinal barrier function: Modulation of intracellular signaling, and organization of tight junctions. *Am. J. Physiol. Cell Physiol.* **2017**, *312*, C438–C445. [CrossRef]
90. Pan, M.H.; Lin-Shiau, S.Y.; Lin, J.K. Comparative studies on the suppression of nitric oxide synthase by curcumin and its hydrogenated metabolites through down-regulation of IkappaB kinase and NFkappaB activation in macrophages. *Biochem. Pharm.* **2000**, *60*, 1665–1676. [CrossRef]
91. Yang, J.Y.; Zhong, X.; Kim, S.J.; Kim, D.H.; Kim, H.S.; Lee, J.S.; Yum, H.W.; Lee, J.; Na, H.K.; Surh, Y.J. Comparative effects of curcumin and tetrahydrocurcumin on dextran sulfate sodium-induced colitis and inflammatory signaling in mice. *J. Cancer Prev.* **2018**, *23*, 18–24. [CrossRef] [PubMed]
92. Sugimoto, K.; Hanai, H.; Tozawa, K.; Aoshi, T.; Uchijima, M.; Nagata, T.; Koide, Y. Curcumin prevents and ameliorates trinitrobenzene sulfonic acid-induced colitis in mice. *Gastroenterology* **2002**, *123*, 1912–1922. [CrossRef] [PubMed]
93. Sanyal, A.J. Past, present and future perspectives in nonalcoholic fatty liver disease. *Nat. Rev. Gastroenterol. Hepatol.* **2019**, *16*, 377–386. [CrossRef] [PubMed]
94. Ihekweazu, F.D.; Versalovic, J. Development of the pediatric gut microbiome: Impact on health and disease. *Am. J. Med. Sci.* **2018**, *356*, 413–423. [CrossRef] [PubMed]

95. Mandato, C.; Di Nuzzi, A.; Vajro, P. Nutrition and liver disease. *Nutrients* **2017**, *10*, 9. [CrossRef] [PubMed]
96. Nikkola, J.; Laukkarinen, J.; Lahtela, J.; Seppanen, H.; Jarvinen, S.; Nordback, I.; Sand, J. The long-term prospective follow-up of pancreatic function after the first episode of acute alcoholic pancreatitis: Recurrence predisposes one to pancreatic dysfunction and pancreatogenic diabetes. *J. Clin. Gastroenterol.* **2017**, *51*, 183–190. [CrossRef] [PubMed]
97. Das, S.L.; Kennedy, J.I.; Murphy, R.; Phillips, A.R.; Windsor, J.A.; Petrov, M.S. Relationship between the exocrine and endocrine pancreas after acute pancreatitis. *World J. Gastroenterol.* **2014**, *20*, 17196–17205. [CrossRef] [PubMed]
98. Hollemans, R.A.; Hallensleben, N.D.L.; Mager, D.J.; Kelder, J.C.; Besselink, M.G.; Bruno, M.J.; Verdonk, R.C.; van Santvoort, H.C. Pancreatic exocrine insufficiency following acute pancreatitis: Systematic review and study level meta-analysis. *Pancreatology* **2018**, *18*, 253–262. [CrossRef] [PubMed]
99. Das, S.L.; Singh, P.P.; Phillips, A.R.; Murphy, R.; Windsor, J.A.; Petrov, M.S. Newly diagnosed diabetes mellitus after acute pancreatitis: A systematic review and meta-analysis. *Gut* **2014**, *63*, 818–831. [CrossRef]

15

Management of Glucose Control in Noncritically Ill, Hospitalized Patients Receiving Parenteral and/or Enteral Nutrition

Céline Isabelle Laesser [1], Paul Cumming [2,3], Emilie Reber [1], Zeno Stanga [1], Taulant Muka [4] and Lia Bally [1,*]

1. Department of Diabetes, Endocrinology, Clinical Nutrition, and Metabolism, Inselspital, Bern University Hospital, University of Bern, 3010 Bern, Switzerland
2. Department of Nuclear Medicine, Inselspital, Bern University Hospital, University of Bern, 3010 Bern, Switzerland
3. School of Psychology and Counselling and IHBI, Queensland University of Technology, Brisbane, QLD 4059, Australia
4. Institute of Social and Preventive Medicine, University of Bern, 3012 Bern, Switzerland

* Correspondence: lia.bally@insel.ch

Abstract: Hyperglycemia is a common occurrence in hospitalized patients receiving parenteral and/or enteral nutrition. Although there are several approaches to manage hyperglycemia, there is no consensus on the best practice. We systematically searched PubMed, Embase, Cochrane Central, and ClinicalTrials.gov to identify records (published or registered between April 1999 and April 2019) investigating strategies to manage glucose control in adults receiving parenteral and/or enteral nutrition whilst hospitalized in noncritical care units. A total of 15 completed studies comprising 1170 patients were identified, of which 11 were clinical trials and four observational studies. Diabetes management strategies entailed adaptations of nutritional regimens in four studies, while the remainder assessed different insulin regimens and administration routes. Diabetes-specific nutritional regimens that reduced glycemic excursions, as well as algorithm-driven insulin delivery approaches that allowed for flexible glucose-responsive insulin dosing, were both effective in improving glycemic control. However, the assessed studies were, in general, of limited quality, and we see a clear need for future rigorous studies to establish standards of care for patients with hyperglycemia receiving nutrition support.

Keywords: glucose control; hyperglycemia; parenteral nutrition; enteral nutrition; nutritional support; insulin

---

1. Introduction

Hyperglycemia is frequently encountered during parenteral (PN) and/or enteral (EN) nutrition in hospitalized patients with and without pre-existing diabetes [1,2]. Indeed, it is estimated that more than 50% of patients on PN and 30% of patients on EN experience hyperglycemia whilst in the hospital [3,4]. Hyperglycemia arises in these patients due to one or more of the following factors: (1) diminished insulin sensitivity due to inflammation, stress hormones, and sedentarism [5]; (2) increased carbohydrate provision [6]; and (3) side-effects of medication such as glucocorticoids that interfere with glucose metabolism [7]. In patients totally reliant on PN, these factors are compounded by the loss of the physiological incretin effect on insulin release, as occurs when entirely bypassing the gastrointestinal tract with intravenous nutrient supply [8]. Furthermore, the diminished glucose-stimulated insulin secretion in diabetic patients with some residual beta-cell function increases their requirement for exogenous insulin.

Evidence from several observational studies suggests that emergent hyperglycemia during nutrition support is associated with increased morbidity and mortality [1,9]. There is an apparently linear relationship between the incidence of adverse outcomes and mean glucose levels once glycaemia surpasses a threshold of 6.3 mM [10]. In individuals on PN, the risk of any complication increases by a factor of 1.58 for each 1 mM increase in glycaemia above this threshold [11]. Conversely, treatment of hyperglycemia is shown to improve clinical outcomes [12–15]. However, striving for tight glucose control inherently increases the risk of hypoglycemia, which is similarly associated with adverse clinical outcomes [16,17].

PN and EN nutrition support are provided in a number of ways, ranging from continuous to cyclic regimens, often in combination with unpredictable and variable oral intake or additional intravenous glucose administration. Maintaining glycemic control is even more demanding in patients with unanticipated interruptions of their feeding (e.g., due to emergency surgery), or if nutrition support is suspended due to accidental removal or obstruction of tubing. Guidelines such as those from the American Diabetes Society [18] and the Endocrine Society [19] recommend that random blood glucose levels be maintained below 10.0 mM, provided that this target can be safely achieved. According to these guidelines, the mainstay of hyperglycemia management in the hospital is the administration of insulin, given its high efficacy, flexibility, and lack of interference with most other pharmacotherapies or organ dysfunctions.

Although there are some recommendations for insulin dosing tailored to the needs of patients receiving PN and/or EN, there is a lack of evidence-based support for specific insulin regimens. Insulin can be delivered via intravenous or subcutaneous routes, or in patients receiving PN, insulin may simply be mixed in the nutrition solution [20]. Intravenous insulin infusion at a rate continuously adjusted according to regular capillary blood glucose measurements helps to maintain glucose levels within the recommended limits. However, implementation of intravenous protocols imposes considerable demand on nursing staff, calling for two hours of direct nursing daily per patient [21], which substantially increases the workload of ward staff. Noncritical care nurses have to manage several patients, and staff levels are reduced at nighttime, which does not encourage constant vigilance of blood glucose and manual adjustment of insulin infusion rates. Thus, for practical and safety considerations in noncritical care settings, subcutaneous administration is the favored route for insulin delivery. However, the formulation of PN and EN support can also influence glucose levels in patients on nutrition support. Whereas glucose is the only carbohydrate source in standard PN solutions, the glycemic impact can be modulated by changing the caloric contributions of carbohydrates versus monounsaturated fatty acids (MUFAs), or by using alternate carbohydrates such as fructose. Furthermore, the addition of fibers to EN formulae can delay carbohydrate absorption, thereby attenuating the glycemic impact [22,23]. An overview of the different management strategies is provided in Figure 1.

Diabetes technology has progressed greatly over the past decade, bringing considerable improvements to the care of outpatients with type 1 and type 2 diabetes. Notably, recent development of continuous glucose monitoring (CGM) systems that measure interstitial fluid glucose concentration every few minutes allow to depict glucose profiles in higher resolution, thereby facilitating adjustment of insulin dosages [24]. CGM systems also project trends for glucose levels and feature customizable hypo- and hyperglycemia alerts. There is a growing interest in the use of this technology in hospital settings given the abundance of additional information that can guide therapy adjustments.

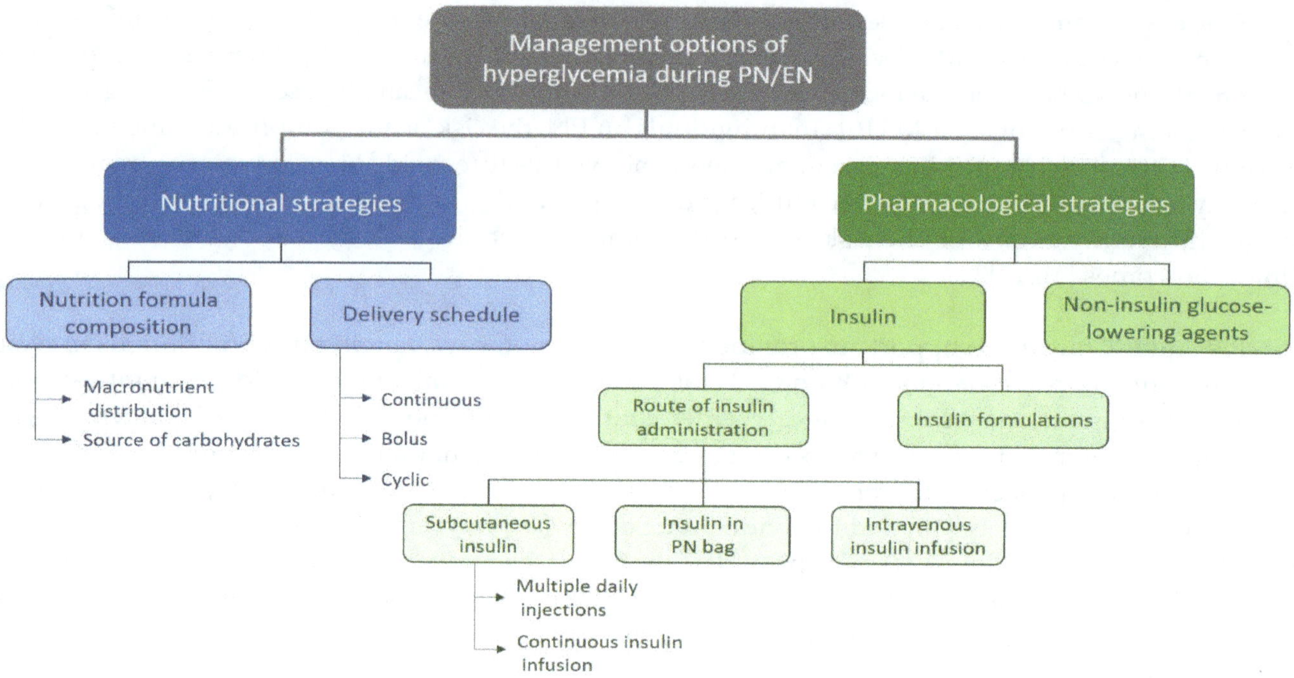

Figure 1. Management options of hyperglycemia during PN/EN. PN = parenteral nutrition, EN = enteral nutrition.

An important variable in the control of glycaemia is the modulation of insulin to meet with the continuously changing metabolic needs. Due to its inherent flexibility of insulin dose adjustment, the predominant mode of delivery in patients with type 1 diabetes is via a subcutaneous insulin pump, also known as continuous subcutaneous insulin infusion [25]. Here, a portable pump infuses rapid-acting insulin at a rate that can be altered on demand or preset to change at fixed times. This flexible adaptation of the insulin delivery profile makes the approach particularly attractive for patients under cyclic nutrition regimens who may receive large amounts of carbohydrates within predefined time windows. The combination of real-time glucose measurements from a CGM device with a control algorithm that directs insulin delivery via an insulin pump constitutes a closed-loop system, also known as the artificial pancreas [26,27]. Closed-loop systems automatically adjust insulin delivery every 10–12 min according to real-time glucose measurements. The autonomy and glucose feedback-regulation obtained through closed-loop systems hold promise in the particular context of hyperglycemia, arising along with nutritional support, while sparing an excess burden on nursing staff.

Our aim in the present review is to provide an overview of the current status and future outlook of glucose management strategies for noncritical care patients receiving PN and/or EN nutrition support.

2. Materials and Methods

2.1. Literature Search

This review was conducted and reported in accordance with the PRISMA and MOOSE guidelines [28,29]. Completed checklists can be found in Supplementary Tables S5 and S6. PubMed and Embase databases were used to identify relevant records over the past 20 years. The Cochrane Central Register of Controlled Trials and ClinicalTrials.gov were searched for published and ongoing studies. The search strategies for the databases are summarized in Supplementary Tables S1–S4. Two reviewers independently evaluated the titles and abstracts according to the selection criteria. For each potentially eligible study, two reviewers assessed the full-text. In cases of disagreement, a decision was made by consensus or, if necessary, a third reviewer was consulted.

2.2. *Study Selection Criteria*

Studies were included if they met the following criteria: (i) were published or registered in English language between 10 April 1999 and 10 April 2019 (date last searched); (ii) were clinical studies evaluating new treatment approaches against a comparator; (iii) included adult (age ≥ 18 years) noncritical care inpatients receiving PN and/or EN nutrition; (iv) investigated strategies to manage blood glucose control; and (v) had outcomes reflecting glucose control. Exclusion criteria were pregnancy, breast feeding, case reports, abstracts, guidelines, or literature reviews. The selection process is shown in Figure 2.

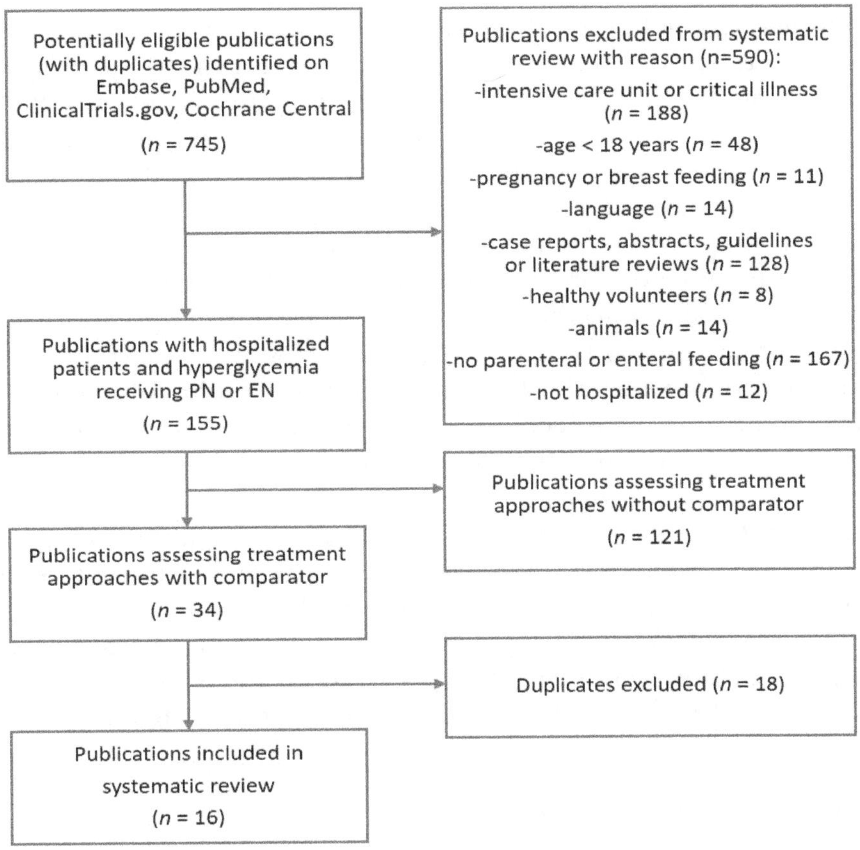

Figure 2. Flowchart illustrating the study selection process.

2.3. *Data Extraction*

Two reviewers extracted data independently using a predesigned form, including study design, sample size, glucose management strategy, primary outcome, and main results. If no primary outcome was specified, we obtained the endpoints deemed most relevant.

2.4. *Quality Assessment*

The quality of clinical trials was evaluated by two reviewers based on the "Cochrane Risk of Bias tool" [30]. According to this tool, studies are judged to be of low or high risk for bias based on criteria to evaluate random sequence generation, allocation concealment, blinding of participants/personnel and outcome assessment, incomplete outcome data, and selective reporting. Since retrospective publications have an inherently high risk of bias in most domains, and there is not a standardized assessment tool available, we refrained them from quality evaluation.

3. Results

3.1. Study Identification and Selection

We identified in total 745 potentially eligible records. Following screening based on titles and abstracts, 34 citations were selected for detailed full-text evaluation. Of those, 16 articles met the selection criteria and were included in the review (Figure 2). One ongoing study was eligible for inclusion.

3.2. Characteristics of the Included Studies

The included published publications comprised 1170 participants from 15 clinical studies, of which 11 were clinical trials (9 randomized and 2 nonrandomized) and 4 were retrospective observational studies. One study was an ongoing registered study. Seven studies were conducted in Europe, three in North America, and five in Asia. Only three studies included more than one center. The study population represented medical (20%), surgical (27%), or mixed medical and surgical (53%) noncritical care inpatients. Three studies explicitly stated the inclusion of patients with type 1 diabetes, three studies explicitly excluded patients with type 1 diabetes, five studies exclusively recruited patients with type 2 diabetes, whereas the remainder did not further characterize the diabetic state of study participants or the reason for hyperglycemia ($n = 4$). Nutrition support comprised PN in six studies, EN in seven studies, and PN and/or EN in two studies. Regarding glucose management strategies, 4 studies investigated nutritional approaches, and 11 studies explored insulin interventions. No studies were found that explored noninsulin pharmacological strategies. The study duration ranged from 36 h to 46 days. Study characteristics and findings are summarized in Tables 1 and 2.

Four of the clinical trials were considered of medium quality, indicating a low risk of bias in all domains except for performance and detection bias, which was deemed reasonable with a near impossibility of blinding [31–34]. The other studies were deemed to be of limited quality, with high risk of bias in the domains of lack of primary outcome definition and selective or incomplete reporting (Supplementary Figure S1). Since retrospective publications have an inherently high risk of bias in most domains, we refrained from a quality evaluation of the four such studies.

3.3. Studies Examining Nutritional Strategies

Four studies examined nutritional strategies to manage glycaemia in patients receiving nutrition support. The use of EN formulae with lower glycemic impacts were contrasted against conventional products in two clinical trials [35,36]. In a nonrandomized crossover study involving inpatients with type 2 diabetes, Tiyapanjanit et al. tested a formula compounded in-house to contain 50% of calories as carbohydrates, thereof 67% as fructose, in comparison with an iso-energetic control formula (53% of calories as carbohydrates and 15% as fructose). Over the study period of 36 h, lower mean glucose was achieved with the high-fructose formula compared to control (6.8 ± 1.5 vs. 8.0 ± 2.1 mM, $p = 0.022$). No insulin or antidiabetic medication was administered in these patients [35]. Similarly, a four-center randomized controlled parallel trial conducted in 104 inpatients with type 2 diabetes found a lower nutrition-induced relative change from baseline glycaemia with the use of lower glycemic impact enteral vs. standard enteral nutrition formula (10% vs. 21%, $p = 0.006$). The investigated EN formula contained a reduced amount of carbohydrates (9.4 vs. 12.5 g/100 mL, p = n/a) and higher amounts of MUFAs (3.8 vs. 1.0 g/100 mL, p = n/a) [36]. Similarly, an ongoing randomized clinical trial (GlyENStroke, NCT03422900) evaluates the efficacy of a diabetes-specific enteral nutrition formula to reduce hyperglycemia (glucose levels > 8.3 mM) in nondiabetic patients with hyperglycemia on nutrition support after stroke [37].

Table 1. Overview of clinical trials.

Author, Year	Study Design [1]	Sample Size	Population	Nutrition Therapy	Interventions	Primary Outcome {Study Period}	Main Results	Risk of Bias [3]
					Insulin adaptation			
Boughton et al., 2019 [31]	RCT, parallel, two-center	43	Non-T1D surgical and medical	PN and/or EN	Fully automated s.c. closed-loop insulin delivery (closed loop, $n = 21$)	% time in target (5.6–10.0 mM) based on CGM values {Up to 15 d or discharge}	% time in target higher in closed-loop vs. control (68% vs. 36%, $p < 0.0001$); hypoglycemia (<3.9 mM) infrequent and similar between closed-loop and control (0.5% for both), p = ns)	Low
					Conventional s.c. insulin therapy according to local practice (control, $n = 22$)			
Olveira et al., 2019 [32]	RCT, parallel, multi-center (26 sites)	161	T2D surgical and medical	TPN	100% regular insulin in PN bag (100% in bag, $n = 80$)	Mean glucose based on capillary POC BG values {Up to 15 d or until PN stop}	Mean glucose during TPN 9.2 vs. 9.6 mM 100% in bag vs. 50% in bag (ns); mean glucose 48 h post-TPN higher in 100% in bag vs. 50% in bag (8.9 vs. 7.9 mM, $p = 0.024$); number of patients with hypoglycemia (≤3.9 mM) lower in 100% in bag vs. 50% in bag (9 vs. 22, $p = 0.016$)	Medium
					50% s.c. glargine + 50% regular insulin in PN bag (50% in bag, $n = 81$)			
Li et al., 2018 [38]	RCT, parallel, single-center	102	T2D surgical	PN (cyclic)	Continuous s.c. insulin infusion (CSII, $n = 50$)	mean amplitude of glycemic excursion (MAGE) based on CGM {4 d}	MAGE lower in CSII vs. basbol (3.7 vs. 6.2 mM, $p < 0.05$), no hypoglycemia events (<3.9 mM) occurred	High
					S.c. basal–bolus glargine/aspart (basbol, $n = 52$)			
Hakeam et al., 2017 [33]	RCT, parallel, single-center	67	Non-T1D surgical (non-cardiac)	PN	S.c. glargine (scGlarg, $n = 35$)	Mean glucose based on capillary POC BG values from day 5 on PN and % of patients who achieved target glycaemia (7.8–10.0 mM) {9 d}	Comparable mean BG in scGlar vs. RIbag, % of values in target 52% in scGlar vs. 48% in RIbag ($p = 0.06$); no significant difference in hypoglycemic (<3.9 mM) events	Medium
					Regular insulin added to PN bag (RIbag, $n = 32$)			
Yuan et al., 2015 [12]	RCT, parallel, single-center	212	T2D surgical (gastrectomy for gastric cancer)	EN (continuous)	VRII (short-acting insulin NOS) (VRII, $n = 106$)	PO not specified; mean glucose based on capillary POC BG values, infective and noninfective complications {8–10 d}	Mean BG lower in VRII vs. s.c.Ins. (5.4 vs. 9.5 mM, $p < 0.001$); higher rate of severe hypoglycemia (≤2.2 mM) in VRII vs. s.c.Ins. (8% vs. 1%, $p = 0.035$)	High
					S.c. conventional insulin therapy (s.c.Ins., $n = 106$)			
Kruyt et al., 2010 [39]	Single-arm intervention with historical control	23	Hyperglycemic patients (excluded patients with previous insulin use)medical (stroke unit)	EN	Continuous feeding with computerized VRII group (continuous, $n = 10$)	% of capillary POC BG values in target range (4.4–6.1 mM){5 d}	Higher % values in target and mean glucose in continuous vs. inter group (55% vs. 19%, $p < 0.005$ and 5.8 vs. 7.6 mM, $p < 0.005$)	Medium
					Bolus feeding with regular i.v. insulin adaptation intermediate group (inter, $n = 13$)			

Table 1. *Cont.*

Author, Year	Study Design [1]	Sample Size	Population	Nutrition Therapy	Interventions	Primary Outcome {Study Period}	Main Results	Risk of Bias [3]
Korytkowski et al., 2009 [40]	RCT, parallel, single-center	50	Diabetes NOS surgical and medical	EN	S.c. SSI (regular insulin) every 4–6 h (SSRI, $n = 25$); (NPH initialized if persistent BG > 10.0 mM) S.c. SSRI plus s.c. glargine (basalPLUS, $n = 25$)	PO not specified; mean glucose based on capillary POC BG values {8 d}	mean BG similar in SSRI and basalPLUS (8.9 vs. 9.2 mM, p = ns); NPH initialized in 55% of those on SSRI	High
					Nutrition adaptation			
Tiyapanjanit et al., 2014 [35]	Non-randomized cross-over (no washout)	10	T2D (BG < 10 mM wo antidiabetic medication) medical	EN (continuous)	In-house prepared EN formula with 50% CHO thereof 67% fructose, (inhouse, $n = 10$) Standard diabetic EN formula with 53% CHO thereof 15% fructose and 57% maltodextrin (standard, $n = 10$)	PO not specified; mean glucose based on capillary POC BG values; glycemic variability based on CGM {3 d, each formula for 36 h)	Mean glucose lower in inhouse vs. standard group (6.8 vs. 8.0 mM, $p = 0.022$); glucose variability comparable	High
Lidder et al., 2009 [34]	RCT, parallel, single-center	30	Prediabetes (fasting BG < 7 mM) surgical (esophagectomy for esophageal cancer)	PN with or wo EN	100% of energy covered by PN (PN, $n = 14$) 70% covered by PN + 30% covered by EN (PN + EN, $n = 16$)	Mean glucose values based on CGM values {surgery until postoperative day 5}	Mean glucose comparable over entire study period, lower from day 3 post-surgery to day 5 post-surgery in PN + EN vs. PN ($p = 0.002$)	Medium
Léon-Sanz et al., 2005 [36]	RCT, parallel, multi-center (4 sites)	104	T2D surgical and medical	EN (continuous)	Low-CHO high-MUFA nutrition formula (lowCHO, $n = 51$) Energy-matched high-CHO nutrition formula (highCHO, $n = 53$)	Mean glucose based on capillary POC BG values and mean daily insulin dose {2 weeks}	BG increase from baseline lower in lowCHO than highCHO after 7 d on EN (10% vs. 21%, $p = 0.006$); mean BG identical (12.7 vs. 12.7 mM[2])	Medium
Valero et al., 2001 [41]	RCT, parallel, double-blind, single-center	138	T1D (21%) and T2D (79%) surgical and medical	TPN (continuous)	Standard TPN containing glucose (PN_G, $n = 71$) Energy-matched TPN containing glucose:fructose:xylitol 2:1:1 (PN_GFX, $n = 67$)	PO not specified; number of patients with target glycaemia (capillary POC BG values 8.3–11.1 mM) at end of TPN {TPN duration 5–46 d)	BG < 11.1 mM at end of TPN reached in 75% vs. 85% in PN_G and PN_GFX respectively [2]	High

RCT = randomized controlled trial, T1D = type 1 diabetes, EN = enteral nutrition, PN = parenteral nutrition, s.c. = subcutaneous, CGM = continuous glucose monitoring, T2D = type 2 diabetes, TPN = total parenteral nutrition, POC = point of care, BG = blood glucose, (ns) = not significant, CSII = continuous subcutaneous insulin infusion, VRII = variable rate intravenous insulin, excl = exclusion, NOS = not otherwise specified, PO = primary outcome, SSI = sliding scale insulin, SSRI = sliding-scale regular insulin, NPH = neutral protamine Hagedorn insulin, wo = without, i.v. = intravenous, CHO = carbohydrates, h = hours, d = day(s) and MUFA = monounsaturated fatty acids. [1] Open-label if not stated otherwise. [2] No p-value available. [3] Overall quality assessment; specific domains can be found in Supplementary Figure S1.

Table 2. Overview of observational, retrospective studies.

Author, Year	Study Design	Sample Size	Population	Nutrition Therapy	Interventions	Primary Outcome {Study Period}	Main Results
					Insulin adaptation		
Truong et al., 2019 [42]	Retrospective observational, single-center	102	Hyperglycemic patients (≥ 2 BG values > 10.0 mM, including T1D and T2D) surgical and medical	PN (continuous or cyclic)	Regular insulin added to PN bag (100% bag, $n = 78$) S.c. insulin glargine (scGlarg, $n = 35$)	% of patients with ≥5/6 capillary POC BG values per day <10.0 mM for ≥2 consecutive days {during PN or until target reached}	Higher % of patients with target achieved in 100%bag vs. scGlarg (72% vs. 49%, $p = 0.017$); ≥2 hypoglycemic events (<3.9 mM) in 9% of 100%bag and 17% of scGlarg group (p = ns); lower need for corrective insulin less in 100%bag vs. scGlarg (28 vs. 57% of patients, $p = 0.003$)
Hijaze et al., 2017 [43]	Retrospective observational, single-center	53	Non-T1D medical	EN (continuous)	S.c. NPH insulin 3×/day (NPH, $n = 26$) (Rescue bolus with 6 units rapid insulin analoga if BG > 16.7 mM) S.c. basal–bolus insulin analoga therapy (basbol, $n = 27$)	PO not specified; mean glucose based on capillary POC BG values and % of values in the target range (7.8–10 mM) {until discharge or stop EN}	mean BG comparable in NPH vs. basbol (10.6 vs. 11.1 mM, p = ns), 24% and 22% of values in range (p = ns)
Neff et al., 2014 [44]	Retrospective observational, single-center	53	Hyperglycemic patients (BG > 10 mM including T1D and T2D) surgical and medical	PN	Protocol-driven VRII (VRII, $n = 32$) S.c. basal–bolus insulin (basbol, $n = 21$)	PO not specified; mean glucose based on POC BG values and % of values in target range (4.0–10.0 mM) {until stop PN}	Mean glucose lower and % values in target range higher in VRII vs. basbol (9.6 vs. 11.2 mM, $p = 0.009$ and 62% vs. 43%, $p = 0.008$)
Hsia et al., 2011 [45]	Retrospective observational, single-center	22	Diabetes NOS surgical and medical	EN (continuous)	S.c. basal–bolus with glargine/lispro (basbol, $n = 8$) S.c. 70/30 premixed insulin 2×/day (mixed2, $n = 8$) S.c. 70/30 pre-mixed insulin 3×/day (mixed3, $n = 6$)	PO not specified; mean glucose based on POC BG values, % of values in target range (7.8–10.0 mM) {72 h}	mean glucose comparable, % of values in target range higher in mixed3 vs. mixed2 and basbol (69% vs. 22% vs. 24%, $p < 0.01$); patients with hypoglycemic events (<3.9 mM) in basbol vs. mixed2 and mixed3 (5 vs. 2 vs. 1)

BG = blood glucose, vs. = versus, T1D = type 1 diabetes, T2D = type 2 diabetes, PN = parenteral nutrition, s.c. = subcutaneous, POC = point of care, EN = enteral nutrition, NPH = Neutral Protamine Hagedorn, ns = not significant, VRII = variable rate intravenous insulin, PO = primary outcome, and NOS = not otherwise specified.

There was only one study examining a modified nutritional formula in abdominal surgery patients that were entirely parenterally fed. In this randomized parallel double-blind single-center study, Valero et al. contrasted a PN formula with glucose as a sole carbohydrate source with an iso-energetic PN formulation containing a 2:1:1 glucose:fructose:xylitol carbohydrate mixture. The study population consisted of patients with type 1 diabetes (21%) or type 2 diabetes (79%). Both formulae provided a similar total amount of carbohydrates (2.9 ± 0.5 vs. 2.9 ± 0.7 g/kg/day), but the test formula under investigation contained less glucose (2.9 ± 0.5 vs. 1.5 ± 0.4 g/kg/day). Protein and fat quantity were similar. The time until attaining target glycaemia (8.3–11.1 mM) did not significantly differ (2.5 ± 1.7 vs. 2.4 ± 2.1 day, p = ns), nor did the percentage of patients attaining values below 11.1 mM (75% vs. 85%, p = ns) and total daily insulin dose (45 ± 19 vs. 45 ± 26 U/day, p = ns). However, when stratified according to the occurrence of sepsis, the nonseptic patients showed lower insulin requirements with the glucose–fructose–xylitol regime (37 ± 17 vs. 44 ± 17 U/day, $p = 0.026$) [41].

Managing glycaemia during PN is more demanding than during EN. In this context, the combination of PN with EN, in addition to its well-established trophic benefits on gastrointestinal function, may also confer glycemic advantages. This was shown by a randomized controlled parallel study performed by Lidder et al. in patients undergoing esophagectomy who received nutrition support for up to five days post-surgery. The study contrasted the coverage of 30% of energy needs by EN and 70% by PN feeds with 100% coverage by PN. Although no effect was seen in mean glucose over the five-day study period, the combined use of EN and PN lead to lower glycaemia three days after surgery ($p = 0.002$) [34].

3.4. Studies Examining Insulin Strategies

Eleven studies examined insulin-based strategies to manage glucose in patients receiving nutrition support (five with PN, five with EN, and one with combined PN/EN). A randomized controlled single-center parallel study involving 212 type 2 diabetic patients who had undergone gastrectomy for gastric cancer compared protocol-driven intravenous insulin therapy with conventional subcutaneous sliding scale insulin delivery over 8–10 days of continuous EN. Mean glucose levels were lower (5.4 ± 1.2 vs. 9.5 ± 1.8 mM, $p < 0.001$), and mean daily insulin doses were higher (55 ± 15 vs. 32 ± 16 U/day, $p < 0.001$) in patients receiving intravenous insulin compared with subcutaneous insulin. However, in the group receiving intravenous insulin, eight participants experienced episodes of severe hypoglycemia (defined as blood glucose < 2.2 mM), versus only one participant in the subcutaneous group ($p = 0.010$). Additionally, this study reported outcomes extending beyond glycemic control, finding a reduced incidence of surgical site infection in the intravenous insulin group [12].

A second randomized controlled trial (RCT) evaluating different insulin treatments during EN included 50 patients with non-type 1 diabetes who were randomly assigned to receive sliding scale subcutaneous regular insulin either with or without once daily subcutaneous glargine. In the group without glargine administration, subcutaneous neutral protamine Hagedorn (NPH, isophane) was given as a rescue medication when glucose levels exceeded 10.0 mM. Mean glucose as the primary outcome was comparable between groups, as were the number of hypoglycemic events and total daily insulin dose. However, NPH was required in 48% of the control participants, as their glucose levels were not sufficiently controlled with the regular sliding scale subcutaneous insulin alone [40].

A single-arm trial evaluated the efficacy of a computerized variable rate insulin infusion rate protocol in previously insulin-naïve stroke patients on continuous EN over five days. Compared to a historical control population who received enteral bolus feeds accompanied by intravenous insulin coverage, the intervention resulted in a higher percentage of values in the target range of 4.4–6.1 mM (55% vs. 19%, $p < 0.005$) [39].

Additionally, two retrospective observational studies evaluated insulin-based strategies to treat hyperglycemia in hospitalized patients receiving EN. Hijaze et al. found comparable mean glucose values, and similar times with glucose values within the target range (7.8–10 mM), in patients receiving subcutaneous NPH insulin thrice daily vs. basal–bolus insulin therapy with insulin analogues [43].

In the second such study, Hsia et al. retrospectively evaluated glucose control using three different insulin regimens in patients with diabetes of type not otherwise specified during at least three days of continuous EN. Treatment consisted of (1) 70/30 biphasic insulin (NPH/regular) every 8 h ($n = 6$), (2) 70/30 biphasic insulin every 12 h ($n = 8$), and (3) a basal–bolus regimen (glargine and lispro, $n = 8$). The 8 h 70/30 biphasic insulin group had the highest proportion of glucose values falling within the target range (7.8–10.0 mM) (69% vs. 22% vs. 24%, $p < 0.01$). Hypoglycemic events (<3.9 mM) occurred five times in glargine/lispro group, twice in the twice-daily biphasic group, and once in the thrice-daily biphasic group [45]. In patients receiving PN, two randomized controlled parallel trials evaluated strategies that involved the addition of regular insulin to the PN feeding bag. Olveira et al. recently compared the use of 100% coverage of insulin needs by regular insulin added to the PN bag with 50% coverage by regular insulin added to the PN bag and 50% administered subcutaneously as insulin glargine in a total of 161 mixed surgical and medical patients with type 2 diabetes recruited at 26 different sites. The glucose values of participants were evaluated while receiving total PN (maximum of 15 days) and two days after cessation of total PN. Mean glucose levels during total PN did not significantly differ between groups (9.2 ± 2.0 vs. 9.6 ± 2.4 mM, p = ns); however, mean glucose two days after cessation of total PN was higher in the group that had received 100% of their exogenous insulin requirements added to the PN feeding bag (8.9 ± 2.5 vs. 7.9 ± 2.4 mM, $p = 0.024$). The authors did not provide any details on the requirement for insulin therapy after cessation of nutrition support [32]. Another randomized controlled clinical trial of PN patients contrasted two different basal insulin regimens. Hakeam et al. compared subcutaneous basal–bolus therapy (insulin glargine + short-acting insulin analogue) with the addition of regular insulin to the PN bag in a total of 67 non-type 1 diabetic patients. Both groups received additional corrective regular subcutaneous insulin according to a sliding scale. Basal insulin delivery dose was titrated based on glucose values by a daily 40%–60% dose increase if glucose values were still above target. The percentage of glucose values within the glycemic target range (7.8–10.0 mM) tended to be higher in the group who received s.c. insulin glargine compared to those who received regular insulin added to the PN bag (52% vs. 48%, $p = 0.06$). Mean glucose levels and number of hypoglycemic events did not differ between treatment groups [33].

In contrast to these prospective findings in PN patients, a retrospective evaluation performed by Truong et al. in 102 patients on PN showed superior glucose control defined as percentage of patients with ≥5 of 6 glucose values <10 mM over 2 days in those who had received 100% of required insulin added to the PN bag ($n = 78$), compared with those treated with subcutaneous insulin glargine ($n = 35$) (72% vs. 49%, $p = 0.017$). Additionally, fewer patients receiving insulin via the PN bag experienced two or more hypoglycemic events compared to those with subcutaneous administration (9% vs. 17.1%, p = ns) [42].

As reviewed above in patients receiving EN, a protocol-driven intravenous insulin delivery approach has proven to confer glycemic benefits in PN patients, according to a retrospective analysis performed by Neff et al. A total of 53 surgical and medical patients requiring insulin therapy whilst in the hospital were treated either with protocol-driven variable rate intravenous insulin ($n = 32$), or received basal–bolus subcutaneous insulin therapy ($n = 21$). The insulin infusion group compared to the group receiving subcutaneous basal–bolus insulin therapy showed lower mean glucose levels (9.6 ± 2.1 vs. 11.2 ± 2.6 mM, $p = 0.009$) and a higher percentage of glucose values within the glycemic target of 4.0–10.0 mM (62% vs. 43%, $p = 0.008$), without increased risk of hypoglycemia [44].

Two recently performed randomized controlled parallel design trials evaluated insulin pump therapy, also known as continuous subcutaneous insulin infusion (CSII), in patients receiving nutrition support. The study performed by Li et al. compared the use of CSII ($n = 50$) to basal–bolus therapy using insulin glargine in combination with insulin aspart ($n = 52$) in patients receiving PN. Study treatment was initialized before surgery, and PN began on day 1 after surgery, with comparison of glucose control with CGM from postoperative day 1 to day 5. Glycemic variability was assessed by mean amplitude of glucose excursion (MAGE) as the primary outcome. CSII reduced glycemic variability compared to basal–bolus injection therapy (3.7 ± 2.8 vs. 6.2 ± 3.0 mM, $p < 0.05$). No hypoglycemic events occurred in either treatment group [38].

The second study evaluated CSII as part of a fully automated subcutaneous closed-loop glucose control ($n = 21$) against conventional subcutaneous insulin therapy according to local practice ($n = 22$) in two different hospitals. Randomization was stratified according to BMI, prestudy total daily insulin dose, and type of nutrition support to ensure to demographic balance between groups. The closed-loop system consisted of a subcutaneous insulin pump, a CGM device, and a control algorithm, which adjusted insulin delivery every 12 min based on real-time CGM values. An example of such fully automated closed-loop insulin delivery is illustrated in Figure 3. Participants were recruited from medical and surgical wards and received PN ($n = 13$), EN ($n = 27$), or combined PN/EN ($n = 3$). The primary outcome was the proportion of time when sensor glucose was within the target range (5.6–10.0 mM). Participants were followed for up to 15 days or until hospital discharge. The closed-loop system nearly doubled the proportion of time spent in the glycemic target range compared to control (68% ± 16% vs. 36% ± 27%, $p < 0.0001$). Time spent above target, mean glucose level, and glucose variability were all significantly lower in the closed-loop group. Hypoglycemia was infrequent in both arms, and its incidence did not differ significantly. The substantially better glycemic control in the closed-loop compared to the control group was achieved with a similar total daily insulin dose (53.9 vs. 40.3 U, p = ns) [31].

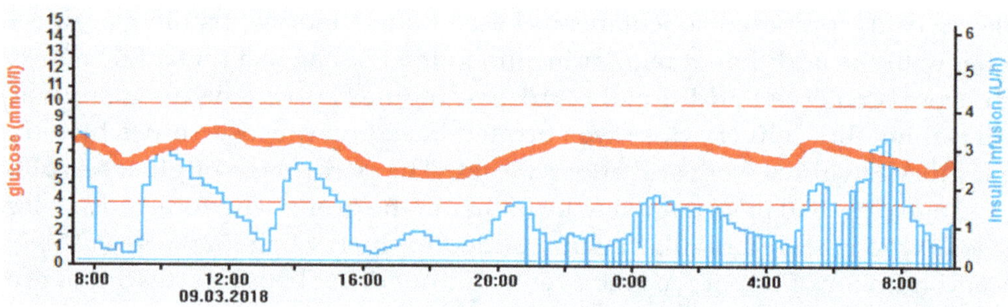

Figure 3. Profile of fully automated subcutaneous closed-loop insulin delivery over 24 h in a noncritical care patient [31]. A control algorithm modulates subcutaneous insulin delivery via an insulin pump (denoted in blue) according to interstitial sensor glucose values (denoted in red). (Kindly provided by Professor Roman Hovorka, University of Cambridge, UK).

4. Discussion

Hyperglycemia is a common occurrence in hospitalized patients receiving PN and/or EN, and its management in noncritical care settings is challenging. The present review summarized the available evidence for strategies to improve glucose control in this vulnerable population. Improved glucose control can be achieved either by lowering the glycemic impact of nutrition supply and/or matching the nutrition-induced glycemic excursions with a tailored pharmacokinetic profile of a given insulin preparation. Both approaches have been evaluated in a limited number of randomized and nonrandomized clinical trials and observational studies over the past 20 years.

Altering the macronutrient distribution (an increase of calories as MUFAs at the expense of carbohydrates) and the use of nonglucose carbohydrate sources along with high fiber content to delay absorption in EN formulae have proven effective in various studies as well as in meta-analyses [22,23]. The use of diabetes-specific enteral formulae is therefore supported by the expert group of the European Society of Clinical Nutrition and Metabolism (ESPEN) for patients with a history of diabetes [46]. With respect to PN formulae, glucose substitutes such as fructose or xylitol to lower the glycemic impact are no longer used in clinical practice. This may relate to previously reported metabolic side effects of parenteral xylitol and fructose such as formation of oxalate crystals in the kidney and lactate accumulation [47–49]. To make matters worse, life-threatening metabolic complications can occur in patients with undeclared hereditary fructose intolerance [50]. There is currently no data on the efficacy and safety of PN formulations with reduced carbohydrate content (and consequently higher protein or lipid fractions) in noncritically ill patients with hyperglycemia. In critically ill patients, however, lipid-based, compared to iso-energetic glucose-based, PN formulae showed more favorable metabolic effects [51]. Additionally, lowering the overall carbohydrate and energy provision has proven effective in reducing hyperglycemia in critically ill patients [52,53].

As an alternative to conventional routes of insulin administration, algorithm-driven intravenous insulin titration protocols during both PN and EN achieved superior glucose control compared to subcutaneous approaches with either sliding scale or basal–bolus insulin therapy. However, this approach poses logistical challenges for ward staff, given the need for frequent glucose draws and insulin dose adjustments, which are either impractical or simply unfeasible in noncritical care settings with low nurse-to-patient ratios. Regarding subcutaneous insulin regimens, administering basal plus supplemental short-acting insulin analogues showed superior efficacy compared to a sliding scale approach with short-acting insulin. The administration of intermediate or long-acting insulins can thus be recommended for PN/EN patients receiving subcutaneous insulin therapy. No data exist with regard to the use of recently introduced ultra-long acting insulins (e.g., degludec). Of note, the required time to reach steady state insulin levels with ultra-long acting formulations imposes certain constraints on the titration method, and prediposes to dysglycemia. There is a practical consideration that administering long-acting insulin in previously insulin-naïve patients brings a risk of hypoglycemia if feeding tubes are accidentally pulled or obstructed.

The admixture of insulin into the PN feeding bag is a safe and effective alternative to using short- or rapid-acting subcutaneous insulin. Moreover, further advantages lie in the lesser need for nursing time, the concomitant discontinuation of insulin delivery upon PN interruption, and the consequently lower risk of hypoglycemic events. The latter is particularly relevant for patients in whom the transient need for exogenous insulin is primarily a result of their nutrition support. However, the need for strict aseptic conditions may render the procedure impractical or not permissible. Furthermore, reservations exist regarding the diminished or highly variable efficacy of PN insulin due to interference from PN ingredients or bag surface material [54,55].

Irrespective to the chosen approach for insulin administration, a limiting factor in obtaining tight glucose control is the risk of inadvertent hypoglycemia [17]. As is the case for hyperglycemia, iatrogenic hypoglycemia is associated with increased cost and adverse medical outcomes [16]. In this context, there is an increasing interest in the use of noninsulin glucose-lowering agents (without hypoglycemia risk) for the treatment of inpatient hyperglycemia. The recent SITA-HOSPITAL randomized controlled study investigated 279 noncritical care patients with type 2 diabetes and showed that oral sitagliptin plus basal insulin led to similar glycemic control than the more labor-intensive basal–bolus insulin regimen [56]. However, challenging patients such as those with high insulin requirements, renal failure, or use of glucocorticoids were excluded from the study. Currently, there are no data on the inpatient use of noninsulin glucose-lowering treatments for hyperglycemia in noncritical care patients on PN and/or EN. Reservations apply to the common side effects of noninsulin treatments (e.g., incretin-based therapies) on the gastrointestinal tract, which is often the primary pathophysiology calling for nutrition support. Further research is needed to explore the potential risks and benefits of noninsulin pharmacotherapy for managing glucose levels in noncritical care settings with EN/PN.

The high prevalence of hyperglycemia amongst noncritical care patients on PN and/or EN support, in conjunction with the increasing workload burden placed on hospital staff, brings an urgent need for innovative approaches to improve the efficacy, efficiency, and safety of healthcare delivery in this context. The advent of novel technologies such as automated closed-loop systems that titrate insulin delivery based on real-time sensor glucose measurements could potentially address this need, whilst reducing staff workload burden. Uncertainties remain with respect to interference with certain medications and inaccurate glucose readouts related to compromised microcirculation. In addition, we concede that there are short-term costs to purchase, install, and train staff in the use of any novel technology. Ongoing studies will further document the potential role of this technology and the obstacles to its integration into clinical practice without disrupting the usual workflow.

The present systematic review turned up rather few randomized controlled trials and a limited number of retrospective observational studies addressing hyperglycemia in noncritical care patients on PN and/or EN. The studies were highly heterogeneous in terms of study population, nutrition regimen, study endpoints, and glucose measurement techniques. Patients with pre-existing diabetes already on insulin treatment before their admission to the hospital and those receiving steroids or showing impaired renal function clearly have different optimal insulin delivery profiles compared to patients without pre-existing diabetes and/or with stress-induced hyperglycemia. The particular nutrition regime (i.e., the EN/PN feeding schedule and any additional oral intake) leads to variable carbohydrate exposures with relevant impact on insulin requirements. The few studies that utilized CGM more comprehensively assessed both hyper- and hypoglycemic excursions, whilst studies adopting intermittent (i.e., six-hourly) point-of-care measurements may have missed important events such as postprandial transients. Most studies were conducted in patients on continuous PN and/or EN, which may be less demanding for insulin management compared to the less common bolus or cyclic feeding practices. The scarce evidence and the many factors (e.g., patient comorbidity, staffing level, hospital guidelines, and policies) that determine the ability and capacity to treat hyperglycemia effectively and safely challenge the provision of generalizable treatment recommendations. In Figure 4, we propose a workflow recommendation considering both nutritional and insulin adaptation to manage hyperglycemia in the noncritical care population receiving nutrition support.

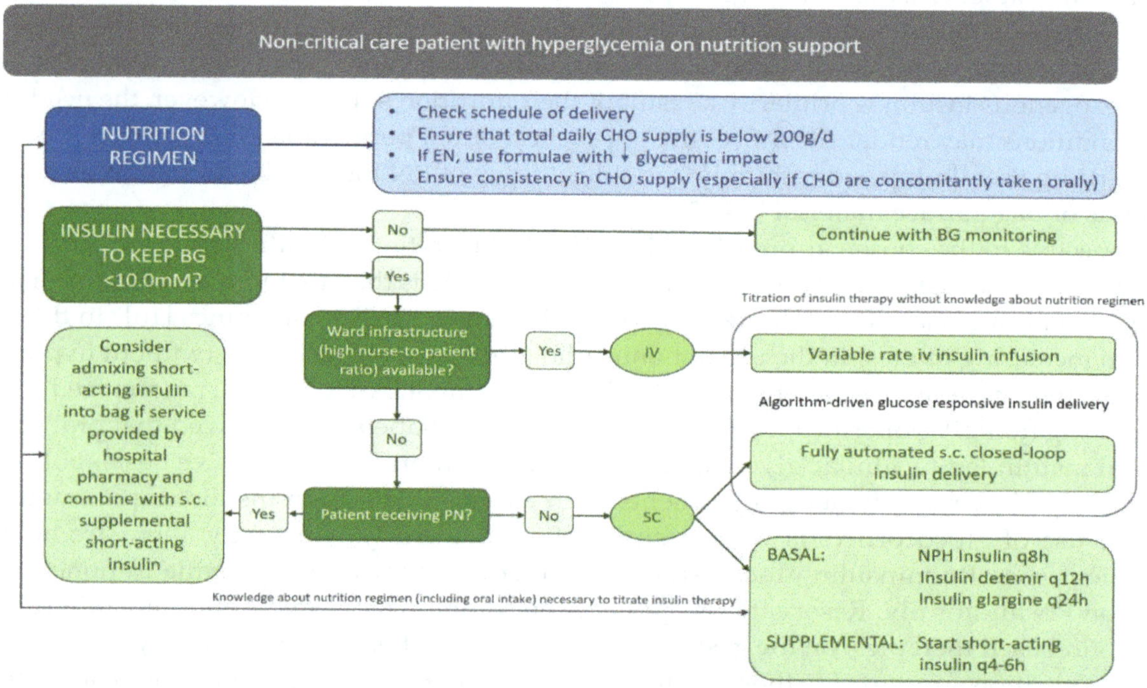

Figure 4. Approach to the management of hyperglycemia in patients receiving enteral or parenteral nutrition. CHO = carbohydrates, EN = enteral nutrition, BG = blood glucose, IV = intravenous, PN = parenteral nutrition, SC = subcutaneous, and q8h = dosing every 8 h.

The majority of the included studies scored poorly in methodology, with a high or unclear risk of biases according to Cochrane criteria. Undoubtably, it is sometimes difficult or unethical to undertake double-blind RCTs with standardized protocols. Also, some studies did not correct for multiple testing, which may have overestimated outcomes. The included retrospective observational studies were not evaluated for quality given the known risk of outcome overestimation and confounding biases inherent in that design. However, we chose to report these studies in this review to cover the widest possible range of different management possibilities.

Small sample sizes and short study durations of some studies may have led to an underestimation of effect sizes, thus hindering the sensitivity to ascertain the efficacy of potential methods to improve glycemic control or indeed to confirm the impact of superior glucose control on patient outcomes. There is clearly a need for further research in the form of well-designed and adequately powered multicenter trials of sufficient duration aiming to examine effects of glucose management strategies on glucose control, clinical outcome, and also optimization of nutritional status in patients receiving PN and/or EN.

5. Conclusions

The management of hyperglycemia in patients receiving PN and/or EN presents unique clinical challenges for both diabetic and nondiabetic hospitalized patients with hyperglycemia. Coherent approaches to this problem are important to avoid potential complications. Obtaining a better match between the carbohydrate dose and the insulin supply is likely to improve glucose control. Granting more attention to the glycemic impact of nutrition regimes in conjunction with deploying novel technologies such as CGM and glucose-responsive automation of insulin delivery through closed-loop systems may address these needs without increasing staff workload. Supplemental or alternate use of noninsulin pharmacological approaches may further open up new lines of research. Well-designed and adequately powered randomized controlled trials are necessary to define the optimal management of hyperglycemia and consequent clinical benefits in patients receiving nutrition support.

Author Contributions: Conceptualization and methodology, L.B.; design and conduction of the search: C.I.L. and L.B.; writing—original draft preparation; C.I.L. and L.B.; writing—reviewing and editing: C.I.L., P.C., E.R., Z.S., T.M. and L.B; supervision: L.B.

Acknowledgments: We would like to thank Heidrun Janka for her help in improving the search strategies and Kai Holtmann for his help in improving the design of the figures.

References

1. Pasquel, F.J.; Spiegelman, R.; McCauley, M.; Smiley, D.; Umpierrez, D.; Johnson, R.; Rhee, M.; Gatcliffe, C.; Lin, E.; Umpierrez, E.; et al. Hyperglycemia during total parenteral nutrition: An important marker of poor outcome and mortality in hospitalized patients. *Diabetes Care* **2010**, *33*, 739–741. [CrossRef] [PubMed]
2. Davidson, P.; Kwiatkowski, C.A.; Wien, M. Management of Hyperglycemia and Enteral Nutrition in the Hospitalized Patient. *Nutr. Clin. Pract.* **2015**, *30*, 652–659. [CrossRef] [PubMed]
3. Pleva, M.; Mirtallo, J.M.; Steinberg, S.M. Hyperglycemic events in non-intensive care unit patients receiving parenteral nutrition. *Nutr. Clin. Pract.* **2009**, *24*, 626–634. [CrossRef] [PubMed]
4. Pancorbo-Hidalgo, P.L.; Garcia-Fernandez, F.P.; Ramirez-Perez, C. Complications associated with enteral nutrition by nasogastric tube in an internal medicine unit. *J. Clin. Nurs.* **2001**, *10*, 482–490. [CrossRef] [PubMed]
5. McCowen, K.C.; Malhotra, A.; Bistrian, B.R. Stress-Induced Hyperglycemia. *J. Clin. Nurs.* **2001**, *17*, 107–124. [CrossRef]
6. Herrmann, C.; Göke, R.; Richter, G.; Fehmann, H.C.; Arnold, R.; Göke, B. Glucagon-Like Peptide-1 and Glucose-Dependent Insulin-Releasing Polypeptide Plasma Levels in Response to Nutrients. *Digestion* **1995**, *56*, 117–126. [CrossRef] [PubMed]
7. Andrews, R.C.; Walker, B.R. Glucocorticoids and insulin resistance: Old hormones, new targets. *Clin. Sci.* **1999**, *96*, 513–523. [CrossRef] [PubMed]

8. Marathe, C.S.; Rayner, C.K.; Bound, M.; Checklin, H.; Standfield, S.; Wishart, J.; Lange, K.; Jones, K.L.; Horowitz, M. Small intestinal glucose exposure determines the magnitude of the incretin effect in health and type 2 diabetes. *Diabetes* **2014**, *63*, 2668–2675. [CrossRef] [PubMed]
9. Olveira, G.; Tapia, M.J.; Ocón, J.; Cabrejas-Gómez, C.; Ballesteros-Pomar, M.D.; Vidal-Casariego, A.; Arraiza-Irigoyen, C.; Olivares, J.; Conde-García, M.e.C.; García-Manzanares, A.; et al. Parenteral nutrition-associated hyperglycemia in non-critically ill inpatients increases the risk of in-hospital mortality (multicenter study). *Diabetes Care* **2013**, *36*, 1061–1066. [CrossRef] [PubMed]
10. Lin, L.Y.; Lin, H.C.; Lee, P.C.; Ma, W.Y.; Lin, H.D. Hyperglycemia correlates with outcomes in patients receiving total parenteral nutrition. *Am. J. Med Sci.* **2007**, *333*, 261–265. [CrossRef] [PubMed]
11. Cheung, N.W.; Napier, B.; Zaccaria, C.; Fletcher, J.P. Hyperglycemia is associated with adverse outcomes in patients receiving total parenteral nutrition. *Diabetes Care* **2005**, *28*, 2367–2371. [CrossRef] [PubMed]
12. Yuan, J.; Liu, T.; Zhang, X.; Si, Y.; Ye, Y.; Zhao, C.; Wang, Q.; Shen, X. Intensive Versus Conventional Glycemic Control in Patients with Diabetes During Enteral Nutrition After Gastrectomy. *J. Gastrointest. Surg.* **2015**, *19*, 1553–1558. [CrossRef] [PubMed]
13. Murad, M.H.; Coburn, J.A.; Coto-Yglesias, F.; Dzyubak, S.; Hazem, A.; Lane, M.A.; Prokop, L.J.; Montori, V.M. Glycemic Control in Non-Critically Ill Hospitalized Patients: A Systematic Review and Meta-Analysis. *J. Clin. Endocrinol. Metab.* **2012**, *97*, 49–58. [CrossRef] [PubMed]
14. Kang, Z.-Q.; Huo, J.-L.; Zhai, X.-J. Effects of perioperative tight glycemic control on postoperative outcomes: A meta-analysis. *Endocr. Connect.* **2018**, *7*, R316–R327. [CrossRef] [PubMed]
15. Umpierrez, G.E.; Smiley, D.; Zisman, A.; Prieto, L.M.; Palacio, A.; Ceron, M.; Puig, A.; Mejia, R. Randomized Study of Basal-Bolus Insulin Therapy in the Inpatient Management of Patients with Type 2 Diabetes (RABBIT 2 Trial). *Diabetes Care* **2007**, *30*, 2181. [CrossRef] [PubMed]
16. Turchin, A.; Matheny, M.E.; Shubina, M.; Scanlon, J.V.; Greenwood, B.; Pendergrass, M.L. Hypoglycemia and clinical outcomes in patients with diabetes hospitalized in the general ward. *Diabetes Care* **2009**, *32*, 1153–1157. [CrossRef]
17. Finfer, S.; Chittock, D.R.; Su, S.Y.; Blair, D.; Foster, D.; Dhingra, V.; Bellomo, R.; Cook, D.; Dodek, P.; Henderson, W.R.; et al. Intensive versus Conventional Glucose Control in Critically Ill Patients. *N. Engl. J. Med.* **2009**, *360*, 1283–1297. [CrossRef] [PubMed]
18. Association, A.D. 15. Diabetes Care in the Hospital. *Diabetes Care* **2019**, *42*, S173–S181. [CrossRef] [PubMed]
19. Umpierrez, G.E.; Hellman, R.; Korytkowski, M.T.; Kosiborod, M.; Maynard, G.A.; Montori, V.M.; Seley, J.J.; Van den Berghe, G.; Society, E. Management of hyperglycemia in hospitalized patients in non-critical care setting: An endocrine society clinical practice guideline. *J. Clin. Endocrinol. Metab.* **2012**, *97*, 16–38. [CrossRef] [PubMed]
20. McCulloch, A.; Bansiya, V.; Woodward, J.M. Addition of Insulin to Parenteral Nutrition for Control of Hyperglycemia. *JPEN* **2018**, *42*, 846–854. [CrossRef] [PubMed]
21. Aragon, D. Evaluation of nursing work effort and perceptions about blood glucose testing in tight glycemic control. *Am. J. Crit. Care* **2006**, *15*, 370–377. [PubMed]
22. Elia, M.; Ceriello, A.; Laube, H.; Sinclair, A.J.; Engfer, M.; Stratton, R.J. Enteral nutritional support and use of diabetes-specific formulas for patients with diabetes: A systematic review and meta-analysis. *Diabetes Care* **2005**, *28*, 2267–2279. [CrossRef] [PubMed]
23. Ojo, O.; Brooke, J. Evaluation of the role of enteral nutrition in managing patients with diabetes: A systematic review. *Nutrients* **2014**, *6*, 5142–5152. [CrossRef] [PubMed]
24. Rodbard, D. Continuous Glucose Monitoring: A Review of Recent Studies Demonstrating Improved Glycemic Outcomes. *Diabetes Technol. Ther.* **2017**, *19*, S25–S37. [CrossRef] [PubMed]
25. Pickup, J.C. Insulin-pump therapy for type 1 diabetes mellitus. *N. Engl J. Med.* **2012**, *366*, 1616–1624. [CrossRef] [PubMed]
26. Bally, L.; Thabit, H.; Hovorka, R. Closed-loop for type 1 diabetes—an introduction and appraisal for the generalist. *BMC Med.* **2017**, *15*, 14. [CrossRef] [PubMed]
27. Bally, L.; Thabit, H.; Hovorka, R. Glucose-responsive insulin delivery for type 1 diabetes: The artificial pancreas story. *Int. J. Pharm.* **2017**. [CrossRef] [PubMed]
28. Moher, D.; Liberati, A.; Tetzlaff, J.; Altman, D.G.; Group, P. Preferred reporting items for systematic reviews and meta-analyses: The PRISMA statement. *Int. J. Surg.* **2010**, *8*, 336–341. [CrossRef] [PubMed]

29. Stroup, D.F.; Berlin, J.A.; Morton, S.C.; Olkin, I.; Williamson, G.D.; Rennie, D.; Moher, D.; Becker, B.J.; Sipe, T.A.; Thacker, S.B.; et al. Meta-analysis of Observational Studies in EpidemiologyA Proposal for Reporting. *JAMA* **2000**, *283*, 2008–2012. [CrossRef]
30. Higgins, J.P.T.; Altman, D.G.; Gøtzsche, P.C.; Jüni, P.; Moher, D.; Oxman, A.D.; Savović, J.; Schulz, K.F.; Weeks, L.; Sterne, J.A.C. The Cochrane Collaboration's tool for assessing risk of bias in randomized trials. *BMJ* **2011**, *343*, d5928. [CrossRef]
31. Boughton, C.K.; Bally, L.; Martignoni, F.; Hartnell, S.; Herzig, D.; Vogt, A.; Wertli, M.M.; Wilinska, M.E.; Evans, M.L.; Coll, A.P.; et al. Fully closed-loop insulin delivery in inpatients receiving nutritional support: A two-center, open-label, randomized controlled trial. *Lancet Diabetes Endocri.* **2019**, *7*, 368–377. [CrossRef]
32. Olveira, G.; Abuin, J.; Lopez, R.; Herranz, S.; Garcia-Almeida, J.M.; Garcia-Malpartida, K.; Ferrer, M.; Cancer, E.; Luengo-Perez, L.M.; Alvarez, J.; et al. Regular insulin added to total parenteral nutrition vs. subcutaneous glargine in non-critically ill diabetic inpatients, a multicenter randomized clinical trial: INSUPAR trial. *Clin. Nutr.* **2019**. [CrossRef] [PubMed]
33. Hakeam, H.A.; Mulia, H.A.; Azzam, A.; Amin, T. Glargine Insulin Use Versus Continuous Regular Insulin in Diabetic Surgical Noncritically Ill Patients Receiving Parenteral Nutrition: Randomized Controlled Study. *JPEN* **2017**, *41*, 1110–1118. [CrossRef] [PubMed]
34. Lidder, P.; Flanagan, D.; Fleming, S.; Russell, M.; Morgan, N.; Wheatley, T.; Rahamin, J.; Shaw, S.; Lewis, S. Combining enteral with parenteral nutrition to improve postoperative glucose control. *Br. J. Nutr.* **2010**, *103*, 1635–1641. [CrossRef] [PubMed]
35. Tiyapanjanit, T.; Boonyavarakul, A. Comparative study between the Phramongkutklao's diabetic blenderized diets and commercial diabetic diets on glycemic variability in continuous tube fed patients with type 2 diabetes. *J. Med. Assoc. Thai.* **2014**, *97*, 1151–1156. [PubMed]
36. Leon-Sanz, M.; Garcia-Luna, P.P.; Sanz-Paris, A.; Gomez-Candela, C.; Casimiro, C.; Chamorro, J.; Pereira-Cunill, J.L.; Martin-Palmero, A.; Trallero, R.; Martinez, J.; et al. Glycemic and lipid control in hospitalized type 2 diabetic patients: Evaluation of 2 enteral nutrition formulas (low carbohydrate-high monounsaturated fat vs. high carbohydrate). *JPEN* **2005**, *29*, 21–29. [CrossRef]
37. Hyperglycemia in Patients with Stroke and Indication of Enteral Nutrition. Available online: https://ClinicalTrials.gov/show/NCT03422900 (accessed on 20 May 2019).
38. Li, F.F.; Zhang, W.L.; Liu, B.L.; Zhang, D.F.; Chen, W.; Yuan, L.; Chen, M.Y.; Zhai, X.F.; Wu, J.D.; Su, X.F.; et al. Management of glycemic variation in diabetic patients receiving parenteral nutrition by continuous subcutaneous insulin infusion (CSII) therapy. *Sci. Rep.* **2018**, *8*, 5888. [CrossRef]
39. Kruyt, N.D.; Biessels, G.J.; Vriesendorp, T.M.; Devries, J.H.; Hoekstra, J.B.; Elbers, P.W.; Kappelle, L.J.; Portegies, P.; Vermeulen, M.; Roos, Y.B. Subjecting acute ischemic stroke patients to continuous tube feeding and an intensive computerized protocol establishes tight glycemic control. *Neurocrit. Care* **2010**, *12*, 62–68. [CrossRef]
40. Korytkowski, M.T.; Salata, R.J.; Koerbel, G.L.; Selzer, F.; Karslioglu, E.; Idriss, A.M.; Lee, K.K.; Moser, A.J.; Toledo, F.G. Insulin therapy and glycemic control in hospitalized patients with diabetes during enteral nutrition therapy: A randomized controlled clinical trial. *Diabetes Care* **2009**, *32*, 594–596. [CrossRef]
41. Valero, M.A.; Leon-Sanz, M.; Escobar, I.; Gomis, P.; de la Camara, A.; Moreno, J.M. Evaluation of nonglucose carbohydrates in parenteral nutrition for diabetic patients. *Eur. J. Clin. Nutr.* **2001**, *55*, 1111–1116. [CrossRef]
42. Truong, S.; Park, A.; Kamalay, S.; Hung, N.; Meyer, J.G.; Nguyen, N.; Momenzadeh, A. Glycemic Control in Adult Surgical Patients Receiving Regular Insulin Added to Parenteral Nutrition vs. Insulin Glargine: A Retrospective Chart Review. *Nutr. Clin. Pract.* **2019**. [CrossRef] [PubMed]
43. Hijaze, D.; Szalat, A. Retrospective Evaluation of Glycemic Control with Basal-Bolus or Neutral Protamine Hagedorn Insulin Regimens in Patients Receiving Continuous Enteral Nutrition Therapy in Medicine Wards. *Nutr. Clin. Pract.* **2017**, *32*, 557–562. [CrossRef] [PubMed]
44. Neff, K.; Donegan, D.; MacMahon, J.; O'Hanlon, C.; Keane, N.; Agha, A.; Thompson, C.; Smith, D. Management of parenteral nutrition associated hyperglycemia: A comparison of subcutaneous and intravenous insulin regimen. *Ir. Med. J.* **2014**, *107*, 141–143. [PubMed]
45. Hsia, E.; Seggelke, S.A.; Gibbs, J.; Rasouli, N.; Draznin, B. Comparison of 70/30 biphasic insulin with glargine/lispro regimen in non-critically ill diabetic patients on continuous enteral nutrition therapy. *Nutr. Clin. Pract.* **2011**, *26*, 714–717. [CrossRef] [PubMed]

46. Dardai, E. Basics in clinical nutrition: Nutritional support in the diabetic patient. *e-SPEN* **2009**, *4*, e304–e307. [CrossRef]
47. Woods, H.F.; Alberti, K.G. Dangers of intravenous fructose. *Lancet* **1972**, *2*, 1354–1357. [CrossRef]
48. Thomas, D.W.; Edwards, J.B.; Gilligan, J.E.; Lawrence, J.R.; Edwards, R.G. Complications following intravenous administration of solutions containing xylitol. *Med. J. Aust.* **1972**, *1*, 1238–1246.
49. Thomas, D.W.; Gilligan, J.E.; Edwards, J.B.; Edwards, R.G. Lactic acidosis and osmotic diuresis produced by xylitol infusion. *Med. J. Aust.* **1972**, *1*, 1246–1248.
50. Keller, U. The sugar substitutes fructose and sorbite: An unnecessary risk in parenteral nutrition. *Schweiz Med. Wochenschr.* **1989**, *119*, 101–106.
51. Tappy, L.; Schwarz, J.M.; Schneiter, P.; Cayeux, C.; Revelly, J.P.; Fagerquist, C.K.; Jequier, E.; Chiolero, R. Effects of isoenergetic glucose-based or lipid-based parenteral nutrition on glucose metabolism, de novo lipogenesis, and respiratory gas exchanges in critically ill patients. *Crit. Care Med.* **1998**, *26*, 860–867. [CrossRef]
52. Ahrens, C.L.; Barletta, J.F.; Kanji, S.; Tyburski, J.G.; Wilson, R.F.; Janisse, J.J.; Devlin, J.W. Effect of low-calorie parenteral nutrition on the incidence and severity of hyperglycemia in surgical patients: A randomized, controlled trial. *Crit. Care Med.* **2005**, *33*, 2507–2512. [CrossRef] [PubMed]
53. Lee, H.; Koh, S.O.; Park, M.S. Higher dextrose delivery via TPN related to the development of hyperglycemia in non-diabetic critically ill patients. *Nutr. Res. Pract.* **2011**, *5*, 450–454. [CrossRef] [PubMed]
54. Forchielli, M.L.; Bongiovanni, F.; Platé, L.; Piazza, G.; Puggioli, C.; D'Alise, A.; Bersani, G. Insulin Instability in Parenteral Nutrition Admixtures. *JPEN* **2018**, *42*, 907–912. [CrossRef] [PubMed]
55. Mühlebach, S.; Franken, C.; Stanga, Z.; Working group for developing the guidelines for parenteral nutrition of The German Association for Nutritional Medicine. Practical handling of AIO admixtures-Guidelines on Parenteral Nutrition, Chapter 10. *Ger. Med. Sci.* **2009**, *7*, Doc18. [CrossRef]
56. Pasquel, F.J.; Gianchandani, R.; Rubin, D.J.; Dungan, K.M.; Anzola, I.; Gomez, P.C.; Peng, L.; Hodish, I.; Bodnar, T.; Wesorick, D.; et al. Efficacy of sitagliptin for the hospital management of general medicine and surgery patients with type 2 diabetes (Sita-Hospital): A multicentre, prospective, open-label, non-inferiority randomized trial. *Lancet Diabetes Endocrinol* **2017**, *5*, 125–133. [CrossRef]

16

Hospital Malnutrition, a Call for Political Action: A Public Health and Nutrition Day Perspective

Michael Hiesmayr [1,*], Silvia Tarantino [1], Sigrid Moick [1], Alessandro Laviano [5], Isabella Sulz [2], Mohamed Mouhieddine [1], Christian Schuh [2], Dorothee Volkert [6], Judit Simon [3] and Karin Schindler [4]

1. Division Cardio-thoracic and Vascular Anesthesia and Intensive Care, Medical University Vienna, 1090 Vienna, Austria; silvia.tarantino@meduniwien.ac.at (S.T.); sigrid.moick@gmail.com (S.M.); mohamed.mouhieddine@meduniwien.ac.at (M.M.)
2. Center for Medical Statistics, Informatics and Intelligent Systems, Medical University Vienna, 1090 Vienna, Austria; isabella.sulz@meduniwien.ac.at (I.S.); christian.schuh@meduniwien.ac.at (C.S.)
3. Department of Health Economics, Center for Public Health, Medical University Vienna, 1090 Vienna, Austria; judit.simon@meduniwien.ac.at
4. Department of Internal Medicine III, Medical University Vienna, 1090 Vienna, Austria; karin.schindler@meduniwien.ac.at
5. Department of Translational and Precision Medicine, Università degli Studi di Roma "La Sapienza", 00185 Roma, Italy; alessandro.laviano@uniroma1.it
6. Institute for Biomedicine of Ageing, Friedrich-Alexander Universität Erlangen-Nürnberg, 90408 Nürnberg, Germany; dorothee.volkert@fau.de

* Correspondence: michael.hiesmayr@meduniwien.ac.at

Abstract: Disease-related malnutrition (DRM) is prevalent in hospitals and is associated with increased care needs, prolonged hospital stay, delayed rehabilitation and death. Nutrition care process related activities such as screening, assessment and treatment has been advocated by scientific societies and patient organizations but implementation is variable. We analysed the cross-sectional nutritionDay database for prevalence of nutrition risk factors, care processes and outcome for medical, surgical, long-term care and other patients (n = 153,470). In 59,126 medical patients included between 2006 and 2015 the prevalence of recent weight loss (45%), history of decreased eating (48%) and low actual eating (53%) was more prevalent than low BMI (8%). Each of these risk factors was associated with a large increase in 30 days hospital mortality. A similar pattern is found in all four patient groups. Nutrition care processes increase slightly with the presence of risk factors but are never done in more than 50% of the patients. Only a third of patients not eating in hospital receive oral nutritional supplements or artificial nutrition. We suggest that political action should be taken to raise awareness and formal education on all aspects related to DRM for all stakeholders, to create and support responsibilities within hospitals, and to create adequate reimbursement schemes. Collection of routine and benchmarking data is crucial to tackle DRM.

Keywords: malnutrition; hospital; nutrition care; continuity of care; mortality; process indicators; benchmarking; disease related malnutrition.

---

1. Introduction

Disease-related malnutrition (DRM) is highly prevalent in hospitalized patients and associated with complications and poor outcome [1–3]. Malnutrition in hospitals originates from imbalances, either deficiencies or excesses, in nutrients intake compared with body needs. Nutritional status and needs may be modified acutely or chronically by the disease process itself. Further deterioration may occur due to hospitalization, thus making the population of hospitalized patients very different from the general population. Prolonged nutrients imbalance is associated with change in body mass index (BMI). Association between body mass index (BMI) and mortality is U-shaped in the general population and J-shaped in patients, especially with chronic diseases, meaning that mortality is higher if BMI is low and lower in patients with increased lean body mass and even obesity [4,5]. This observation called "obesity paradox" underscores the importance of a "good" nutrition status for patients with illnesses for short and long-term outcomes.

Malnutrition in hospitalized patients often addresses an evident poor nutritional status (low BMI and low muscle mass) whereas being at risk of malnutrition is derived from a set of risk factors typically associated with a loss in lean body mass persisting over a certain period of time [6]. Nutrition care in hospitals is a treatment for patients with malnutrition and a preventive intervention for patients at risk of malnutrition. Nevertheless, nutrition care is still an underrated field when compared to medical diagnostics procedures, or pharmacological and technological interventions in hospitals.

There are several reasons why nutrition care has received so little attention in acute care hospitals. There is a common knowledge deficit reflected in a lack of proper education in university curricula for healthcare professionals (doctors, nurses, care assistants) combined with patients and relatives giving low value to nutrition as part of a successful therapy of the primary disease. Since no immediate effects of nutrition can be expected during a short hospital length of stay, the attention for nutrition related issues is often low. Standard nutrition care processes such as screening, assessment, planning and monitoring together with documentation and continuity of care are not regular parts of care on all hospital wards [7]. Moreover, food provision and related tasks are not considered part of healthcare responsibilities. Food provision is not part of the medical budget but usually of the administrative budget of a hospital where cost reduction is not considered to influence directly patient care. Inadequate management of food provision might affect food quality, presentation [8] and composition and, subsequently, patient care. Food costs are to be added to the overall malnutrition related costs. Patients with malnutrition usually stay longer in hospitals, are more often re-hospitalized or transferred to long-term care [9–12]. Each of these, together with the reimbursement schemes, do create additional costs for the healthcare system. Insights on improved hospital nutrition care processes and reduced healthcare costs come from the Swiss EFFORT study.

In patients with risk of malnutrition, nutrition intake was improved with enriched meals or oral nutritional supplements, food intake was monitored and was associated with better outcomes and reduced healthcare costs [11].

These multiple barriers and the lack of proper attention to DRM and nutrition care in hospitals has been formally addressed at a political level by a resolution of the European Council in 2003 but was not followed by national regulatory actions [3].This lack of action led to several independent initiatives. The European Society for Clinical Nutrition and Metabolism (ESPEN) (www.espen.org) together with the Medical University of Vienna developed a tailored action to tackle malnutrition in hospitals and healthcare institutions [4]. The resulting project "nutritionDay" aimed to generate more awareness on DRM with a yearly one-day data collection on patient's malnutrition risk factors, outcomes and quality indicators of nutrition care (www.nutritionday.org). In the nutritionDay analysis, several nutrition related risk factors, such as low BMI, recent weight loss and reduced food intake (in the week before nutritionDay or on nutritionDay itself), were found to be independently associated with death within 30 days in hospital [4]. In an another analysis that led to the development of the PANDORA score for prediction of death in hospital within 30 days after nutritionDay, decreased food intake was identified among the seven most important risk factors as it contributed 3–12 points out of a maximum of 75 points to the final score [5]. nutritionDay rapidly became a worldwide benchmarking tool for monitoring and improving nutrition care in hospital wards [13–15]. Patient related risk factors for decreased eating have a similar pattern in all world regions [16] and nutrition care processes implementation appears highly variable [7].

A multi-stakeholder initiative to promote screening for risk of disease-related malnutrition/undernutrition and implement nutritional care across Europe "Optimal Nutritional Care for All" has started an annual meeting with national nutrition societies and political representatives in 2008 [17]. The last meeting in Sintra, Portugal in 2018 involved representatives from 18 countries that had already joined the initiative and had the motto: "Optimal Nutrition Care across Europe: Fair Access and Shared Decision Making". The decision was taken together with the European Patient Forum [18] to translate relevant guidelines into a lay version to increase the possibility for patients to take informed responsibility [19].

The human right for proper nutrition care was acknowledged in the Cartagena declaration [20] and signed on 3rd May 2019 by all presidents of the Latin American Federation of Nutritional Therapy, Clinical Nutrition (FELANPE). The declaration includes 13 principles, such as patient empowerment, dignity, ethical principles, justice and equity and urges the United Nations and the Human Rights Council to recognize the Right to Nutrition Care as a human right in line with the "Sustainable Development Goals" [21].

The worldwide Global Leadership Initiative on Malnutrition (GLIM) composed by the major nutrition societies aims at defining universally accepted criteria for DRM [22]. This process is still ongoing with planned steps of validation and regular updating. Current recommendations from scientific societies emphasize that it is mandatory to identify the malnourished as well as those at risk early during hospitalization to trigger proper treatment or a set of preventive measures [19]. The recommended three step process consists of screening, assessing and developing a nutrition care plan. A further important and less appreciated step is that nutrition care needs to be monitored and adapted to the patient's changing condition. Finally, proper documentation and communication of a comprehensive care plan to the next sector, "extramural health care", and the patients themselves are essential to ensure continuity of care. To be efficient, responsibilities need to be cleared delineated and all relevant stakeholder (Table 1) involved.

Table 1. List and role of important stakeholders.

1. Within the hospital	
a. Patients and their relatives	
b. Care persons	
i. Nurses	Screening, diet ordering, documentation
ii. Physicians	Assessment, ordering, documentation, information
iii. Dieticians	Assessment, documentation
iv. Physiotherapists	Effect monitoring
v. Speech Therapists	Swallowing disorders
vi. Pharmacists	Clinical nutrition supply and counselling
c. Kitchen/Catering services	
i. Administrators	Budget
ii. Chefs	Standards, variety, quality control
iii. Kitchen aids	Presentation
iv. Delivering staff	Monitoring
d. Hospital administration	Budget, planning, controlling
2. Outside the hospital	
a. Patients and relatives	
b. Extramural medical services/family medicine/primary health care centres	
c. Extramural care services/mobile nursing	
d. Services for disabled and dependent persons	
e. Local food producers	
f. Medical food producing industries	

Table 1. *Cont.*

3. Scientific societies and stakeholder associations	
a. Medical	Guidelines, standards
b. Nursing	Guidelines, standards
c. Dietician	Guidelines, standards
d. Nutrition science	Research, standards
e. Patient organizations	Guidelines
4. Policy maker	
a. Health care system	Reimbursement
b. Social affairs	Equity
c. Agriculture	Local production integration
d. Environmental affairs	Sustainable planning, waste prevention
5. Payers	
a. Reimbursement of the nutrition care process in the whole health care system	
b. Public procurement of food supply and services	

This study aims to determine in the medical patients of the nutritionDay database 2006–2018, first, the prevalence of simple nutrition related risk factors and their association with outcome and, second, to determine the routine use of recommended nutrition care procedures such as screening, nutrition intake monitoring and documentation in patients with and without risk factors.

Based on the findings we will propose several options for political action to tackle malnutrition in hospitals.

2. Experimental Section

The nutritionDay audit is a cross-sectional international data collection in hospitalized patients with 30 days in hospital outcome assessment. The nutritionDay project was approved by the Ethical Committee of the Medical University of Vienna (EK407/2005) and it has been amended annually. In accordance with national regulations, the project was also submitted to national or local ethical committees in each participating country. This trial was registered at clinicaltrials.gov as NCT02820246. We analysed the complete nutritionDay database 2006–2015 for the association between nutrition related risk factors and 30 days hospital mortality. We assessed the 2016–2018 nutritionDay database for nutrition care process indicators newly introduced in 2016.

We included all adult patients with the exception of women before or after giving birth. Patients were divided into four groups: group surgical (patients admitted to a surgical unit or waiting for surgery or after surgery on any medical/other ward), group medical (all patients admitted to general medical, cardio, gastro, hepatology, nephrology, infectiology or oncology), group long-term (geriatric or long-term care wards) and others (all other specialties such as ear-nose-throat, gynecology, obstetrics, trauma, orthopedics, etc.). Risk factors were age, gender, BMI, weight change in the last three months, decreased eating during the previous week and on nutritionDay, fluid status (as intravascular or tissue fluid overload or depletion as observed by a clinician), reduced mobility and whether patients have been admitted to an intensive care unit at any time before nutritionDay during this index admission. In addition we included in the multivariate analysis the diagnostic categories derived from the 17 ICD 10 top categories (brain and nerves, eye and ear, nose and throat, heart and circulation, lung, liver, gastrointestinal tract, kidney/urinary tract/female genital tract, endocrine system, skeleton/bone/muscle, blood/bone marrow, skin, ischemia, cancer, infection, pregnancy, others) and six comorbidities (diabetes, stroke, COPD, myocardial infarction, cardiac failure and others), each one used as a unique variable as condition being present versus not present. All factors were used as categorical variables and included a missing category according to the STROBE guidelines [23]. Reference categories were either the "normal" category or the group including the median or the largest subgroup as appropriate. Age was divided into eight groups spanning 10 years with 60–70 years as reference; BMI was divided into 6 WHO groups with normal BMI 18.5–25 used as a reference [24].

Sensitivity analysis included only patients from units fulfilling quality criteria, such as >60% recruitment of admitted patients and outcome reporting for >80% of included patients. In addition a second sensitivity analysis was done for the multivariate modelling of the association between risk indicators and outcome after exclusion of all cases with missing values. The sensitivity study population includes 82,993 patients compared with 153,470 in the full study population.

Descriptive statistics report frequencies and median with interquartile range. Comparison of proportions were done with the χ^2 test and corrected for multiple testing. All associations between mortality and risk factors were done with logistic regression based on general linear models with units as clusters and weighting of patients to compensate for time-based bias from cross-sectional data acquisition [25]. In short, patients with a longer observed length of stay had less weight because they were more likely to be included in the study sample than short stay patients. We used univariate analysis for all risk factors and included all significant factors in the multivariate analysis. The effect of risk factors was also analysed within all four patient groups separately in the multivariate model (STATA 15.1, Statacorp, College Station, TX, USA). To show the extent of use of selected nutrition care processes, they are shown as percentages within different risk categories. Significant differences to each reference group were tested with a proportions test, comparisons were considered significant when $p < 0.005$ as we accounted for multiple tests for each reference category.

3. Results

Medical patients in the nutritionDay database (n = 59,126/153,470) (39%) represent the second largest group after surgical patients (n = 63,289/153,470) (41%). Patients were admitted in 61 countries and 19 countries recruited more than 1000 patients.

Medical patients were four years older than surgical patients (65.2 years SD 17.2 versus 61.2 years SD 18.0). The proportion of female was 48.3 in medical and 48.1 in surgical patients. Weight (71.3 kg SD 19.4 versus 71.9 kg SD 18.1) and height (166.1 cm SD 10.3 versus 166.5 cm SD 10.2) were similar in both groups. BMI was nearly identical (25.7 SD 6.3 versus 25.8 SD 5.8) ($p = 0.02$). Based on WHO categories (www.who.int) both groups have a similar proportion of obese with BMI > 30 (17.7% versus 17.4%) but the proportion with low BMI < 18.5 was significantly higher in medical than in surgical patients (7.5% versus 6%) ($p < 0.0001$).

3.1. *Prevalence of Nutrition Risk Factors*

Nutrition risk factors such as weight loss during the last three months (26,790, 45%), not eating normally in the previous week (28,950, 49%) and did not eat all food served on nutritionDay (30,965, 52%) were highly prevalent in the medical patients of the cohort 2006–2015 (Figure 1) and in the three other patient groups (Table 2).

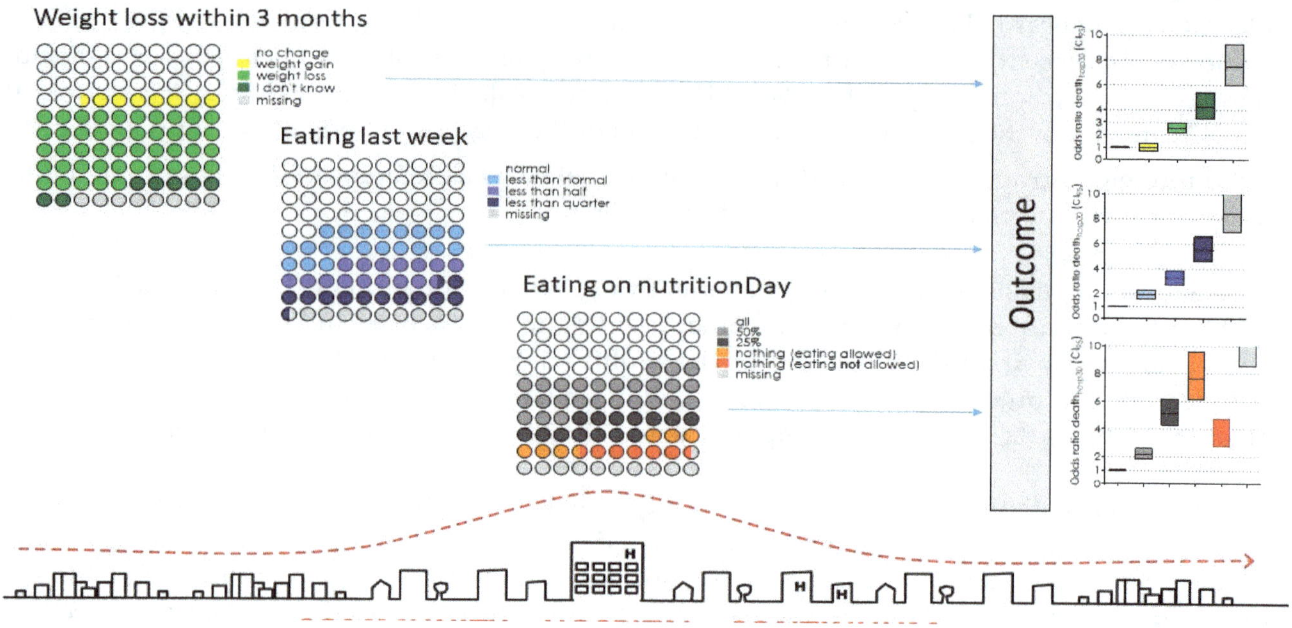

Figure 1. Prevalence of risk factors and association with odds ratio for death in hospital within 30 days after nutritionDay in medical patients. Prevalence is indicated by dots. Each dot represents 1% of the total population. All risk indicators are collected on one single day, the nutritionDay 2006–2015. Odds ratio are indicated with 95% confidence intervals and colours according to risk indicator categories Graph of Community–Hospital–Continuum from Magdalena Maierhofer's architectural diploma thesis: A Hospital is not a Tree (2016).

Table 2. Demographic characteristics and prevalence of nutrition risk factors of patients in the nutritionDay cohort 2006–2015, in the four studied groups.

	Medical		Surgical		Long-Term Care		Others	
Characteristics	***n* (%)**	**Mean ± SD**	***n* (%)**	**Mean ± SD**	***n* (%)**	**Mean ± SD**	***n* (%)**	**Mean ± SD**
Age (year)	59,046	65.1 ± 17.2		61.2 ± 18.0		80.7 ± 12.4		61.2 ± 18.8
Gender (female)	28,535 (49%)		30,445 (49%)		6937 (62%)		9992 (51%)	
Weight (kg)	52,735 (89%)	71.3 ± 19.4		71.9 ± 18.1		66.4 ± 16.9		71.8 ± 18.3
Height (cm)	52,735	166.1 ± 10.3		166.6 ± 10.2		163.0 ± 9.5		166.7 ± 10.4
BMI * (kg·cm^{-2})	52,735	25.7 ± 6.3		25.8 ± 5.8		24.9 ± 5.8		25.7 ± 5.9
Weight change within three months								
Unchanged *	19,139 (32%)		25,164 (40%)		3153 (28%)		7338 (37%)	
Increase	4335 (7.3%)		4997 (8%)		671 (6%)		1990 (10%)	
Loss	26,790 (45%)		24,928 (39%)		4989 (44%)		7356 (37%)	
Do not know	4020 (6.8%)		3679 (6%)		1339 (12%)		1205 (6%)	
Missing	4842 (8.2%)		4521 (7%)		1127 (10%)		1887 (10%)	
Eating last week								
Normal *	24,679 (42%)		29,898 (47%)		4731 (42%)		9973 (50%)	
Less than normal	12,613 (21%)		12,618 (20%)		2526 (22%)		4047 (20%)	
Less than a half	8979 (15%)		7894 (12%)		1628 (14%)		2262 (11%)	
Less than a quarter	7358 (12%)		7691 (12%)		1076 (9%)		1433 (7%)	
Missing	5497 (9.3%)		5188 (8%)		1318 (12%)		2061 (10%)	

Table 2. *Cont.*

	Medical		Surgical		Long-Term Care		Others	
Eating on nutritionDay								
All *	22,046 (37%)		22,232 (35%)		4131 (37%)		8496 (43%)	
Half	15,327 (26%)		15,141 (24%)		3363 (30%)		5054 (26%)	
Quarter	8256 (14%)		7262 (11%)		1592 (14%)		2206 (11%)	
Nothing (eating allowed)	3696 (6.3%)		3666 (6%)		698 (6%)		927 (5%)	
Nothing (eating not allowed)	3686 (6.2%)		8717 (14%)		372 (3%)		875 (4%)	
Missing	6115 (10%)		6271 (10%)		1123 (10%)		2218 (11%)	
Mobility on nutritionDay								
Normal	35,846 (61%)		37,439 (59%)		3731 (33%)		12,227 (62%)	
With help	12,299 (21%)		14,110 (22%)		4557 (40%)		3838 (19%)	
Bedridden	5587 (9.4%)		6832 (11%)		1841 (16%)		1732 (9%)	
Missing	5394 (9.1%)		4908 (8%)		1150 (10%)		1979 (10%)	
Fluid status on nutritionDay								
Normal *	28,499 (48%)		3619 (6%)		1147 (10%)		1284 (6%)	
Overload	6214 (11%)		33,636 (53%)		5836 (51%)		1142 (58%)	
Deficit	3267 (6%)		2723 (4%)		985 (9%)		886 (4%)	
Missing	21,146 (36%)		23,311 (37%)		3311 (29%)		6178 (31%)	
Any Intensive Care Stay before nutritionDay	4143 (7.0%)		10,465 (17%)		564 (5%)		1464 (8%)	
Medical specialty								
General internal medicine	29,173 (49%)		3958 (6%)					
Oncology	11,412 (19%)		1953 (3%)					
Gastroenterology/ Hepatology	9744 (16%)		1350 (2%)					
Cardiology	5401 (9.1%)		1405 (2%)					
Nephrology	1785 (3.0%)		370 (1%)					
Infectiology	1611 (2.7%)		149 (0%)					
Neurology			592 (1%)				4442 (22%)	
Psychiatry			17 (0%)				1409 (7%)	
ENT			2195 (3%)				1272 (6%)	
General surgery			28,310 (45%)					
Cardiothorcic surgery			2013 (3%)					
Characteristics	***n* (%)**	**Mean ± SD**	***n* (%)**	**Mean ± SD**	***n* (%)**	**Mean ± SD**	***n* (%)**	**Mean ± SD**
Orthopaedic surgery			7803 (12%)					
Trauma			2160 (3%)					
Neurosurgery			1717 (3%)					
Gynecology			1198 (2%)				1151(6%)	
Long-term care			526 (1%)		9885 (88%)			
Other			5955 (9%)				11,401(58%)	
Pediatrics			46 (0%)				101 (1%)	
Geriatrics			1572 (2%)		1785 (12%)			

* indicates the reference categories.

There is some overlap between risk categories. Two third of patients (17,497/26,790) with weight loss reported not eating normal in the previous week and a similar proportion did not eat all served on nutritionDay (16,681/26,790).

Nearly 40% of patients (9551/24,679) that did eat normally in the previous week were eating less than all meal served on nutritionDay indicating a new nutrition risk associated with hospitalization.

In most patients (80%) all four nutrition risk factors, low BMI, weight loss, reduced eating during the previous week and on nutritionDay could be evaluated. 91% had no more than one risk factor missing. Only 32,216/140,418 (23%) of patients had no single nutrition related risk factor, 31% had one risk factor, 28% two risk factors and 16% had three risk factors.

3.2. Nutrition Care

3.2.1. Food provision

Oral diet, either normal hospital food or special diet, was mostly used in medical patients (Table 3). Two third of oral diets were given as hospital food and one third as special diet. Oral nutritional supplements were given to 9.3% of patients whereas enteral nutrition was used in 7.1% and parenteral nutrition in 3.5% (Table 3). Surprisingly, the use of enteral or parenteral nutrition only increased by a factor of three between patients who reported having eaten their full meal and those who had eaten nothing. Two-thirds of patients reporting eating nothing were on oral diet. The use of enteral and parenteral nutrition was not differentiating much in patients who have eaten nothing regardless of being allowed to eat or not.

Table 3. Nutrition care versus amount eaten on nutritionDay according to the patients in the four studied groups.

		Oral	ONS	EN	PN	Othercomb
Medical n = 59,126	all	19,484 (88.4%)	1651 (7.5%)	1154 (5.2%)	289 (1.3%)	794 (3.6%)
	half	13,657 (89.1%)	1560 (10.2%)	770 (5%)	311 (2%)	544 (3.5%)
	quarter	7176 (87%)	1132 (13.7%)	426 (5.2%)	354 (4.3%)	332 (4%)
	nothing_a	2760 (74.7%)	448 (12.1%)	428 (11.6%)	306 (8.3%)	278 (7.5%)
	nothing_na	2391 (65%)	226 (6.1%)	329 (8.9%)	417 (11.3%)	521 (14.1%)
	missing	3377 (55.2%)	462 (7.6%)	1083 (17.7%)	381 (6.2%)	323 (5.3%)
	Total	48,845 (82.6%)	5479 (9.3%)	4190 (7.1%)	2058 (3.5%)	2792 (4.7%)
Surgical n = 63,289	all	19,368 (87.1%)	1468 (6.6%)	1286 (5.8%)	429 (1.9%)	1184 (5.3%)
	half	13,106 (86.6%)	1294 (8.5%)	913 (6%)	506 (3.3%)	906 (6%)
	quarter	6066 (83.5%)	779 (10.7%)	472 (6.5%)	381 (5.2%)	536 (7.4%)
	nothing_a	2384 (65%)	324 (8.8%)	448 (12.2%)	415 (11.3%)	573 (15.6%)
	nothing_na	4611 (53%)	301 (3.5%)	810 (9.3%)	1535 (17.6%)	1906 (21.9%)
	missing	3596 (57.3%)	392 (6.3%)	819 (13.1%)	605 (9.6%)	689 (11%)
	Total	49,131 (77.6%)	4558 (7.2%)	4748 (7.5%)	3871 (6.1%)	5794 (9.2%)
Longterm n = 11,279	all	3480 (84.3%)	824 (19.9%)	370 (9%)	15 (0.4%)	135 (3.3%)
	half	2858 (85%)	790 (23.5%)	268 (8%)	29 (0.9%)	113 (3.4%)
	quarter	1312 (82.4%)	482 (30.3%)	130 (8.2%)	28 (1.8%)	70 (4.4%)
	nothing_a	473 (67.8%)	225 (32.2%)	111 (15.9%)	41 (5.9%)	53 (7.6%)
	nothing_na	200 (53.8%)	75 (20.2%)	85 (22.8%)	46 (12.4%)	43 (11.6%)
	missing	672 (59.8%)	177 (15.8%)	247 (22%)	36 (3.2%)	45 (4%)
	Total	8995 (79.7%)	2573 (22.8%)	1211 (10.7%)	195 (1.7%)	459 (4.1%)
Others n = 19,776	all	7435 (87.5%)	509 (6%)	672 (7.9%)	70 (0.8%)	392 (4.6%)
	half	4398 (87%)	380 (7.5%)	403 (8%)	84 (1.7%)	258 (5.1%)
	quarter	1885 (85.4%)	267 (12.1%)	147 (6.7%)	78 (3.5%)	118 (5.3%)
	nothing_a	628 (67.7%)	84 (9.1%)	160 (17.3%)	68 (7.3%)	90 (9.7%)
	nothing_na	544 (62.2%)	49 (5.6%)	100 (11.4%)	101 (11.5%)	131 (15%)
	missing	1214 (54.7%)	124 (5.6%)	355 (16%)	91 (4.1%)	128 (5.8%)
	Total	16,104 (81.4%)	1413 (7.1%)	1837 (9.3%)	492 (2.5%)	1117 (5.6%)

Percentages are indicated within each eating category. Multiple entries in the nutrition type for one patient are possible. Patients who ate nothing on nutritionDay were divided into those who did not eat even if they were allowed to (nothing_a) and those who did not eat because they were told not to eat by the doctor (nothing_na) as, for instance, before planned surgery or diagnostic tests. Combined enteral and parenteral nutrition was used in less than 2.5% of patients in any patient category and is not shown.

3.2.2. Process indicators

A total of 1415 units reported in 2016–2018 about the screening tool utilised (Figure 2). The majority, used a formal tool such as NRS-2002 (Nutrition Risk Screening 2002), MUST (Malnutrition Universal Screening Tool), MST (Malnutrition Screening Tool), or a local tool. Only 10% of the units did not have a routine screening nor fixed screening criteria. Patients identified as malnourished were overall 3340/28,100 (11.9%), with the highest proportion identified with an informal tool 722/4793 (15.1%) or NRS-2002 1169/8453 (13.8%) followed by MUST 134/1210 (11.1%), MST 269/2269 (11.9%) and visual experience 197/1666 (11.8%) whereas the proportion of identified malnourished patients was lower with no implemented routine 204/2154 (9.5%). The proportion of patients identified at nutritional risk was overall 4944/28,100 (17.6%). Of those, the highest proportion, 22.4% was identified with an unspecified tool while only 14–16% of patients were identified at risk when no routine, only visual appearance or MST was used. Only 28.9% of malnourished patients had a BMI below 18.5, 49.8% a normal BMI, 21.4% were overweight or obese. Being identified as malnourished was associated with unintentional weight loss within the last three months in 85% of patients, with reduced nutrient intake before admission in 57% of patients and with not eating a full lunch in hospital in 65% of patients. Not being identified as malnourished or at risk of malnutrition was associated with unintentional weight loss within the last three months in 47% of patients, with reduced nutrient intake before admission in 28% of patients and with not eating a full lunch in hospital in 48% of patients. The proportion of patients with two or more nutrition risk factors was 50% in the 2016–2018 cohort.

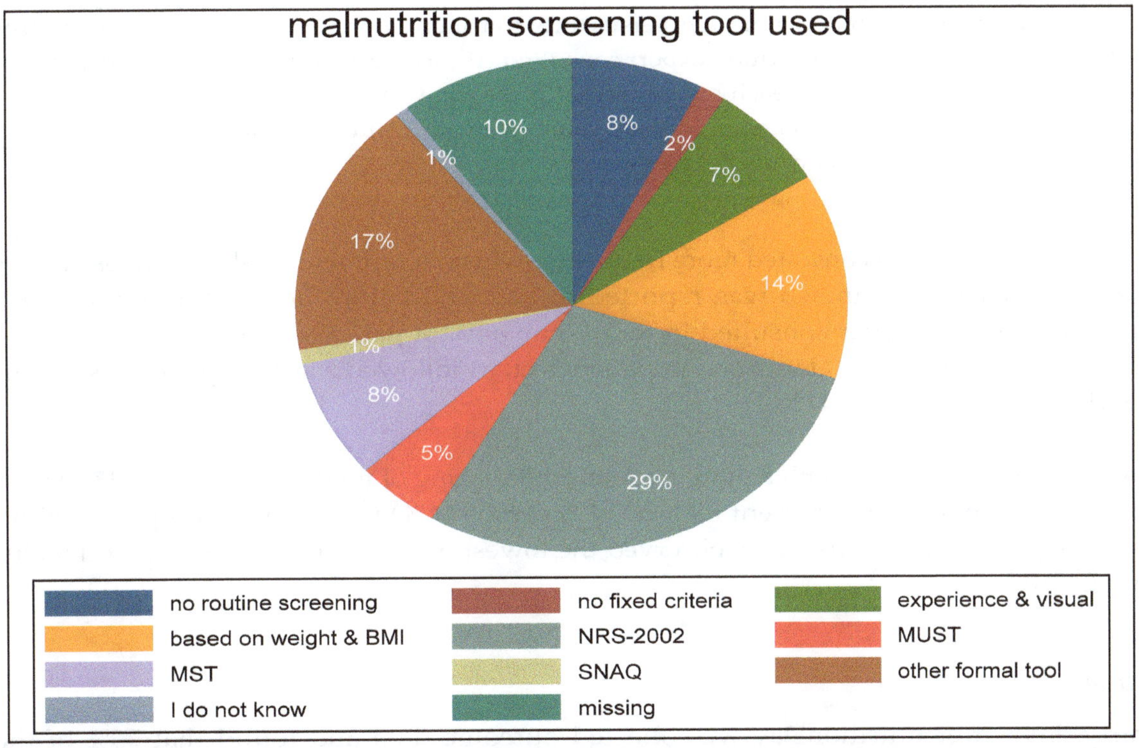

Figure 2. Proportion of different methods/approaches used for malnutrition screening in 1415 units from 46 countries in the nutritionDay cohort 2016–2018. NRS-2002 (nutrition risk screening 2002); MUST (Malnutrition Universal Screening Tool); MST (Malnutrition Screening Tool); SNAQ (Short Nutritional Assessment Questionnaire).

Nutrition intake monitoring was more frequent in patients with unintentional weight loss than in patients with stable weight (52% versus 41%) (Figure 3). Still, nearly 50% of patients with a history of weight loss did not have their nutrition intake monitored while in hospital. Similarly, history of poor nutrition intake before admission triggered more frequent monitoring compared with history of normal eating but intake was never monitored in more than 50% of patients with a history of poor nutritional intake. Actual poor food intake did not have any effect on monitoring of food intake.

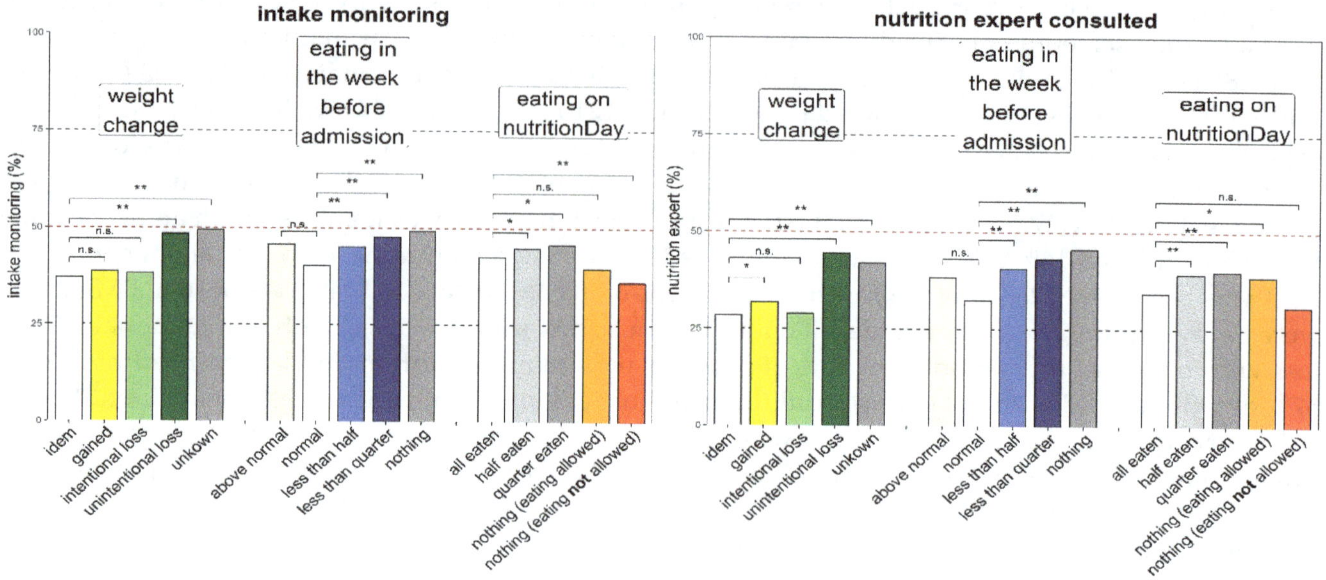

Figure 3. Nutrition care process indicators versus three nutrition associated risk factors. Daily nutrition intake monitoring (**left**) and nutrition expert consulted (**right**). Bars indicate percentage answering "yes", significant differences to each reference group are shown with * $p < 0.005$ and ** $p < 0.00001$, 'n.s.' indicates no significant difference. Missing values were <7.5% in all subcategories. Colour coding similar to Figure 1 (the empty bar is the reference).

A nutrition expert was consulted more frequently when an unintentional weight loss was reported by patients or when food intake was reported as reduced before hospital admission (Figure 3). A nutrition expert was never consulted in more than 46% of patients even when risk factors were reported. Documentation of malnutrition in patient's chart followed a similar pattern as consulting an expert and was always below 41%.

Low BMI was associated with a more frequent monitoring of intake (58% versus 47%) ($p < 0.0001$) and malnutrition reporting in patient record (52% versus 36%) ($p < 0.0001$) compared with normal BMI. In obese patients (BMI 30–35) we observed the lowest intake monitoring (40%) and malnutrition reporting (27%).

3.3. Outcome

Thirty days after nutritionDay we collected outcome data and found that 73% of the study patients had been discharged home, 11.8% had been transferred to another health care facility, hospital, long-term care or rehabilitation; 9.4% were still in the same hospital and 5.5% had died (Table 4). Similar results were observed in the sensitivity analysis. In medical patients, death was observed more than twice as frequently as in surgical patients (4.6% versus 1.7%, $p < 0.0001$) and was similar to the groups geriatrics and long-term care (4.6% versus 4.8%, $p < 0.0001$).

The group "other", which includes patients from neurology, psychiatry and non-operative patients in gynecology and ENT, has a lower mortality (2.6% versus 4.6%) ($p < 0.0001$) a lower proportion discharged home $p > 0.0001$) at day 30 after nutritionDay than medical patients (Table 4).

Table 4. Outcomes in hospital within 30 days after nutritionDay in the four patient groups.

Outcome	Surgery	Medical	Longterm	Other
in hospital	5740 (9.1%)	4639 (7.8%)	1560 (13.8%)	2303 (11.6%)
transfer other hospital	1500 (2.4%)	1343 (2.3%)	290 (2.6%)	390 (2%)
transfer longterm care	1424 (2.2%)	2109 (3.6%)	1471 (13%)	574 (2.9%)
transfer rehabilitation	1967 (3.1%)	1341 (2.3%)	441 (3.9%)	535 (2.7%)
discharge home	39,705 (62.7%)	36,439 (61.6%)	4710 (41.8%)	11,049 (55.9%)
death within 30 days	1053 (1.7%)	2721 (4.6%)	541 (4.8%)	512 (2.6%)
other destination	948 (1.5%)	1033 (1.7%)	322 (2.9%)	376 (1.9%)
missing	10,952 (17.3%)	9501 (16.1%)	1944 (17.2%)	4037 (20.4%)

Nutrition risk factors were associated with death in hospital within 30 days in a univariate analysis with odds ratios 2.6 CI 95 [2.2–3.0] for weight loss, 5.5 CI 95 [4.6–6.6] for eating less than a quarter of their meals in the previous week and 7.6 CI 95 [6.1–9.6] if eating nothing on nutritionDay despite being allowed to eat. The prevalence of individual risk categories for weight loss, decreased eating last week and on nutritionDay were associated with significantly worse outcomes (Figure 1), while increasing BMI was associated with decreasing odds ratios for death.

Other risk factors such as increasing age and male gender were also associated with poor outcome. The largest univariate association with hospital death was observed in patients with reduced mobility or those who were bedridden. Mortality within 30 days after nutritionDay increased with the number of nutrition risk factors present from 0.9% for no risk factor, 1.68% for one risk factor, 3.55% for two risk factors, 8.13% for three risk factors and 13% for four risk factors.

Multivariate Outcome Analysis

All risk factors that were significantly associated with 30 days hospital death in the univariate analysis were also significant in the multivariate analysis (Figures 4 and 5) including all affected organs and comorbidities that could be estimated. Most estimates indicated a reduced strength of the association of the individual risk factors compared with univariate analysis, which indicates confounding. In the multivariate analysis, history of decreased eating before hospital admission was associated with higher odds ratio for death in surgical patients than in medical patients, weight loss was associated with similar odds ratio. History of a stay in intensive care during the hospitalization before nutritionDay was found to be significantly associated with death only in medical patients. "Eating less than normal in the previous week" is associated with death 30 days after nDay in medical, surgical and long-term care patients but not in the "other" group. Weight loss is only associated with poor outcome in medical and surgical patients. Higher BMI was associated with better outcome in medical, surgical and "other" patients, an observation called "reverse epidemiology" and low BMI with worse outcome but not in long-term care patients. Higher age is in all groups associated with worse outcome. Abnormal fluid status, identified as either overloaded or dehydrated, based on clinical judgment, was a robust risk indicator in all patient groups. Decreased food intake on nutritionDay was always associated with worse outcome. A clear difference between eating nothing while not being allowed (nil by mouth) or being allowed is only found in the surgical patient group whereas in all three other groups there was no clear difference. A very robust risk indicator is "reduced mobility" in all patient groups (Figure 4). Having had an ICU stay before nutritionDay was only associated with worse outcome in medical patients.

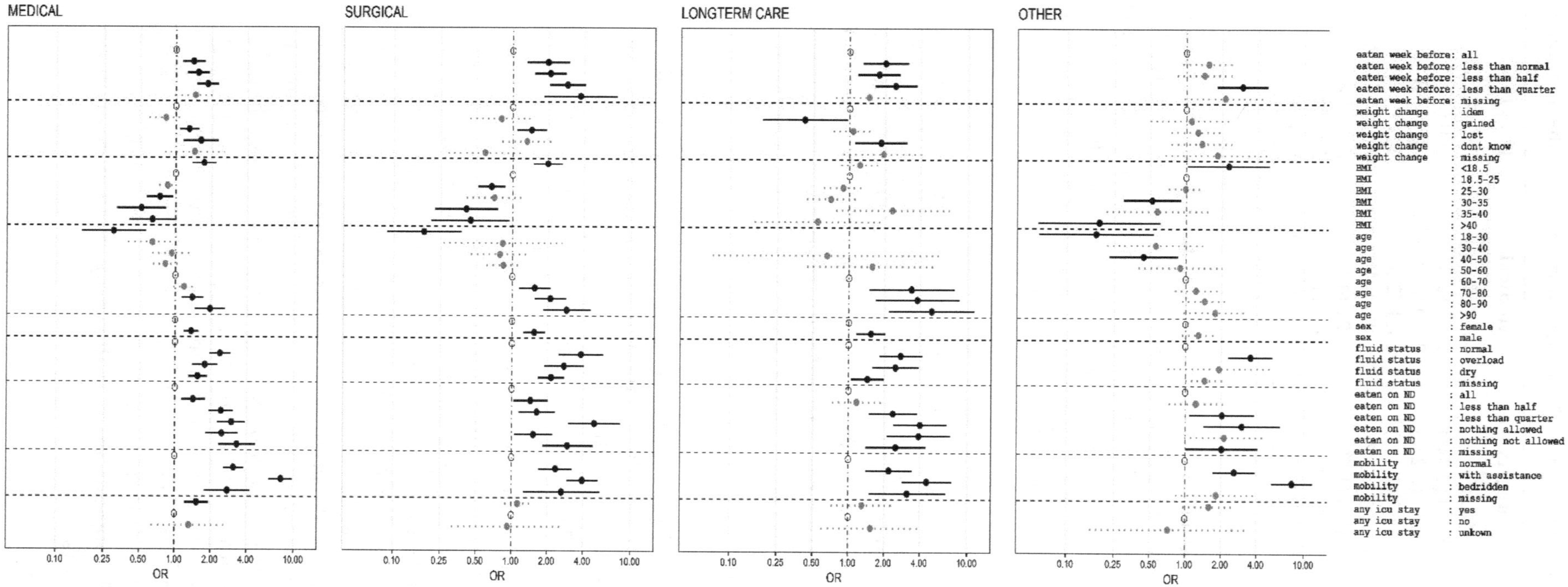

Figure 4. Multivariate analysis of association between demographic and nutrition related risk factors and death in hospital within 30 days after nutritionDay for medical, surgical, long-term care and other patient groups with the general linear model for logistic regression with wards as clusters and weighting of individual patients for sampling probability [25] and including all diagnostic categories and comorbidities (see Figure 5). Odds ratios (OR) with 95% confidence intervals indicated by horizontal line. Reference categories are indicated by an open symbol. Missing values are included in the model as individual categories.

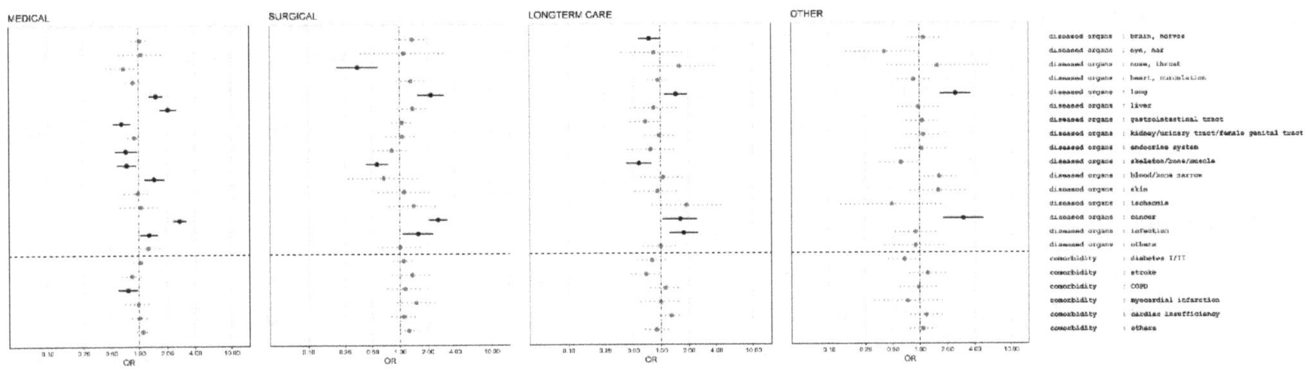

Figure 5. Multivariate analysis of association between organ related disease categories from ICD 10 as well as comorbidities and death in hospital within 30 days after nutritionDay for medical, surgical, long-term care and other patient groups with the general linear model for logistic regression with wards as clusters and weighting of individual patients for sampling probability [25] and including demographic and nutrition related risk factors (see Figure 4). Odds ratios (OR) with 95% confidence intervals indicated by horizontal line. Multiple entries are possible. Missing values are included in the model as individual categories.

The association between affected organs as derived from ICD 10 categories is very different for medical and surgical patients (Figure 5). No comorbidities had a negative prognostic effect in the multivariate analysis.

4. Discussion

This analysis of medical/surgical patients from the nutritionDay cohort 2006–2015 showed that individual nutrition risk indicators such as low BMI, weight loss in last three months, poor eating before admission and low nutrient intake in hospital are highly prevalent in hospitalized patients and are associated with poor hospital outcome within 30 days after nutritionDay. Each additional risk indicator observed was associated with a nearly two-times higher mortality in the overall population.

All four risk indicators were independently associated with death in the hospital within 30 days after nutritionDay in the multivariate analysis (Figure 4) in the two largest groups medical and surgical patients. There is no clear indication that a single risk indicator can be ignored because the presence of each risk indicator is associated with a higher rate of dying by nearly a factor of two for these two groups. Surprisingly recent weight-loss and lower BMI was not associated with worse prognosis in long-term care whereas only weight-loss was not associated with worse outcome for the group of non-medical and non-surgical patients including neurological and psychiatric disorders.

Three risk indicators emerge similarly for all four patient groups, poor eating in hospital, reduced mobility and altered fluid status. All three had also being found as individual risk indicators in the PANDORA risk scoring system whereas recent weight loss and history of poor eating were not included [5]. These robust factors may also serve as indicators that may trigger more consistent observation and initiation of treatments that have proven to efficacious [26].

In recent years (2016–2018) healthcare teams identified only half of the patients as having nutrition related risk factors such as being malnourished or at risk of malnutrition in comparison to the nutritionDay indicators 8701/28,013 (31%) versus 21,070/28,100 (75%) such as unintentional weight loss, low BMI or decreased food intake. Thus, it appears that a large group of patients with nutrition related risk factors is not identified in standard care practice. This observed gap may originate from the different type of data collected from patients during routine clinical practice and the targeted data collection of the nutritionDay audit.

The efficiency of interventions may depend on the size of risk of the individual patient. It has recently been demonstrated that patients identified at high risk of malnutrition by the Nutritional Risk Screening (NRS-2002) risk system benefit from an integrated intervention [26]. It is unknown, however, whether the large group of patients with moderate risk, which account for almost half of the hospitalized patients on any given day, would also benefit from some targeted interventions. Interventions effective for the moderate risk group may be less complex and costly, and potentially integrated in to routine care processes, and could lead to better outcomes and reduced hospital length of stay and better patient outcomes.

4.1. Nutrition Care

Nutrition care processes such as screening, prescribing nutrition treatment, monitoring daily nutrition intake and recording of malnutrition status are applied in less than 50% of patients. These observations may again arise from identification issues, from lack of a systematic screening processes which then lead to a weak targeting even in the presence of nutrition risk factors. Educational gaps of healthcare professionals in the field of nutrition, as well as the importance given to nutrition care might also be considered crucial to fight DRM. Recent results from a large randomized trial [26] from a Swiss team could demonstrate that a systematic approach to patients with nutrition risk factors is associated with a decreased short and long-term mortality.

Our data suggest that a systematic care for patients with nutrition related risk factors in hospitals is currently missing. Reception and dissemination of current recommendations from major clinical nutrition societies such as ESPEN and ASPEN requires further efforts to reach all the involved stakeholders, not only those directly involved in nutrition care but also those in management and decision making.

4.2. Political Action Derived from Observations

A structured approach to tackle the challenges of disease related malnutrition needs to include all involved stakeholders to implement universal screening for risk factors, apply systematically supportive nutrition care, monitor the effect in individual patients and take measures to promote continuity of care after discharge from acute care hospitals.

4.3. Limitations of the Study

A limitation of such a cross-sectional international data collection may be that clinical observations and their evaluation are not matching the same clinical pattern. Participants are provided with a document explaining all collected variables in English and with questionnaires which were translated and checked by clinicians in order to achieve as much as possible consistency between answers. Great care was taken to utilize a simple and self-explanatory wording. This was also essential because the patient questionnaires are intended to be answered by patients independently of their education level. For such factors as fluid status, overloaded or dehydrated, we had to accept the data as clinically evaluated.

Such large databases with participating centres from more than 60 countries carry also the risk of missing data and non-homogeneous data reporting. Over the years we found stable proportions of missing data in the individual risk indicators. Surprisingly, this missingness does not appear to be at random as missing data were often associated with a poor outcome and not with an intermediate outcome from the various strata of a variable. We have addressed this issue by including missing categories in all variables as recommended by the STROBE statement [23] and have performed in addition a sensitivity analysis with complete cases without missing data that yielded quite similar results.

In addition, large databases may identify risk indicators with a minimal clinical relevance despite a large univariate effect. We have, thus, selected to present multivariate analysis where spurious associations are less likely.

A further limitation is that cross-sectional observational data from a convenience sample are not appropriate to determine a causal association between risk indicators and outcome. Nevertheless only observational studies can identify risk indicators because risk indicators cannot be randomised (Table 5).

Table 5. Problem areas and suggested options for political action.

Problem Area	Political Action
Education of all healthcare professionals directly involved in patient care in disease related malnutrition and nutrition care insufficient.	Mandatory inclusion of disease related malnutrition and nutrition care processes in curriculum for nurses, doctors, dieticians, etc.
Limited awareness of the importance of nutrition in disease states in the public especially the population at risk.	National nutrition care campaigns targeting the general population, residents of nursing homes and also targeted nutrition campaigns run through general practitioners. Availability of an education platform for patients and families.
Nomination of responsible person or team for patient nutrition care missing. No monitoring of nutrition care processes part of hospital quality control.	Mandatory designation of a nutrition team/responsible person in each hospital with a threefold responsibility: coordination of expertise, definition of processes and regular benchmarking of applications of processes through initiatives like nutritionDay, the Dutch nutrition benchmarking program, the British malnutrition awareness week and the analysis of electronic patients records.
Inconsistent screening and collection of data. Missing documentation of nutrition risk factors and communication of nutrition status and care at discharge to the next sector.	Mandatory inclusion of data in a nutrition care benchmarking program. Definition and inclusion of mandatory harmonized fields for a systematic collection and documentation of nutrition risks factors and nutrition care processes in the electronic patient record. Inclusion of planned nutrition treatment recorded in patient's discharge letter/information to patients and relatives.
Missing patients and families empowerment due to insufficient communication of nutrition status and care to the patients and their families.	Mandatory monitoring of communication processes in quality assurance programs.
Lack of a harmonized reimbursement schemes for nutrition related processes such as screening, assessment and treatment such as oral nutritional supplements, enteral or parenteral nutrition.	Clear reimbursement schemes.
Missing a partnership for hospital food provision and of a positive image for hospital food.	Creation of a public best practice platform for food provision in hospitals. Supported use of local food in hospital kitchen for the creation of wealth not only for the community using the hospital but also for the local community.

5. Conclusions

In summary the analysis and dissemination of the nutritionDay data helps to increase awareness of nutrition related issues in hospitals and provides discussion for potential political actions. There are many options for political action. The key points appear to be the raised awareness about all the described aspects related to DRM to all stakeholders, as well as the proposal of easy and standardized nutrition care processes, defined responsibilities within hospitals, and the establishment of adequate reimbursement schemes. Collection of data is crucial to allow monitoring of DRM as well as food provision at all levels and to allow benchmarking and discussion within the teams. DRM is unlikely to disappear from hospitals because disease acts as a strong driver towards malnutrition. Appropriate nutrition care should be continued after discharge to prevent further deterioration in patient's autonomy, quality of life and poor outcome. A systematic approach to DRM in hospitals and an adequate continuity of care may lead to better outcomes [11,12,26]. nutritionDay in this regard has served and it will keep serving as a tool to monitor changes in clinical practice and associated outcome.

Author Contributions: Conceptualization: M.H., S.T., D.V., J.S. and K.S.; data curation: M.M. and C.S.; formal analysis: M.H. and I.S.; funding acquisition: M.H., S.T., D.V. and J.S.; investigation: S.M.; methodology: M.H., J.S. and K.S.; project administration: S.T., S.M. and D.V.; resources: M.H. and D.V.; software: M.M. and C.S.; supervision: A.L. and J.S.; validation: M.H. and I.S.; visualization: M.H., S.T. and I.S.; writing—original draft: M.H., S.T., D.V., J.S. and K.S.; writing—review and editing: M.H., S.T., A.L., I.S., D.V., J.S. and K.S.

Acknowledgments: We acknowledge the nutritionDay national coordinators and the Austrian Society for Clinical Nutrition (AKE) for logistic support. We acknowledge all national coordinators contributing to nutritionDay: Jean-Charles Preiser and Brigitte Croix (Belgium), M. Cristina Gonzalez (Brazil), Luiza Kent-Smith (Canada), Angélica María Pérez Cano and Olga Lucía Pinzón Espitia (Colombia), Dina Ljubas (Croatia), Evelyn Frias Toral (Ecuador), Elina Ioannou (Cyprus), Frantisek Novak (Czech Republic), José Gutiérrez (El Salvador), Ulla Siljamäki-Ojansuu (Finland), Stéphane Schneider (France), Elke-Tatjana Schütz (Germany), Meropi Kontogianni and Kalliopi-Anna Poulia (Greece), Laszlo Harsányi (Hungary), Hartono (Indonesia), Pierre Singer (Israel), Marcello Maggio and Pietro Vecchiarelli (Italy), Hiroyoshi Takemoto (Japan), Laila Meija and Ilze Jagmane (Latvia), Gintautas Kekstas and Edita Gaveliene (Lithuania), Cora Jonkers-Schuitema (The Netherlands), Hugo Nilssen (Norway), Kinga Kupczyk (Poland), Paula Alves and Luis Matos (Portugal) Ioana Grintescu and Liliana Mirea (Romania), Vanessa Kotze (South Africa), Katja Kogovšek (Slovenia), Rosa Burgos (Spain), Barbara Hürlimann (Switzerland), Sonqsri Keawtanom (Thailand), Sadik Kilicturgay (Turkey), Sergii Dubrov and Olesia Gavrilenko (Ukraine), Kate Hall (United Kingdom) and Gail Gewirtz (USA).

References

1. Butterworth, C.E., Jr. Editorial: Malnutrition in the hospital. *JAMA* **1974**, *230*, 879. [CrossRef]
2. Bistrian, B.R.; Blackburn, G.L.; Vitale, J.; Cochran, D.; Naylor, J. Prevalence of malnutrition in general medical patients. *JAMA* **1976**, *235*, 1567–1570. [CrossRef]
3. Council of Europe Committee of Ministers. Resolution ResAP (2003) 3 on Food and Nutritional Care in Hospitals. Available online: https://search.coe.int/ (accessed on 18 November 2019).
4. Hiesmayr, M.; Schindler, K.; Pernicka, E.; Schuh, C.; Schoeniger-Hekele, A.; Bauer, P.; Laviano, A.; Lovell, A.D.; Mouhieddine, M.; Schuetz, T.; et al. Decreased food intake is a risk factor for mortality in hospitalised patients: The NutritionDay survey 2006. *Clin. Nutr.* **2009**, *28*, 484–491. [CrossRef]
5. Hiesmayr, M.; Frantal, S.; Schindler, K.; Themessl-Huber, M.; Mouhieddine, M.; Schuh, C.; Pernicka, E.; Schneider, S.; Singer, P.; Ljunqvist, O.; et al. The Patient- And Nutrition-Derived Outcome Risk Assessment Score (PANDORA): Development of a Simple Predictive Risk Score for 30-Day In-Hospital Mortality Based on Demographics, Clinical Observation, and Nutrition. *PLoS ONE* **2015**, *10*, e0127316. [CrossRef]
6. Kondrup, J.; Rasmussen, H.H.; Hamberg, O.; Stanga, Z. Nutritional risk screening (NRS 2002): A new method based on an analysis of controlled clinical trials. *Clin. Nutr.* **2003**, *22*, 321–336. [CrossRef]
7. Schindler, K.; Pernicka, E.; Laviano, A.; Howard, P.; Schutz, T.; Bauer, P.; Grecu, I.; Jonkers, C.; Kondrup, J.; Ljungqvist, O.; et al. How nutritional risk is assessed and managed in European hospitals: A survey of 21,007 patients findings from the 2007–2008 cross-sectional nutritionDay survey. *Clin. Nutr.* **2010**, *29*, 552–559. [CrossRef] [PubMed]
8. Navarro, D.A.; Boaz, M.; Krause, I.; Elis, A.; Chernov, K.; Giabra, M.; Levy, M.; Giboreau, A.; Kosak, S.; Mouhieddine, M.; et al. Improved meal presentation increases food intake and decreases readmission rate in hospitalizd patients. *Clin. Nutr.* **2016**, *35*, 1153–1158. [CrossRef]
9. Correia, M.I.; Waitzberg, D.L. The impact of malnutrition on morbidity, mortality, length of hospital stay and costs evaluated through a multivariate model analysis. *Clin. Nutr.* **2003**, *22*, 235–239. [CrossRef]
10. Lim, S.L.; Ong, K.C.; Chan, Y.H.; Loke, W.C.; Ferguson, M.; Daniels, L. Malnutrition and its impact on cost of hospitalization, length of stay, readmission and 3-year mortality. *Clin. Nutr.* **2012**, *31*, 345–350. [CrossRef] [PubMed]
11. Reber, E.; Norman, K.; Endrich, O.; Schuetz, P.; Frei, A.; Stanga, Z. Economic Challenges in Nutritional Management. *J. Clin. Med.* **2019**, *8*, 1005. [CrossRef]

12. Reber, E.; Strahm, R.; Bally, L.; Schuetz, P.; Stanga, Z. Efficacy and Efficiency of Nutritional Support Teams. *J. Clin. Med.* **2019**, *8*, 1281. [CrossRef] [PubMed]
13. Bendavid, I.; Singer, P.; Theilla, M.; Themessl-Huber, M.; Sulz, I.; Mouhieddine, M.; Schuh, C.; Mora, B.; Hiesmayr, M. NutritionDay ICU: A 7 year worldwide prevalence study of nutrition practice in intensive care. *Clin. Nutr.* **2017**, *36*, 1122–1129. [CrossRef] [PubMed]
14. Schindler, K.; Pichard, C.; Sulz, I.; Volkert, D.; Streicher, M.; Singer, P.; Ljungqvist, O.; Van Gossum, A.; Bauer, P.; Hiesmayr, M. nutritionDay: 10 years of growth. *Clin. Nutr.* **2017**, *36*, 1207–1214. [CrossRef] [PubMed]
15. Streicher, M.; Themessl-Huber, M.; Schindler, K.; Sieber, C.C.; Hiesmayr, M.; Volkert, D. nutritionDay in Nursing Homes-The Association of Nutritional Intake and Nutritional Interventions With 6-Month Mortality in Malnourished Residents. *J. Am. Med. Dir. Assoc.* **2017**, *18*, 162–168. [CrossRef]
16. Schindler, K.; Themessl-Huber, M.; Hiesmayr, M.; Kosak, S.; Lainscak, M.; Laviano, A.; Ljungqvist, O.; Mouhieddine, M.; Schneider, S.; de van der Schueren, M.; et al. To eat or not to eat? Indicators for reduced food intake in 91,245 patients hospitalized on nutritionDays 2006–2014 in 56 countries worldwide: A descriptive analysis. *Am. J. Clin. Nutr.* **2016**, *104*, 1393–1402. [CrossRef]
17. Man, F.D. Optimal Nutrition Care for All (ONCA). Available online: https://european-nutrition.org (accessed on 21 August 2019).
18. European Patient Forum. Available online: http://www.eu-patient.eu/ (accessed on 21 August 2019).
19. Kondrup, J.; Allison, S.P.; Elia, M.; Vellas, B.; Plauth, M. ESPEN guidelines for nutrition screening 2002. *Clin. Nutr.* **2003**, *22*, 415–421. [CrossRef]
20. Cardenas, D.; Bermudez, C.; Barazzoni, R. The Cartagena Declaration: A call for global commitment to fight for the right to nutritional care. *Clin. Nutr.* **2019**. [CrossRef]
21. United Nations. *Sustainable Development Goals*; United Nations: New York, NY, USA, 2015.
22. Cederholm, T.; Jensen, G.L.; Correia, M.; Gonzalez, M.C.; Fukushima, R.; Higashiguchi, T.; Baptista, G.; Barazzoni, R.; Blaauw, R.; Coats, A.; et al. GLIM criteria for the diagnosis of malnutrition—A consensus report from the global clinical nutrition community. *Clin. Nutr.* **2019**, *38*, 1–9. [CrossRef]
23. Von Elm, E.; Altman, D.G.; Egger, M.; Pocock, S.J.; Gotzsche, P.C.; Vandenbroucke, J.P.; Initiative, S. The Strengthening the Reporting of Observational Studies in Epidemiology (STROBE) statement: Guidelines for reporting observational studies. *Lancet* **2007**, *370*, 1453–1457. [CrossRef]
24. World Health Organisation. Body Mass Index. Available online: http://www.euro.who.int/en/health-topics/disease-prevention/nutrition/a-healthy-lifestyle/body-mass-index-bmi (accessed on 10 September 2019).
25. Frantal, S.; Pernicka, E.; Hiesmayr, M.; Schindler, K.; Bauer, P. Length bias correction in one-day cross-sectional assessments—The nutritionDay study. *Clin. Nutr.* **2016**, *35*, 522–527. [CrossRef]
26. Schuetz, P.; Fehr, R.; Baechli, V.; Geiser, M.; Deiss, M.; Gomes, F.; Kutz, A.; Tribolet, P.; Bregenzer, T.; Braun, N.; et al. Individualised nutritional support in medical inpatients at nutritional risk: A randomised clinical trial. *Lancet* **2019**, *393*, 2312–2321. [CrossRef]

Permissions

All chapters in this book were first published by MDPI; hereby published with permission under the Creative Commons Attribution License or equivalent. Every chapter published in this book has been scrutinized by our experts. Their significance has been extensively debated. The topics covered herein carry significant findings which will fuel the growth of the discipline. They may even be implemented as practical applications or may be referred to as a beginning point for another development.

The contributors of this book come from diverse backgrounds, making this book a truly international effort. This book will bring forth new frontiers with its revolutionizing research information and detailed analysis of the nascent developments around the world.

We would like to thank all the contributing authors for lending their expertise to make the book truly unique. They have played a crucial role in the development of this book. Without their invaluable contributions this book wouldn't have been possible. They have made vital efforts to compile up to date information on the varied aspects of this subject to make this book a valuable addition to the collection of many professionals and students.

This book was conceptualized with the vision of imparting up-to-date information and advanced data in this field. To ensure the same, a matchless editorial board was set up. Every individual on the board went through rigorous rounds of assessment to prove their worth. After which they invested a large part of their time researching and compiling the most relevant data for our readers.

The editorial board has been involved in producing this book since its inception. They have spent rigorous hours researching and exploring the diverse topics which have resulted in the successful publishing of this book. They have passed on their knowledge of decades through this book. To expedite this challenging task, the publisher supported the team at every step. A small team of assistant editors was also appointed to further simplify the editing procedure and attain best results for the readers.

Apart from the editorial board, the designing team has also invested a significant amount of their time in understanding the subject and creating the most relevant covers. They scrutinized every image to scout for the most suitable representation of the subject and create an appropriate cover for the book.

The publishing team has been an ardent support to the editorial, designing and production team. Their endless efforts to recruit the best for this project, has resulted in the accomplishment of this book. They are a veteran in the field of academics and their pool of knowledge is as vast as their experience in printing. Their expertise and guidance has proved useful at every step. Their uncompromising quality standards have made this book an exceptional effort. Their encouragement from time to time has been an inspiration for everyone.

The publisher and the editorial board hope that this book will prove to be a valuable piece of knowledge for researchers, students, practitioners and scholars across the globe.

List of Contributors

Jana Kopčeková, Mária Holovičová, Martina Gažarová, Jana Mrázová, Marta Habánová and Lucia Mečiarová
Department of Human Nutrition, Faculty of Agrobiology and Food Resources, Slovak University of Agriculture in Nitra, 949 01 Nitra, Slovakia

Monika Bronkowska
Department of Human Nutrition, Faculty of Biotechnology and Food Science, Wroclaw University of Environmental and Life Sciences, 51-630 Wroclaw, Poland

Tamara Sorić and Mladen Mavar
Psychiatric Hospital Ugljan, Otočkih dragovoljaca 42, 23275 Ugljan, Croatia

Ivana Rumbak
Faculty of Food Technology and Biotechnology, University of Zagreb, 10000 Zagreb, Croatia

Wei-Ning Wang
Department of Food and Nutrition, Taichung Veterans General Hospital, Taichung 40705, Taiwan

Chen-Yu Wang
Department of Critical Care Medicine, Taichung Veterans General Hospital, Taichung 40705, Taiwan
Department of Nursing, Hungkuang University, Taichung 43302, Taiwan

Chiann-Yi Hsu
Biostatistics Task Force of Taichung Veterans General Hospital, Taichung 40705, Taiwan

Pin-Kuei Fu
Department of Critical Care Medicine, Taichung Veterans General Hospital, Taichung 40705, Taiwan
College of Human Science and Social Innovation, Hungkuang University, Taichung 43302, Taiwan
Department of Computer Science, Tunghai University, Taichung 40705, Taiwan

Hang-Tsung Liu, Ching-Hua Tsai, Chi Li, Sheng-En Chou, Wei-Ti Su and Shiun-Yuan Hsu
Department of Trauma Surgery, Kaohsiung Chang Gung Memorial Hospital, Chang Gung University College of Medicine, Kaohsiung City 833, Taiwan

Shao-Chun Wu
Department of Anesthesiology, Kaohsiung Chang Gung Memorial Hospital, Chang Gung University College of Medicine, Kaohsiung City 833, Taiwan

Ching-Hua Hsieh
Department of Plastic Surgery, Kaohsiung Chang Gung Memorial Hospital, Chang Gung University College of Medicine, Kaohsiung City 833, Taiwan

Ulrich Keller
FMH Endocrinology-Diabetology, Fichtlirain 33, CH-4105 Biel-Benken, Basel, Switzerland

Mette M Berger, Olivier Pantet, Antoine Schneider and Nawfel Ben-Hamouda
Service of Adult Intensive Care Medicine and Burns, Lausanne University Hospital (CHUV), BH 08.612, Rue du Bugnon 46, 1011 Lausanne, Switzerland

Peter J.M. Weijs
Department of Nutrition and Dietetics, Amsterdam University Medical Centers, VU University, 1081 HV Amsterdam, The Netherlands
Faculty of Sports and Nutrition, Amsterdam University of Applied Sciences, 1067 SM Amsterdam, The Netherlands

Kris M. Mogensen
Department of Nutrition, Brigham and Women's Hospital, Boston, MA 02115, USA

James D. Rawn
Department of Surgery, Brigham and Women's Hospital, Boston, MA 02115, USA

Kenneth B. Christopher
The Nathan E. Hellman Memorial Laboratory, Division of Renal Medicine, Brigham and Women's Hospital, Boston, MA 02115, USA

Jessica Stirnimann
Division of Diabetology, Endocrinology, Nutritional Medicine and Metabolism, University Hospital Inselspital and University of Bern, 3010 Bern, Switzerland

Guido Stirnimann
University Clinic for Visceral Surgery and Medicine, University Hospital Inselspital and University of Bern, 3010 Bern, Switzerland

Emilie Reber
Department for Diabetes, Endocrinology, Nutritional Medicine and Metabolism, Bern University Hospital, and University of Bern, 3010 Bern, Switzerland

Kristina Norman
Department of Nutrition and Gerontology, German Institute for Human Nutrition Potsdam-Rehbrücke, 14558 Nuthetal, Germany
Research Group on Geriatrics, Charité Universitätsmedizin Berlin, Corporate Member of Freie Universität Berlin, Humboldt-Universität zu Berlin and Berlin Institute of Health, 13347 Berlin, Germany

Olga Endrich
Health Data Management and Health Economics, Medical Directorate, Bern University Hospital, and University of Bern, 3010 Bern, Switzerland

Philipp Schuetz
Medical University Department, Division of General Internal and Emergency Medicine, Kantonsspital Aarau, 5001 Aarau, Switzerland

Andreas Frei
Freelance Health Economist, 4133 Pratteln, Switzerland

An Jacobs, Ines Verlinden, Ilse Vanhorebeek and Greet Van den Berghe
Clinical Division and Laboratory of Intensive Care Medicine, Department of Cellular and Molecular Medicine, KU Leuven University Hospital, 3000 Leuven, Belgium

Emilie Reber
Department for Diabetes, Endocrinology, Nutritional Medicine and Metabolism, Bern University Hospital and University of Bern, 3010 Bern, Switzerland

Markus Messerli
Department of Pharmaceutical Sciences, Pharmaceutical Care Research Group, University of Basel, 4050 Basel, Switzerland

Stefan Mühlebach
Department of Pharmaceutical Sciences, Division of Clinical Pharmacy & Epidemiology/Hospital Pharmacy, University of Basel, 4050 Basel, Switzerland

Marina V. Viana, Arianne Martinez, Eva Favre, Philippe Eckert and Mette M. Berger
Service of Adult Intensive Care Medicine and Burns, Lausanne University Hospital (CHUV), 1011 Lausanne, Switzerland

Geraldine Bagnoud, Mélanie Charrière and Doris Favre
Service of Adult Intensive Care Medicine and Burns, Lausanne University Hospital (CHUV), 1011 Lausanne, Switzerland
Service of Endocrinology, Diabetes and Metabolism, Lausanne University Hospital, 1011 Lausanne, Switzerland

Paweł Więch
Institute of Nursing and Health Sciences, Faculty of Medicine, University of Rzeszów, 35-959 Rzeszów, Poland

Dariusz Bazaliński
Institute of Nursing and Health Sciences, Faculty of Medicine, University of Rzeszów, 35-959 Rzeszów, Poland

Izabela Sałacińska
Institute of Nursing and Health Sciences, Faculty of Medicine, University of Rzeszów, 35-959 Rzeszów, Poland

Monika Binkowska-Bury
Institute of Nursing and Health Sciences, Faculty of Medicine, University of Rzeszów, 35-959 Rzeszów, Poland

Bartosz Korczowski
Pediatric Department, Clinical Provincial Hospital No. 2 in Rzeszów, Faculty of Medicine, University of Rzeszów, 35-301 Rzeszów, Poland

Artur Mazur
Pediatric Department, Clinical Provincial Hospital No. 2 in Rzeszów, Faculty of Medicine, University of Rzeszów, 35-301 Rzeszów, Poland

Maria Kózka
Department of Clinical Nursing, Faculty of Health Sciences, Collegium Medicum, Jagiellonian University, 31-501 Kraków, Poland

Mariusz Dąbrowski
Institute of Nursing and Health Sciences, Faculty of Medicine, University of Rzeszów, 35-959 Rzeszów, Poland
Institute of Nursing and Health Sciences, Faculty of Medicine, University of Rzeszów, 35-959 Rzeszów, Poland

Lena J. Storck and Reinhard Imoberdorf
Kantonsspital Winterthur, Department of Medicine, 8401 Winterthur, Switzerland

Peter E. Ballmer
Kantonsspital Winterthur, Department of Medicine, 8401 Winterthur, Switzerland
Zürcher RehaZentrum Davos, 7272 Davos Clavadel, Switzerland

Céline Isabelle Laesser, Emilie Reber, Zeno Stanga and Lia Bally
Department of Diabetes, Endocrinology, Clinical Nutrition, and Metabolism, Inselspital, Bern University Hospital, University of Bern, 3010 Bern, Switzerland

Paul Cumming
Department of Nuclear Medicine, Inselspital, Bern University Hospital, University of Bern, 3010 Bern, Switzerland
School of Psychology and Counselling and IHBI, Queensland University of Technology, Brisbane, QLD 4059, Australia

Taulant Muka
Institute of Social and Preventive Medicine, University of Bern, 3012 Bern, Switzerland

Michael Hiesmayr, Silvia Tarantino, Sigrid Moick and Mohamed Mouhieddine
Division Cardio-thoracic and Vascular Anesthesia and Intensive Care, Medical University Vienna, 1090 Vienna, Austria

Isabella Sulz and Christian Schuh
Center for Medical Statistics, Informatics and Intelligent Systems, Medical University Vienna, 1090 Vienna, Austria

Judit Simon
Department of Health Economics, Center for Public Health, Medical University Vienna, 1090 Vienna, Austria

Karin Schindler
Department of Internal Medicine III, Medical University Vienna, 1090 Vienna, Austria

Alessandro Laviano
Department of Translational and Precision Medicine, Università degli Studi di Roma "La Sapienza", 00185 Roma, Italy

Dorothee Volkert
Institute for Biomedicine of Ageing, Friedrich-Alexander Universität Erlangen-Nürnberg, 90408 Nürnberg, Germany

Index

www.ingramcontent.com/pod-product-compliance
Lightning Source LLC
LaVergne TN
LVHW060557210926
848485LV00005B/1331